The Human Nervous System
Structure and Function

Fifth Edition

The Human Nervous System
Structure and Function

Fifth Edition

Charles R. Noback, PhD
Professor Emeritus of Anatomy and Cell Biology
College of Physicians and Surgeons
Columbia University
New York, New York

Norman L. Strominger, PhD
Professor of Surgery (Otolaryngology)
The Albany Medical College
Professor of Neuroscience
School of Public Health
State University of New York at Albany
Albany, New York

Robert J. Demarest
Director Emeritus, Medical Illustration
College of Physicians and Surgeons
Columbia University
New York, New York

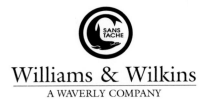

Williams & Wilkins
A WAVERLY COMPANY

BALTIMORE • PHILADELPHIA • LONDON • PARIS • BANGKOK
HONG KONG • MUNICH • SYDNEY • TOKYO • WROCLAW

Executive Editor: Donna Balado
Developmental Editor: Victoria M. Vaughn
Production Coordinator: Marette D. Magargle
Project Editor: Jennifer D. Weir

The cover illustration, *Eye and Hand Coordination* by Robert J. Demarest, highlights two major neural systems perfected during the evolution of the human nervous system. The visual pathway—projecting from the eyes to the visual cortex—is coordinated with the corticospinal pathway and peripheral nerves in the motor control of the complex movements expressed by the fingers, opposable thumb, and upper limb.

Copyright © 1996
Williams & Wilkins
Rose Tree Corporate Center
1400 North Providence Road
Building II, Suite 5025
Media, PA 19063-2043 USA

Accurate indications, adverse reactions, and dosage schedules for drugs are provided in this book, but it is possible they may change. The reader is urged to review the package information data of the manufacturers of the medications mentioned.

Printed in the United States of America

Library of Congress Cataloging-in-Publication Data

Noback, Charles Robert, 1916–
    The human nervous system : structure and function / Charles R.
  Noback, Norman L. Strominger, Robert J. Demarest.—5th ed.
      p.   cm.
    Includes bibliographical references and index.
    ISBN 0-683-06538-6
    1. Neurophysiology. I. Strominger, Norman L. II. Demarest,
  Robert J. III. Title.
    [DNLM: 1. Nervous System—anatomy & histology. 2. Nervous System—
  physiology. WL 101 N744h 1995]
  QP361.N58 1995
  612.8—dc20
  DNLM/DLC
  for Library of Congress   95-10315
                                      CIP

The Publishers have made every effort to trace the copyright holders for borrowed material. If they have inadvertently overlooked any, they will be pleased to make the necessary arrangements at the first opportunity.

96 97 98 99
2 3 4 5 6 7 8 9 10

Reprints of chapters may be purchased from Williams & Wilkins in quantities of 100 or more. Call Isabella Wise, Special Sales Department, (800) 358-3583.

Dedication

This book is dedicated to our grandchildren

Lindsay Barton and Peter Noback
Jessica Anne Strominger
Zoe, Quinn, and Lauren Demarest and Timothy and Brett O'Donnell

Preface

This fifth edition continues to represent the combined efforts of two neuroscientists and a medical illustrator to succinctly present the fundamental principles of the organization, structure, and function of the human nervous system. The book is intended to meet the basic needs primarily of (1) medical and dental students who want to get a general overview of this discipline; (2) beginning students in the allied health sciences and psychology fields who need an introductory, yet reasonably comprehensive, survey of the subject; (3) residents in neurology, neurosurgery, and neuroradiology who wish to review this subject matter; and (4) readers with a background in biology who want to review some general concepts and specific details.

The text is designed so that the students who are getting their first exposure to neuroscience can get an organized view of the bewilderingly and extremely complex human nervous system. The illustrations have been specifically prepared for this book to simplify and clarify items in the text. Clinical correlations and relevant symptoms from lesions are integrated in the text to elucidate important features of the substrate of the brain, spinal cord, and peripheral nervous system. Two chapters specifically deal with *Lesions of the Spinal Nerves and Spinal Cord* and *Lesions of the Brainstem*. Each chapter contains a list of slected references to guide readers who wish to read about topics in greater detail.

The book incorporates many of the significant recent advances made in Neurobiology and Molecular Biology during this "Decade of the Brain." Chapters on *Basic Neurophysiology, Development and Growth of the Nervous System, Auditory and Vestibular Systems, Neurotransmitters as the Chemical Messengers of Certain Circuits and Pathways,* and *Basal Ganglia and Extrapyramidal System* have been substantially expanded and revised. In addition, there are 24 new half tone drawings along with 4 photographs and some examples of CAT scans, magnetic resonance imaging, and positron emission tomography.

We wish to thank our students and colleagues for their many invaluable comments and their input. We especially wish to thank Marilyn Dockum for her tireless and insightful efforts and Robert Strominger, M.D., for his contributions.

Charles R. Noback
Robert J. Demarest
New York, New York

Norman L. Strominger
Albany, New York

Introduction and Terminology

Divisions of the nervous system

Orientation in the brain

Organization of neurons in the CNS: brain and spinal cord

Most students feel a baffling uncertainty when beginning the study of neuroanatomy. Not until many of the facets of the subject blend in the latter half of the course do they feel a gain in their control over the material. To ameliorate the uncertain feeling, you should study the text and examine the figures in the first five chapters (especially Chap. 1) for a general understanding only, then use them later for reference. Chapters 8 through 13 will give you basic information about pathway systems, as well as background knowledge for the remaining chapters in the book.

The nervous system and the endocrine system harmonize the many complex functional activities of the body. The former is the rapid coordinator, whereas the latter is more deliberate in its action.

DIVISIONS OF THE NERVOUS SYSTEM

The nervous system essentially exhibits a bilateral symmetry with those structural features and pathways located on one side of the midline that are also found on the other side. It is subdivided (1) anatomically, into the *central nervous system* and the *peripheral nervous system* and (2) functionally, into the *somatic nervous system* and the *autonomic (visceral) nervous system*.

The central nervous system (CNS) comprises the brain and spinal cord. The brain is encapsulated within the skull and the spinal cord is at the center of the vertebral column. The *peripheral nervous system* (PNS) consists of the nerves emerging from the brain (called cranial nerves) and from the spinal cord (called spinal nerves). The peripheral nerves convey neural messages (1) from the sense organs and sensory receptors in the organism inward to the CNS and (2) from the CNS outward to the muscles and glands of the body.

The *somatic nervous system* comprises those neural structures of the CNS and PNS responsible for (1) conveying and processing conscious and unconscious sensory (*afferent*) information—e.g., vision, pain, touch, and unconscious muscle sense—from the head, body wall, and extremities to the CNS and (2) motor (*efferent*) control of the voluntary (striated) muscles. The *autonomic nervous system* may include the neural structures responsible for (1) conveying and processing sensory input from the visceral organs (e.g., digestive system and cardiovascular system) and (2) motor control of the involuntary (smooth) and cardiac musculature and of glands of the viscera. Most authors, however, consider the autonomic nervous system to be exclusviely concerned with visceral motor activities.

Sensory signals originating in the sensory receptors are transmitted through the nervous system along *sensory pathways*, e.g., pain and temperature pathways and visual pathways. These signals may reach the conscious sphere or may be utilized at unconscious levels. The neural messages for motor activity are conveyed through the nervous system to the muscles and glands along *motor pathways*. Both the sensory (ascending) and motor (descending) pathways include *processing centers* (e.g., ganglia, nuclei, laminae, and cortices) for each pathway located at different anatomic levels of the spinal cord and brain. The processing centers are the "computers" of these complex, high-speed systems.

From the sensory receptors in the body to the highest centers in the CNS, each *sensory pathway system* follows, in a general way, a basic sequence: (1) Sensory receptors, e.g., touch corpuscles of Meissner in the skin, transmit along (2) nerve fibers to (3) processing centers in the spinal cord and brain, from which signals are conveyed by (4) other nerve fibers, which may ascend on the same side of the CNS or may cross the midline (*decussate*) and ascend on the opposite side of the CNS before terminating in (5) higher processing centers; from these centers, (6) other nerve fibers ascend on the same side before terminating in (7) the highest processing centers in the cerebral cortex. Differences in the basic sequence are present in some ascending systems.

In a general way, the motor systems are organized: to receive stimuli from the sensory systems at all levels of the spinal cord and brain and to convey messages via motor pathways to neuromuscular and neuroglandular endings at muscle and gland cells in the head, body, and extremities. The motor pathways include: sequences of processing centers and their fibers conveying neural influences to other processing centers within the CNS and the final linkages extending from the CNS via motor nerves of the PNS to muscles and glands.

ORIENTATION IN THE BRAIN

The long axis through the brain and spinal cord is called the *neuraxis*. It is shaped in the form of a T, with the vertical part being a line passing through the entire spinal cord and brainstem (medulla, pons, and midbrain) and the horizontal part being a line extending from the frontal pole to the occipital pole of the cerebrum (**Fig. 1.2**). In essence, the cerebral long axis is oriented roughly at a right angle to the long axis of the brainstem-spinal cord.

The term *rostral* ("toward the beak") means in the direction of the cerebrum. *Caudal* means in the direction of the coccygeal region. These terms are used in relation to the neuraxis. In this usage, the crebrum is rostral to the brainstem and the frontal pole of the cerebrum is rostral to the occipital lobe. *Horizontal sections* are those cut parallel to the neuraxis. Horizontal sections through the cerebrum are cut from the frontal pole to the occipital pole, parallel to a plane passing through both eyes. Horizontal sections through the brainstem and spinal cord are cut rostrocaudally, parallel to the front and back of the neuraxis. A *sagittal section* is cut in a vertical plane along the midline; it divides the CNS into symmetric right and left halves. *Midsagittal* is sometimes used for sagittal. *Parasagittal sections* are also in the vertical plane, but lateral to the midsagittal section. A *coronal section* of the cerebrum is cut at a right angle to the horizontal plane. An *axial section* of the brainstem and spinal cord is a cut oriented perpendicular to the neuraxis, giving a cross section or transverse section (see **Figs. 7.7 and 13.8**).

Afferent (or *-petal*, as in centripetal) refers to bringing to or into a structure such as a nucleus; afferent is often used for sensory. *Efferent* (or *-fugal*, as in centrifugal) refers to going away from a structure such as a nucleus; efferent is often used for motor.

ORGANIZATION OF NEURONS IN THE CENTRAL NERVOUS SYSTEM: BRAIN AND SPINAL CORD

The CNS comprises gray matter and white matter. The *gray matter* consists of neuronal cell bodies, dendrites, axon terminals, synapses, and glial cells, and is highly vascular. The *white matter* consists of bundles of axons, many of which are myelinated, and oligodendrocytes; the white color comes from the myelin. It lacks neuronal cell bodies and is less vascular than gray matter.

Groupings of neuronal cell bodies and their immediate processes within the gray matter are variously known as a *nucleus, ganglion, lamina, body, cortex, center, formation,* or *horn*. A cortex is a layer of gray matter on the surface of the brain. Two major cortices are recognized: cerebral and cerebellar cortices. The superior and inferior colliculi of the midbrain and the hippocampal formation also form cortex-like structures. The gray matter, when examined under the microscope, resembles a tangle of nerve and glial processes, called the *neuropil;* this is actually a functionally organized entanglement of processes. Bundles of nerve fibers, many myelinated, are given such special names as *tract, fasciculus, brachium, peduncle, lemniscus, commissure, ansa,* and *capsule.* A *commissure* is a bundle of fibers crossing the midline at right angles to the neuraxis; it interconnects similar structures of the two sides of the brain.

Contralateral refers to the opposite side; it is used primarily to indicate, for example, that pain or paralysis occurs on the side opposite to that of the lesion. *Ipsilateral,* or *homolateral,* refers to the same side; it is used primarily to indicate that pain or paralysis occurs on the same side as that of the lesion.

A *modality* refers to the quality of a stimulus and the resulting forms of sensation (e.g., touch, pain, sound, and vision). Some pathways (tracts, nuclei, or areas of cortex) are *somatotopically (topographically) organized;* specific portions of these structures are associated with restricted regions of the body. For example, fibers conveying position sense from the hand are in definite locations within the posterior columns (sensory pathway), and certain areas of the motor cortex regulate movements of the thumb. Some structures of the visual pathway are topographically related to specific regions within the retina (retinotopic organization), and, similarly, some structures of the auditory pathways are organized functionally with respect to different frequencies or tones (tonotopic organization).

Contents

Subdivisions of the brain

Cerebrum

Brainstem—midbrain, pons and medulla

In the average adult human, the brain weighs about 1400 g, approximately 2% of the total body weight. The brain, a gelatinous mass, is invested by a succession of three connective tissue membranes called *meninges* and is protected by an outer capsule of bone, the *skull*. The brain floats in cerebrospinal fluid, which supports it and acts as a shock absorber in rapid movements of the head. The major arteries and veins supplying the brain lie among the meninges.

SUBDIVISIONS OF THE BRAIN

The major subdivisions of the brain *(encephalon)* are derived from vesicles present in the embryo. They are the *telencephalon, diencephalon, mesencephalon, metencephalon*, and *myelencephalon* (Fig. 6.4). The telencephalon develops into the *cerebral hemispheres*, the diencephalon into the *diencephalon* (between brain), the mesencephalon into the *midbrain*, the metencephalon into the *pons* and *cerebellum* and the myelencephalon into the *medulla oblongata* (shortened to *medulla*) (Fig. 1.1).

The brain may be divided into the cerebrum, brainstem, and cerebellum. The term *cerebrum* is generally used to include the pair of cerebral hemispheres and the diencephalon. The *brainstem* comprises the midbrain, pons, and medulla. The cerebellum is located dorsal to the pons. The definitions for these terms have been adopted in this book. The lower brainstem (pons and medulla) is called the *bulb* or *bulbar region*.

These subdivisions are summarized as follows:

Telencephalon	
Diencephalon	} Cerebrum
Mesencephalon (midbrain)	
Metencephalon (pons portion)	} Brainstem
Myelencephalon (medulla)	
Metencephalon (roof portion)	Cerebellum

On the basis of the location of the tentorium (the double layer of inner dura mater located between the cerebellum and cerebral hemispheres) (Fig. 5.1), the brain is separated into *supratentorial* and *infratentorial* divisions. Thus, the cerebrum is located supratentorially, and the brainstem and cerebellum infratentorially. The diencephalon is a supratentorial structure, whereas the brainstem is an infratentorial entity.

The ventricular system (Chap. 5) is a continuous series of cavities within the brain filled with cerebrospinal fluid (CSF). It is subdivided as follows: the paired *lateral ventricles* are the cavities of the telencephalon (cerebral hemispheres); the *third ventricle*, a median structure, is within the diencephalon; the tubelike *cerebral aqueduct of Sylvius* is the midbrain portion, and the *fourth ventricle* is within the pons and medulla (Figs. 5.1 to 5.3).

The ventricular system continues through the caudal medulla and spinal cord as the *central canal*, which terminates without outlet in the coccygeal segments of the latter.

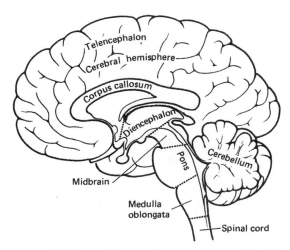

Figure 1.1: The major subdivisions of the central nervous system viewed in sagittal section.

CEREBRUM

The *cerebrum* includes the paired cerebral hemispheres, a small median segment (derived from the telencephalon), and the diencephalon. The surface of each *cerebral hemisphere* is covered by the highly convoluted cerebral cortex that is a 1.5- to 5-millimeter thick layer of gray matter This cortex is subdivided into gyri, sulci, and lobes (**Figs. 1.2 through 1.7, see later**). Underlying the cortex are (1) gray matter structures such as the lenticular nucleus, caudate nucleus, hippocampal formation, and amygdaloid body (amygdala) and (2) white matter structures including the corpus callosum and internal capsule (**Figs. 1.5, 1.7, and 1.8, see later**). The *corpus callosum* is the massive commissure and the *anterior commissure* is the small commissure. Both consist of nerve fibers that inter-

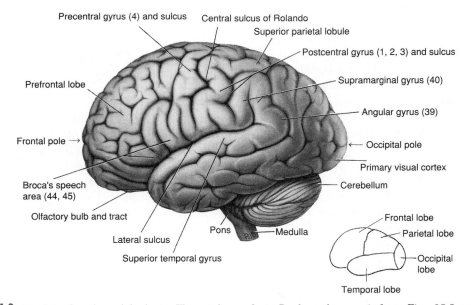

Figure 1.2: The lateral surface of the brain. The numbers refer to Brodmann's areas (refer to Figs. 25.5 and 25.6).

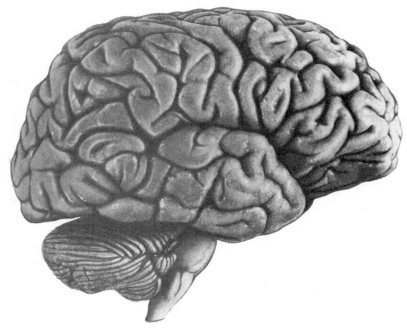

Figure 1.3: Photograph of the lateral surface of the brain. The surface structures can be identified by referring to Figures 1.2 and 25.5. (Courtesy of Dr. Howard A. Matzke, University of Kansas Medical Center.)

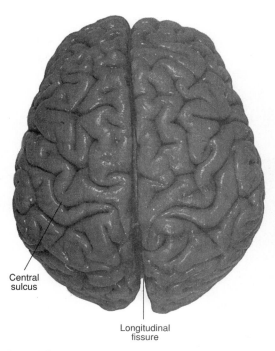

Central sulcus

Longitudinal fissure

Figure 1.4: Photograph of the dorsal surface of the cerebrum. Some gyri and sulci can be identified by referring to Figures 1.2 and 25.5. (Courtesy of Dr. Howard A. Matzke, University of Kansas Medical Center.)

connect the cortices of the two hemispheres (**Figs. 1.1 and 1.5 to 1.8**). The *hippocampal formation* and *amygdala* are structures of the limbic system (**Fig. 1.7**). The unpaired median portion of the telencephalon is a small region in the vicinity of the lamina terminalis and adjacent hypothalamus (**Fig. 1.5**).

Cerebral Topography

The hemispheres are marked on the surface, by slit-like incisures called *sulci* (**Fig. 1.3**). The term *fissure* is sometimes used to designate a particularly deep and constant sulcus. The raised ridge between two sulci is a gyrus. The hemispheres are separated from one another in the midline by the *longitudinal fissure*. Each hemisphere is conventionally divided into six *lobes*: frontal, parietal, occipital, temporal, central (insula or island of Reil), and limbic (**Figs. 1.2 and 1.7**).

Lobes

The lobes are delineated from each other by several major sulci including the lateral sulcus of Sylvius, central sulcus of Rolando, cingulate

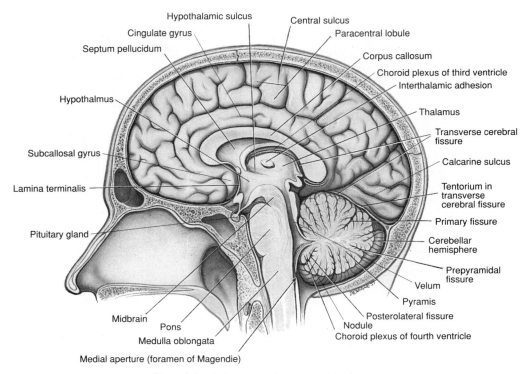

Hypothalamic sulcus
Cingulate gyrus
Septum pellucidum
Central sulcus
Paracentral lobule
Corpus callosum
Choroid plexus of third ventricle
Interthalamic adhesion
Hypothalmus
Thalamus
Transverse cerebral fissure
Subcallosal gyrus
Calcarine sulcus
Lamina terminalis
Tentorium in transverse cerebral fissure
Primary fissure
Pituitary gland
Cerebellar hemisphere
Prepyramidal fissure
Velum
Pyramis
Midbrain
Pons
Posterolateral fissure
Nodule
Medulla oblongata
Choroid plexus of fourth ventricle
Medial aperture (foramen of Magendie)

Figure 1.5: Median sagittal section of the brain.

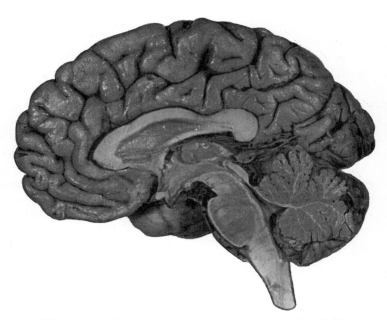

Figure 1.6: Photograph of the midsagittal view of the brain. Structures can be identified by referring to Figures 1.5 and 13.3. (Courtesy of Dr. Howard A. Matzke, University of Kansas Medical Center.)

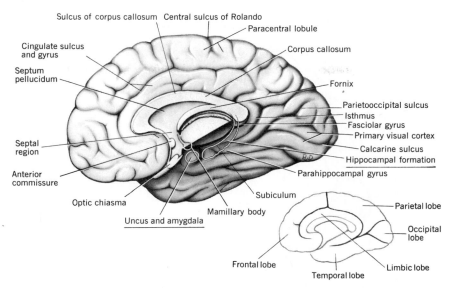

Figure 1.7: The median surface of the cerebral hemisphere. The amygdala and the hippocampal formation are represented by white lines. The amygdala is located within the uncus. The hippocampal formation (hippocampus and dentate gyrus) is located in the floor of the temporal horn of the lateral ventricle (Fig. 1.9).

sulcus, and parietooccipital sulcus. The lateral sulcus is a deep furrow which extends posteriorly from the basal surface of the brain along the lateral surface of the hemisphere to terminate usually as an upward curve within the inferior part of the parietal lobe (**Fig. 1.2**). The central sulcus of Rolando extends obliquely from the region of the lateral sulcus, across the dorsolateral cerebral surface, and, for a short distance, onto the medial surface (**Figs. 1.2 to 1.6**). The cingulate sulcus is a curved cleft on the medial surface extending parallel to the curvature of the corpus callosum. The parietooccipital sulcus is a deep cleft on the medial surface located between the central sulcus and the occipital pole (**Fig. 1.7**).

The boundaries of the lobes on the lateral cerebral surface are as follows: (1) the frontal lobe is located anterior to the central sulcus and above the lateral sulcus; (2) the occipital lobe is posterior to an imaginary line parallel to the parietooccipital sulcus which is on the medial surface; (3) the parietal lobe is located posterior to the central sulcus, anterior to the imaginary parietooccipital line, and above the lateral sulcus and a line extrapolated towards the occipital pole; (4) the temporal lobe is located below the lateral sulcus and anterior to the imaginary pa-

rietooccipital line; and (5) the central lobe is located at the bottom (medial surface) of the lateral sulcus of Sylvius, which is actually a deep fossa (depression). It can be seen only when the temporal and frontal lobes are reflected away from the lateral sulcus.

The boundaries of the lobes on the medial cerebral surface (**Fig. 1.7**) are as follows: (1) the frontal lobe is located rostral to a line formed by the central sulcus; (2) the parietal lobe is between the central sulcus and the parietooccipital sulcus; (3) the temporal lobe is located lateral to the parahippocampal gyrus; (4) the occipital lobe is posterior to the parietooccipital sulcus; and (5) the limbic lobe is a synthetic one formed by parts of the frontal, parietal, and temporal lobes. It is located central to the curved line formed by the cingulate sulcus and the collateral sulcus (the latter is located lateral to the parahippocampal gyrus). The limbic lobe is the ring (limbus) of gyri bordered by this line; it includes the subcallosal area, cingulate gyrus, parahippocampal gyrus, hippocampus, dentate gyrus, and uncus (**Figs. 1.5–1.7, and 1.9**).

Gyri

The *precentral gyrus* is anterior and parallel to the central sulcus of Rolando. The *postcentral*

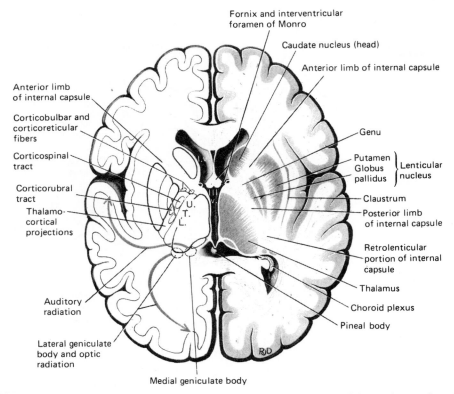

Fornix and interventricular
foramen of Monro

Caudate nucleus (head)

Anterior limb of internal capsule

Anterior limb
of internal capsule

Corticobulbar and
corticoreticular
fibers

Corticospinal
tract

Corticorubral
tract

Thalamo-
cortical
projections

Auditory
radiation

Lateral geniculate
body and optic
radiation

Medial geniculate body

Genu

Putamen
Globus
pallidus

Lenticular
nucleus

Claustrum

Posterior limb
of internal capsule

Retrolenticular
portion of internal
capsule

Thalamus

Choroid plexus

Pineal body

Figure 1.8: Horizontal section through the cerebrum. Note the location of the head of the caudate nucleus, lenticular nucleus, thalamus relative to the ventricles, and the internal capsule. The components of the internal capsule are indicated on the left side. The topographic distribution of the motor pathway from the motor cortex is indicated: U = upper extremity; T = trunk; and L = lower extremity. Note that the right lateral ventricle (l.v.) is represented twice and the third ventricle (III v.) once.

gyrus is posterior and parallel to the central sulcus. The paracentral lobule, on the medial surface, is continuous with the precentral and postcentral gyri on the lateral surface and is partially divided by the central sulcus (**Figs. 1.5 and 1.6**).

The cortex anterior to the central sulcus is motor in function; that posterior to the central sulcus is sensory in function. The postcentral gyrus and the posterior part of the paracentral lobule are known as Brodmann areas 1, 2, and 3 of the cerebral cortex (**Fig. 25.5**). The posterior part of the precentral gyrus and adjacent portion of the paracentral gyrus are called area 4 or the motor cortex. The *transverse gyri of Heschl* located in the upper part of the temporal lobe, facing the lateral sulcus, make up the primary receptive areas for audition (areas 41 and 42). The cortex on either side of the calcarine

sulcus is the primary receptive area for vision (area 17). The areas outside the primary receptive areas are called *association areas*; Broca's area (**Fig. 1.2**), for example, is a cortical area associated with the formulation of speech. The functional aspects of the Brodmann areas are discussed in Chapter 25.

Basal Ganglia

The term *basal ganglia* refers to several groups of subcortical nuclei (**Figs. 1.8 and 24.4**). These are the caudate nucleus, lenticular nucleus, subthalamic nucleus, and substantia nigra. No longer included are the claustrum and amygdala (amygdaloid body or amygdaloid nucleus); the latter is a component of the limbic system (Chap. 23). The *caudate nucleus* and the *lenticular nucleus* are collectively called the

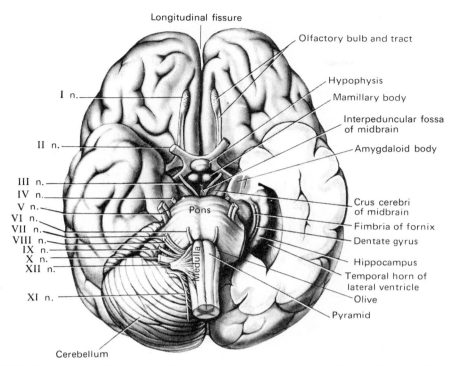

Longitudinal fissure

Olfactory bulb and tract

I n.

Hypophysis

Mamillary body

Interpeduncular fossa
of midbrain

II n.

Amygdaloid body

III n.
IV n.
V n.
VI n.
VII n.
VIII n.
IX n.
X n.
XII n.

Pons

Crus cerebri
of midbrain

Fimbria of fornix

Dentate gyrus

Hippocampus

Temporal horn of
lateral ventricle

XI n.

Medulla

Olive

Pyramid

Cerebellum

Figure 1.9: The basal surface of the brain. Note roots of the cranial nerves. A horizontal section through the left temporal and occipital lobes reveals the hippocampus, dentate gyrus, fimbria of the fornix, and temporal horn of the lateral ventricle. The fimbria of the fornix consists of fibers entering the fornix from the hippocampus. The hypophysis and the mamillary body are components of the diencephalon. n = cranial nerve.

corpus striatum; they are the deep nuclei of the cerebral hemispheres. The *lenticular nucleus* is subdivided into the *putamen* and *globus pallidus* (pallidum, paleostriatum). The *putamen* and the *caudate nucleus* are called the *striatum* (neostriatum). The *subthalamic nucleus* is located within the ventral thalamus (Chap. 23). The *substantia nigra* is a nucleus located within the midbrain (Chap. 13).

The Basal Ganglia*

Lenticular nucleus		
Globus pallidus		
Putamen	} Striatum	} Corpus striatum
Caudate nucleus		
Subthalamic nucleus		
Substantia nigra		

* See Tables 24.1 and 24.2 for further details.

Diencephalon

The *diencephalon*, located in the ventromedial portion of the cerebrum, is continuous caudally

with the midbrain (**Fig. 1.1**). It consists of four subdivisions: epithalamus, thalamus (dorsal thalamus), hypothalamus, and ventral thalamus (subthalamus). The epithalamus, choroid plexus of the third ventricle (**Fig. 1.5**), and the pineal body (**Fig. 1.8**) form the upper margin (roof) of the diencephalon. Ventral to the thalamus is the hypothalamus including the hypophysis (pituitary gland) and mamillary bodies (**Figs. 1.5 and 1.9**). The ventral thalamus is located lateral to the hypothalamus (not seen in Fig. 1.5).

Internal Capsule

The *internal capsule* is a massive bundle of nerve fibers that contains almost all the fibers projecting from subcortical nuclei to the cerebral cortex and from the cerebral cortex to subcortical structures in the cerebrum, brainstem, and spinal cord (**Figs. 13.5 and 23.3**). It is divided into an anterior limb, genu, and posterior limb (**Fig. 1.8**). Retrolenticular and sub-

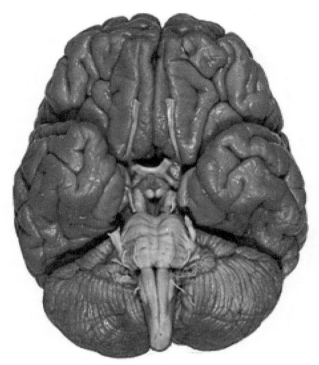

Figure 1.10: Photograph of the basal view of the brain. Structures can be identified by referring to Figures 1.5 and 13.3. (Courtesy of Dr. Howard A. Matzke, University of Kansas Medical Center.)

lenticular parts of the posterior limb are recognized (Figs. 1.8 and 23.3). The *anterior (caudatolenticular) limb* is located between the caudate nucleus and the lenticular nucleus. The *genu (knee)* is located between the anterior and posterior limbs. The *posterior (thalamolenticular) limb* is located between the thalamus and lenticular nucleus. The *retrolenticular (postlenticular)* part of the posterior limb is located lateral to the thalamus and posterior to the lenticular nucleus and the *sublenticular part* is ventral to the lenticular nucleus.

BRAINSTEM—MIDBRAIN, PONS, AND MEDULLA

Several prominent landmarks are present on the anterior surface of the brainstem (Figs. 1.9, 1.10, and 13.4). In the midbrain, the paired crura cerebri are lateral to the interpeduncular fossa through which passes the *oculomotor nerves (third cranial nerve)*. The *trochlear nerve (fourth cranial nerve)* emerges from the lower

aspect of the dorsal surface of the midbrain (Fig. 13.2). The *trigeminal nerve (fifth cranial nerve*, composed of a small motor root and a large sensory root) emerges on the lateral aspect of the massive pons. The pyramids, olives, and roots of seven cranial nerves are features visible on the anterior surface of the medulla. The *pyramids* are formed by the fibers of the pyramidal tracts (corticospinal tract). The *olive* is a protuberance formed by the inferior olivary nucleus (Figs. 13.3 to 13.5). From medial to lateral, the *abducent (sixth), facial (seventh)*, and *vestibulocochlear (eighth) nerves* emerge at the junction of the pons and medulla. The *glossopharyngeal (ninth)* and *vagus (tenth) nerves* emerge as a series of rootlets from the sulcus on the posterior margin of the olive. The *spinal accessory (eleventh) nerve* emerges in the form of rootlets from the medulla and from the spinal cord (between the dorsal and ventral roots of the first six cervical spinal nerves). The *hypoglossal (twelfth) nerve* emerges from the sulcus between the olive and pyramid.

Note that the third, sixth, and twelfth cranial

nerves emerge from the anterior brainstem in a longitudinal line just lateral to the midsagittal plane. The fifth, seventh, ninth, tenth, and eleventh cranial nerves emerge from the lateral aspect of the brainstem.

For a more complete description of the surface anatomy of the brainstem, see Chapter 13.

SUGGESTED READINGS

Angevine J, Cotman C. *Principles of Neuroanatomy*. 2nd ed. New York, NY: Oxford University Press; 1993.

Barr M, Kiernan J. *The Human Nervous System: An Anatomical Viewpoint*. 6th ed. Philadelphia, Pa: JB Lippincott; 1993.

Brodal P. *The Central Nervous System: Structure and Function*. New York, NY: Oxford University Press; 1992.

Burt A. *Textbook of Neuroanatomy*. Philadelphia, Pa: W B Saunders; 1992.

Carpenter M. *Core Text of Neuroanatomy*. 4th ed. Baltimore, Md: Williams & Wilkins; 1991.

Clemente C, ed. *Gray's Anatomy of the Human Body*. 30th ed. Philadelphia, Pa: Lea & Febiger; 1985.

Daube J, Reagen T, Sandok B, Westmoreland B. *Medical Neurosciences, An Approach to Anatomy, Pathology, and Physiology by System and Levels*. 3rd ed. Boston, Mass: Little Brown & Co; 1994.

Gilman S, Newman S. *Manter and Gatz's Essentials of Clinical Neuroanatomy and Neurophysiology*. 8th ed. Philadelphia, Pa: FA Davis Co; 1992.

Haines D. *Neuroanatomy: An Atlas of Structures, Sections, and Systems*. 4th ed. Baltimore, Md: Williams & Wilkins; 1995.

Heimer L. *The Human Brain and Spinal Cord: Functional Neuroanatomy and Dissection Guide*. 2nd ed. New York, NY: Springer-Verlag; 1994.

Kandel E, Schwartz J, Jessell T, eds. Essentials of Neural Science and Behavior. Norwalk, Conn: Appleton & Lange; 1995.

Kuffler S, Nicholls J, Martin A. *From Neuron to Brain: A Cellular Approach to the Function of the Nervous System*. 2nd ed. Sunderland, Mass: Sinauer; 1984.

Lockard I. *Desk Reference for Neuroscience*. New York: Springer-Verlag; 1991.

Martin J. *Neuroanatomy, Text and Atlas*. New York, NY: Elsevier; 1989.

Nauta W, Fertig M. *Fundamental Neuroanatomy*. New York, NY: WH Freeman; 1986.

Netter F. *Atlas of Human Anatomy*. West Caldwell, NJ: Ciba-Geigy; 1989.

Nieuwenhuys R, Voogd R, Hurjzen C. *The Human Central Nervous System*. 4th ed. New York, NY: Springer-Verlag; 1993.

Noback C, Demarest R. *The Human Nervous System. Basic Principles of Neurobiology*. 3rd ed. New York, NY: McGraw-Hill; 1981.

Nolte J. *The Human Brain. An Introduction to Its Functional Anatomy*. 3rd ed. St Louis, Mo: CV Mosby Co; 1993.

Roberts M, Hanaway J, Morest D. *Atlas of the Human Brain in Section*. 2nd ed. Philadelphia, Pa: Lea & Febiger; 1987.

Rowland L, ed. *Merritts Textbook of Neurology*. 9th ed. Baltimore, Md: Williams & Wilkins; 1995.

Shepherd G. *Neurobiology*. 3rd ed. New York, NY: Oxford University Press; 1994.

Thompson R. *The Brain: An Introduction to Neuroscience*. New York, NY: WH Freeman; 1985.

Williams P, Warwick R, Dyson M, Bannister L, eds. Neurology. In: *Gray's Anatomy*. 37th ed. Edinburgh: Churchill Livingstone; 1989:859–1244.

Willis W Jr, Grossman R. *Medical Neurobiology: Neuroanatomical and Neurophysiological Principles Basic to Clinical Neuroscience*. 3rd ed. St Louis, Mo: CV Mosby; 1981.

Many of the above are general references that contain subject matter presented in subsequent chapters.

Neurons and Associated Cells 2

Organelles and components

Trophic effects and nerve growth factor (NGF)

Structure of peripheral nerves and ganglia

Neuroglia (GLIA)

Nerve regeneration

Plasticity and axonal sprouting

Over 100 billion (10^{11}) neurons (nerve cells), as well as many more glial cells, are integrated into the structural and functional fabric that is the brain. They exhibit a wide diversity of forms and sizes. With the exception of a few cell types, each neuron usually consists of a *cell body* (*soma*) from which extends a single nerve process called an *axon* and a variable number of branching processes called *dendrites* (*dendrons*) (Fig. 2.1). Each axon, including its collateral branches, usually terminates as an arbor of fine fibers; each fiber ends as an enlargement called a *bouton*, which is a part of a synaptic junction (see later). At the other end of the neuron, there is the three-dimensional *dendritic field*, which is an arbor formed by the branching of the neuron's dendrites.

The neuron is the basic unit of the nervous system. Each neuron is in synaptic contact through its processes with other neurons, so that each is a segment in the network of which the nervous system is composed. A neuron is designed to react to stimuli; to transmit the resulting excitation rapidly to other portions of the cell; and to influence other neurons, muscle cells, and glandular cells. Neurons are so specialized that most are incapable of reproducing and lose viability if denied just minutes of oxygen.

The term *nerve cell* is a synonym for a neuron, including all of its processes. Its use as the equivalent for *cell body* or *soma* (excluding its processes) is erroneous.

Some idea of the relative proportions of various parts of a neuron can be obtained from this well-known comparison. If the cell body of a lower motoneuron of the spinal cord (Chap. 7) is enlarged to the size of a baseball, the axon would be about 1 mile long, and the dendrites and their branches would arborize throughout a large amphitheater (Fig. 2.1).

ORGANELLES AND COMPONENTS

Each neuron consists of a large nucleus; a plasma (cell) membrane and a cytoplasm consisting of a cytosol (everything except organelles); and a number of organelles including endoplasmic reticulum, Nissl substance, Golgi apparatus, mitochondria, lysosomes, neurotubules (microtubules), and neurofilaments (microfilaments) (Figs. 2.2 to 2.4).

Nucleus

The nucleus is delineated from the cytoplasm by the double layer of unit membrane called the *nuclear envelope*. This membrane is perforated by *nuclear pores*, through which large *macromolecules* synthesized in the nucleus pass into the cytoplasm. The nucleus contains DNA in the form of genes that, along with some proteins, comprise the 46 chromosomes of the human. Some DNA (genes) that encode some functions

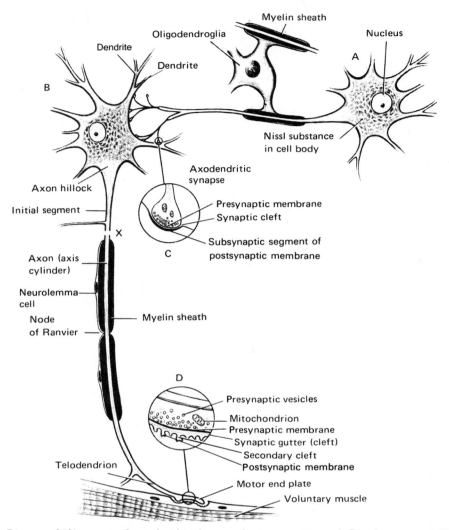

Figure 2.1: Diagram of (**A**) a neuron located within the central nervous system and (**B**) a lower motoneuron located in both the central and peripheral nervous systems. The latter synapses with a voluntary muscle cell to form a motor end plate. Note the similarities, as reconstructed from electron micrographs, between (**C**) a synapse between two neurons, and (**D**) a motor end plate. The X represents the border between the central nervous system (above the X) and the peripheral nervous system (below the X). Note that the myelin sheath of neuron (**A**) is entirely the product of a glial (oligodendroglia) cell, and that of neuron (**B**) is produced by a glial cell while inside the central nervous system and by a Schwann (neurolemma) cell in the peripheral nervous system.

are present in the mitochondria. The *outer layer* of the nuclear envelope is continuous with the membranes of the endoplasmic reticulum. The *inner layer* of the envelope has filaments that attach to the nuclear chromatin and to other structures involved in pore diameter control.

The chromosomes contain sequences of DNA called genes. The genes act by determining, through transcription, the amino acid sequences

of polypeptides and, thus, the structures and properties of proteins. A gene is that portion of the DNA sequence responsible for the primary structure (amino acid sequence) of a particular polypeptide. The *translation* of the *DNA code* into a protein is done by a special ribonucleic acid (RNA) called messenger RNA (mRNA). The mRNA migrates from the nucleus through the nuclear pores to the cytoplasm and becomes associated with a ribosome, which contains another RNA called ribosomal RNA (rRNA). The rRNA acts as a template onto which the amino acids are assembled. Another RNA, called transfer RNA (tRNA) brings the amino acids in the cytosol to the messenger RNA to be synthesized into the peptide. In other words, DNA specifies RNA through the process known as transcription. The RNA then specifies proteins via translation. Thus the information coded into the DNA sequence of the gene is *transcribed* to the mRNA which carries it to the ribosome where it is translated into a specific amino acid sequence to the corresponding peptide. The ribosomes are the sites of protein synthesis.

Like other cells, each neuron synthesizes three classes of proteins, each with a specific physiological role in the neuron. Except for a few proteins encoded by mitochondria, essentially all of the macromolecules of a neuron are made in the cell body from mRNAs. These 3 classes are as follows: (1) *Proteins synthesized in the cytosol by free ribosomes and polysomes and remain in the cytosol of the neuron.* These proteins, distributed by slow axoplasmic transport (see later), include enzymes essential to catalyze metabolic processes of the cytoskeleton. (2) *Proteins synthesized in the cytosol by free ribosomes and polysomes and incorporated into the nucleus, mitochondria, and peroxisomes.* These include enzymes that are involved in the synthesis of RNA, DNA, transcription factors regulating gene expression, and other proteins required by these organelles. Mitochondria are distributed by slow axoplasmic flow. (3) *Proteins synthesized in association with the membrane systems attached to or within the lumen of the endoplasmic reticulum and Golgi Apparatus (GA).* They are disbursed by vesicles that bud off the GA and are distributed, via fast axoplasmic flow, to such organelles as lysosomes and secretory (transmitter containing) vesicles and to the plasma membrane for the maintenance of its protein composition.

The prominent nucleolus within the nucleus of a neuron is a ribosome-producing machine consisting largely of RNA and protein, along with some DNA. It is the site of ribosomal (rRNA) production and initial assembly. The nucleolus is well developed in cells, such as neurons, which are active in protein synthesis.

The brain is conceived of as utilizing more genes than any other organ in the body, maybe as many as 50,000 genes. It is likely that of these, 30,000 may be unique to the neural tissue.

In females, nuclei of cells throughout the body, including neurons, contain a condensation of one of the two X chromosomes (sex chromatin) called a Barr body **(Fig 2.3)**. It appears as a small clump near the nuclear envelope. These structures, first described in cat spinal motoneurons, can be seen in smears of cells inside the mouth (buccal smears). A normal male has an XY constitution and lacks Barr bodies.

Plasma (Cell) Membrane

The *plasma (cell) membrane* is a highly organized and dynamic 8- to 10-nanometer thick organelle. Many cellular processes are initiated as a consequence of molecular reactions within the membrane. It is a flexible, nonstretchable structure consisting of two layers of lipid molecules (bilipid layer of phospholipids) and associated proteins, lipids (cholesterol and glycolipids), and carbohydrates **(Fig. 2.2)**. Its surface area can only be changed by the addition or subtraction of membrane. The lipids are oriented with their hydrophilic (polar) ends facing the outer surface and the hydrophobic (nonpolar) ends projecting to the middle of the membrane. Thus the hydrophilic heads face the water on both sides of the membrane. The membrane proteins (peptide chains) embedded in the bilipid layer are called *integral* or *intrinsic proteins* to which *peripheral proteins* are attached. On the external side of the membrane are carbohydrate chains; those linked to proteins form *glycoproteins* and those linked to lipids form *glycolipids*. These carbohydrates can act as mediators in cell and molecular recognition and of cell adhesion. As a result, the side facing the tissue fluids differs from that facing the interior of the neuron not only structurally, but in function as well.

All biologic membranes are organized (1) to block the diffusion of water soluble molecules; (2) to be selectively permeable to certain molecules via specialized pores or channels (ionophores); and (3) to transduce information by

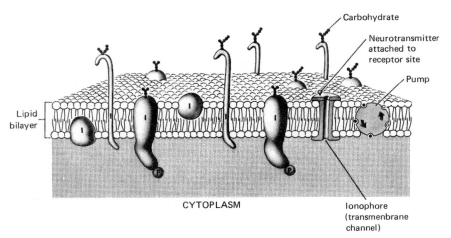

Figure 2.2: Plasma membrane of a neuron. Several types of integral proteins (I) are embedded in the bilipid layer of the 5-nanometer thick plasma membrane. The carbohydrate chains of the glycoproteins are located on the outer membrane surface. The differential distribution of specific proteins is a basis for regional differences in the functional activities expressed by the membrane. The carbohydrate chains of the glycolipids are not illustrated.

At right, integral proteins are schematized as (1) a transmembrane channel (ionophore) with about a 0.5-nanometer wide pore and (2) a coupled sodium-potassium pump (Chap. 3). An ionophore acts as a selective channel for the preferential passage of an ion such as sodium or potassium (Chap. 3). The disk on the outer margin of the ionophore represents the receptor site (receptor protein) acting as a binding subunit for a neurotransmitter, which is represented as an irregular object above the receptor site. The pump is specialized to transport sodium ions (open circles) out of the neuron in exchange for pumping potassium ions (solid circles) into the neuron. Peripheral proteins (P) are attached to the integral proteins.

protein receptors responsive to chemical or physical stimulation by neurotransmitters, hormones (chemical), light, vibrations or pressure (physical) (Chap. 3). The lipid layers act as a barrier to diffusion by being impermeable to ions; the proteins are organized as specific receptors, ion channels, transporters, and carriers that make them quite permeable to particular ions under certain circumstances (Chap. 3).

There is a continuous traffic of small molecules crossing the plasma membrane. This movement involves (1) the regulation of the neuron's concentration of such inorganic ions as Na^+, K^+, CA^{++}, and Cl^- and shifting them one way or another across the plasma membrane; (2) taking in oxygen for cellular respiration and expelling carbon dioxide; and (3) transporting nutrients into and waste products of metabolism out of the cell. Some substances diffuse across the membranes from a region of higher concentration to one of lower concentration. This diffusion down the concentration gradient is called *passive transport*, because the neuron does not expend energy to effect the

movement. The concentration gradient represents the potential energy that powers the diffusion. A form of passive transport is called *facilitated diffusion (transport)* because the ions and molecules diffuse across the membrane with the help of *transport proteins* that span the membrane. In this diffusion, the transport proteins apparently remain in place and help the ions across the membrane by undergoing a subtle change that translocates the binding site from one side of the membrane to the other. These changes can trigger both the binding and the release of the transported ions.

The movement of substances across a semipermeable plasma membrane from sites of low concentration to sites of high concentration ("uphill") occurs by *active transport, exocytosis,* and *endocytosis*. Active transport has a critical role in a neuron to maintain the internal concentration of small molecules that differ from the concentrations in the extracellular environment. The process is called *active transport* because in order to pump the molecules "uphill," the neuron must expend its own energy. The work of active transport is carried out by specific proteins inserted in the membrane, with adenosine triphosphate (ATP) supplying the energy. ATP powers the active transport by transferring its terminal phosphate group directly to the transport ion. This presumably induces the protein to change its configuration in a manner that translocates the ions bound to the protein across the membrane. One such transport system is the sodium-potassium pump, an integral membrane protein, which exchanges sodium for potassium ions across the plasma membrane. This pump transport system drives the ions against steep gradients. The pump oscillates between two conformational states in pumping cycle that translocates three Na^+ ions out of the neuron for every two K^+ ions pumped into the neuron. ATP powers the changes in conformation by transferring a phosphate group to the pump transport protein. The two conformational states differ in their affinity for Na^+ and K^+ and in the directional orienting of the ion binding sites. Prior to phosphorylation, the binding sites face the cytoplasm and only the Na^+ sites are receptive. Sodium binding induces phosphate transfer from ATP to the pump, triggering the conformational change. In its new conformation, the pump's binding sites face the extracellular side of the plasma membrane, and the protein now has a greater affinity for K^+ than it does for Na^+. Potassium binding causes the release of the phosphate, and the pump returns to its original conformation. Because the pump also acts as an enzyme that removes phosphate from ATP, it is also called ATPase.

In the process called *exocytosis*, the neuron releases macromolecules (e.g., neurotransmitters) by the fusion of the vesicles with the plasma membrane (see Synapses at the Motor End Plate, Chap. 3). In the process called *endocytosis*, the neuron takes in macromolecules and particulate matter by forming vesicles derived from the plasma membrane (see Recycling of Synaptic Vesicles, Chap. 3).

Physiologically, the membrane proteins may be characterized in functional terms. These include:

1. *Channels (ionophores)* that allow for the passage of certain ions (such as Na^+, K^+, Cl^-, and Ca^{++}), across the membrane, and down concentration and voltage gradients (Chap. 3). The channels are glycoproteins surrounding continuous pores through the membrane (transmembrane) that allow some ions to flow at rates as high as 100 million ions per second per channel. Some channels are permanently open, others only transiently. The latter are said to be "gated." When the gate opens, ions pass through the channel, and when the gate closes ions do not pass through (Chap. 3). A calculation indicates that a chemically gated acetylcholine channel (a channel that opens in the presence of acetylcholine) will open for 1 millisecond and then close. During the 1 millisecond, about 20,000 Na^+ ions flow into the neuron, and somewhat fewer K^+ ions out of the neuron, through each channel.

2. *Pumps* that serve to transport certain ions (sodium-potassium pump, Chap. 3) or metabolic precursors of macromolecules. Pumps work against an ionic gradient and thus extrude Na^+ from the neuron. Energy for this activity is obtained from the hydrolysis of ATP.

3. Receptor Protein Sites are involved with the recognition of neurotransmitters and hormones. They act as binding sites for these substances on the outer surface of the plasma membrane. The sites initiate the responses of the neuron, muscle fiber, or gland cell to specific stimuli (chemical or mechanical).

4. *Transducer Proteins* are involved in coupling receptors to enzymes following the binding of a ligand, such as a transmitter or a hormone, to the receptor (the term ligand refers to any molecule that binds to a receptor on the surface of a cell). Through the action of a transducer, an enzyme may initiate the action of a *second messenger* such as cyclic adenosine monophosphate (cAMP) (see Second Messenger System, Chap. 3).

5. *Structural Proteins* are those which form junctions with other neurons, such as cell adhesion molecules (CAM). Intercellular recognition among neural cells and their adhesion one to the other in functionally meaningful patterns involves glycoproteins called *neural cell adhesion molecules (NCAM)*. These molecules are present on the cell sur-

face of all developing neural cells where they influence pathways of cell migration and terminal axonal outgrowths. NCAMs also have important roles in adult tissues, where they are responsible for the affinity of nerve terminals to their targets and for the interactions between neurons and other cell types. NCAMs also contribute to the general adherence property of all neural cells. Each is a glycoprotein with a high content of a carbohydrate called sialic acid. It appears that this molecule is important in promoting the outgrowth of the developing axon and to be involved in its response to guidance cues during neural development (Chap. 6). The *NCAMs* and another glycoprotein family called *cadherins* form the basis of cell-specific adhesion where identical molecules on different cells bind to each other. Another glycoprotein family called *integrins* mediate between the neuronal surface and molecules in the extracellular matrix. The NCAM is present in most neural induction and is presumed to contribute to the general adhesive properties of neural cells.

6. *Neurotransmitter Transporter Proteins* are plasma membrane glycoproteins involved with the uptake from the synaptic cleft of such transmitters as serotonin, dopamine, and glutamate for recycling (**Fig 3.9**). The energy stores in the transmembrane electrochemical gradients are utilized to drive these chemical agents into the axon terminal.

The cell membrane has a dynamic fluidity in that the proteins, which are suspended in a "solution of membrane lipids," can shift laterally and even rotate within the bilipid layer unless restrained by the binding of the protein to some underlying cytoplasm.

The movement and addition of acetylcholine (ACh) receptors within the plasma membrane is a graphic example of this fluidity. ACh receptors of the plasma membrane of a muscle fiber are normally clustered and confined in the subsynaptic membrane of the motor end plate (**Fig. 2.4**). Prior to the formation of a motor end plate during early development, ACh receptors are distributed throughout the plasma membrane of the embryonic muscle fiber. Within hours following the contact of an axon with the embryonic muscle a motor end plate commences to

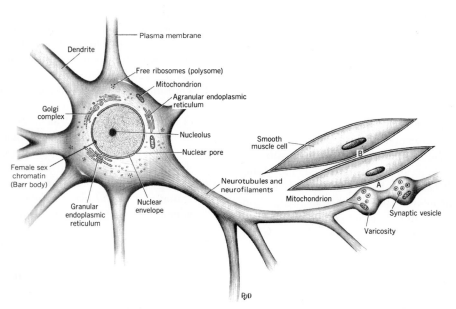

Figure 2.3: Some of the cytoplasmic organelles and associated structures of a postganglionic neuron of the autonomic nervous system. The junction between the varicosity and smooth muscle cell **A** is a typical synapse (Fig. 15–3). The junction between two smooth muscle cells **B** is an electrical synapse (gap junction, nexus). The small circles in the cell body represent lysosomes.

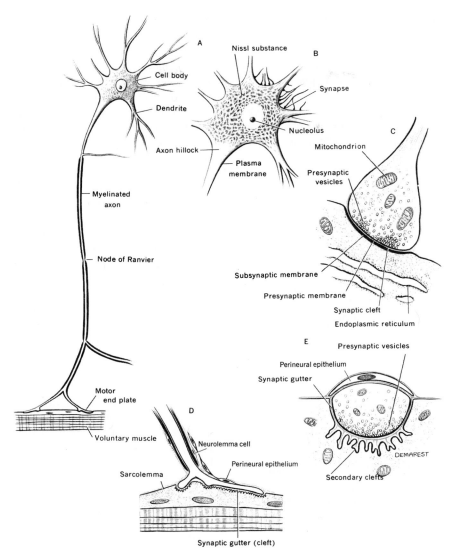

Figure 2.4: A motoneuron (lower motor neuron, alpha motor neuron) of the anterior horn of the spinal cord. **A.** The neuron includes a cell body and its processes (dendrites and axons). Note the axon collateral process branching at a node of Ranvier. **B.** Axons terminate as telodendria; each telodendritic terminal has a bulbous ending, forming either an axosomatic or an axodendritic synapse. **C.** The synapse as reconstructed from electron micrographs. Note similarities between synapse and motor end plate in E. **D.** Motor end plate as visualized with the light microscope. The sarcolemma (plasma membrane of muscle cell) is the postsynaptic membrane of the motor end plate. **E.** Section through motor end plate as based on electron micrographs. Portion of terminal ending fits into synaptic gutter of muscle fiber. Neurolemma (Schwann) cells cover portion of axon not in the gutter. The secondary clefts (junctional folds) are modifications of the sarcolemma. The basal lamina is within the synaptic cleft.

form. ACh receptors accumulate in the subsynaptic membrane by the *migration of some receptors* from non-end plate plasma membrane and largely from the *insertion of newly formed receptors*. This clustering, induced by putative chemotropic factors, is accompanied by the drastic reduction of receptors on the non-end plate plasma membrane. At this stage, the muscle can no longer be innervated by another axon. If the axon is cut and the muscle denervated and allowed to degenerate, there is a reduction in the number of ACh receptors at the former end plate accompanied by their wide distribution all over the plasma membrane. If this muscle is reinnervated, the ACh receptors again accumulate in the new subsynaptic membrane and are reduced in the non-end plate plasma membrane.

Regional differences in the biochemical properties of the plasma membrane result in local functional specializations of the membrane (Chap. 3).

Nissl Bodies and Endoplasmic Reticulum (ER)

The *Nissl bodies* (chromophilic substance) are basophilic aggregates located in the cell body and dendrites of each neuron, but absent in the axon and axon hillock located at the junction of cell body and axon (Fig. 2.1). Each Nissl body is composed of (1) flattened sacs (called cisternae) of *granular endoplasmic reticulum (rough ER)* studded with ribosomes facing the cytosol, (2) *free ribosomes*, and (3) clusters of ribosomes linked together, called *polysomes* (Fig. 2.3). The granular ER is continuous with the smooth ER (ER without ribosomes). The *rough ER* is the organelle involved in the synthesis of neurosecretory proteins, integral membrane proteins of the plasma membrane, and proteins of the lysosomes (see Golgi apparatus later). The free ribosomes and polysomes are associated with the synthesis of the proteins of the cytosol and non-integral proteins of the plasma membrane. The *smooth ER* is the locale where triglycerides, cholesterol, and steroids are synthesized.

Neurons require prodigious amounts of proteins to maintain their integrity and to perform their functional activities. In 1 to 3 days, they synthesize an amount equal to the total protein content of the neuron. Much of it is distributed within the neuron by plasmic transport (see later). Neurons are actually neurotransmitter secretory cells rivaling glandular cells as the most prolific protein synthesizing cells.

Mitochondria and Peroxisomes

Mitochondria are membrane-bound organelles that, as the cell's power plants (Fig. 2.3), are the chief source of energy for each cell. Energy, water, and carbon dioxide are the products of cell respiration and enzymatic activity, mainly of carbohydrates, and, to a lesser degree, of amino acids and fats. The energy released from the oxidation of food is converted to phosphate-bound energy as ATP. ATP-bound energy is essential for several cellular processes including the maintenance of the pumps for the transport of ions across the plasma membrane, muscle contraction, and protein synthesis (Chap. 3).

Neurons, unlike most cells, lack the ability to store glycogen as an energy source. As a consequence, they are dependent for their energy on circulating glucose and oxygen. Glucose is the substrate utilized by mitochondrial enzyme systems of neurons for the aerobic generation of ATP. (Neurons do not utilize fat as a substrate for the process of anaerobic generation of ATP.) This explains why we lose consciousness if the blood supply to the brain is interrupted for a short time.

The mitochondria have a small amount of their own DNA (mtDNA) which enables them to produce some constituent proteins, RNA, and enzymes. Many substances required by the mitochondria are derived from the cytoplasm.

Several developmental neurologic disorders, called *mitochondrial myopathies*, have been attributed to the inheritance of mitochondrial mtDNA abnormalities. Such a congenital myopathy is myoclonic epilepsy with ragged red fibers (with special stains abnormal mitochondria appear red—hence ragged red fibers). Myopathies are conditions in which the symptoms are due to the dysfunction of muscle but with no evidence of nerve degeneration.

Mitochondria are present in the ovum but not in sperm. Thus mtDNA inheritance is said to be matrilinear and independent of nuclear inheritance.

Peroxisomes are organelles that function to detoxify with the enzyme catalase by the hydrolyzing hydrogen peroxide, and thereby protect the neuron from this chemical agent.

Lysosomes

Lysosomes are the membrane-bound vesicles that act as an intracellular digestive system. They contain a variety of hydrolytic enzymes that digest and degrade substances originating both inside and outside the neuron. The hydrolytic enzymes and lysosome membrane are

synthesized in the rough ER and then transferred to the GA for further processing. After
budding from the GA these products are transported via vesicles to the lysosomes. The di-
gested materials include many cell components
such as receptors and membranes, some of
which can be recycled. The so-called yellow
lipofuscin granules found in neurons of advanced age are said to represent the effects of
"wear and tear" and may be insoluble residues
of lysosomal activity.

Golgi Apparatus (GA)

The GA is a complex organelle composed of
stacks of flattened cisternal sacs (**Fig. 2.3**).
Newly ER synthesized protein molecules move
through the ER tubules and then bud off into
vesicles which are transported to the GA (vesicle transport). In turn, the proteins pass by vesicle transport sequentially to and through several
GA cisternal compartments. While passing
through, the proteins are modified and sorted
out before finally emerging from the GA by budding off the cisternal membrane as vesicles containing glycoproteins. These glycoproteins are
then dispersed to their destinations via plasmic
transport (see later) as (1) the integral proteins
of the plasma membrane, (2) the secretory proteins packaged into secretory vesicles that are
released in response to an external signal, and
(3) enzymes of the lysosomes. Each membranous vesicle budded from the GA apparently
has external molecules that recognize "docking
sites" on the surface of the specific organelle
to which they are destined to join.

Neurotubules, Neurofilaments, and Axonal (Plasmic) Transport

Each neuron contains numerous fibrillar organelles called (1) *neurotubules (microtubules)*,
each roughly 20 to 25 nm in diameter; (2) *neurofilaments (microfilaments)*, roughly 10 nm in
diameter; and (3) *actin microfilaments*, each 8
nm in diameter. They comprise the cytoskeleton
of the neuron. Neurotubules and neurofilaments
are found throughout the cytoplasm. The actin
microfilaments primarily are located close to
the plasma membrane. They are critical organelles in growth cones (Chap. 6). These longitudinally oriented organelles are components of

the cytoskeleton present throughout the neuron
and its processes. These tubules and filaments
are of variable length with no single element
extending the entire length of an axon or dendrite. The tubules are polar structures. Within
an axon, the so-called plus end of each tubule
is oriented toward the axon terminus and the
minus end toward the cell body (**Fig. 2.5**). The
polarities of the tubules are mixed within a dendrite, with about one half having the plus end
oriented toward the cell body and the other half
with the minus end toward the cell body. These
organelles are in a dynamic state of flux and are
continuously growing longer or shorter. Each of
these tubules and filaments is actually a polymer of repeating subunits.

The *neurotubules* are unbranched cylinders
composed of polymers of the protein *tubulin*.
They are involved in the transport of membranous organelles throughout the neuron. The
neurofilaments are unbranched cylinders
formed by the globular protein actin and other
proteins. The neurofilament proteins, which are
found only in neurons, are members of a family
of proteins that include intermediate filament
proteins of other cells and a protein in glial cells
called *glial fibrillary acidic protein (GFAP)*.

The special properties of these cytoskeletal
elements enable them to be, depending upon
the need, both stable and plastic structures.
Furthermore, they are able to undergo transi-
tions from stable to dynamic structures. In the
fully differentiated neurons (1) the cytoskeleton
gives each neuron and its processes (axon and
dendrites) mechanical strength and (2) via its
neurotubules, the tracks to transport materials
between the cell body and its fiber terminals.
A highly plastic cytoskeleton is exhibited during the development of a neuron or in nerve
regeneration following the transection of a peripheral nerve. In these situations, growth cones
utilize the cytoskeleton to elongate, retract, or
rapidly change their shape and to act as mobile
sensors (Chap. 6).

*Axonal Transport (Axoplasmic or Axon
Transport or Axoplasmic Flow)*

The distribution of many substances from the
cell body throughout the neuronal processes
and from the processes to the cell body are car-

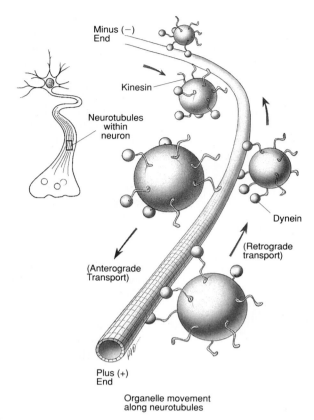

Minus (−)
End

Kinesin

Neurotubules
within
neuron

Dynein

(Anterograde
Transport)

(Retrograde
transport)

Plus (+)
End

Organelle movement
along neurotubules

Figure 2.5: Schema illustrating the anterograde and retrograde transport of synaptic vesicles and other organelles along neurotubules. After their components are synthesized within the endoplasmic reticulum and Golgi apparatus, the *organelles* are assembled within the cell body. While in the cell body, the organelles bind with the motor proteins *kinesin* and *dynein*. Kinesin has the means to power their rapid movement via fast axonal anterograde transport via and to the *plus* (+) end of each neurotubule toward the nerve terminals. The motor is presumed to be transported back to the cell body in an inactive form. The organelle bound kinesin molecules interact transiently with the microtubule during the anterograde transport via the neurotubule. The retrograde motor protein dynein is transported to the terminal in an inactive form, becomes activated, binds to degraded membranes and organelles and then is conveyed by retrograde transport to the *minus* (−) end of the microtubules toward the cell body for disposal. Kinesin appears to have a fan-shaped tail that binds to the organelle to be moved and two globular heads that bind to the neurotubule. A hinge-like site is present midway along the kinesin molecule. The similarities between kinesin and myosin of muscle suggest the movement is produced by the sliding of kinesin molecules along the tracks of the neurotubules. Neurons have adapted an ancient mechanism of transport, in that kinesin and dynein are present in single-celled organisms and eukaryotic cells.

ried out by what is called *axonal transport*. It is called "*anterograde*" or "*orthograde*" *axonal transport* when the transport is away from the cell body into the dendrites and axon and "*retrograde axonal transport*" when the transport is from the dendrites and axon toward the cell body. Transport comprises two general rates (components): (1) a *fast rate (system)* with movement of 200 to 400 mm per day and (2) a *slow rate (system)* of about 1 to 5 mm per day.

These systems are active in all dendrites and axons. There is both anterograde and retrograde fast transport, but only anterograde slow transport. The anterograde fast system conveys mitochondria and the precursors of smooth endoplasmic reticulum, synaptic vesicles, and plasma membrane. The fast retrograde system includes conveying of such structures as mitochondria, "multivesiculate" bodies (may be degradative structures), and vesicles containing such ligands as nerve growth factors (see later) taken up by receptor-mediated endocytosis. Mitochondria travel in both the anterograde and retrograde direction; individual mitochondria can move bidirectionally. The neurotubules in association with certain so-called *force-generating motor proteins* (neurotubule-based motors) act as the intracellular engines for fast transport, also called *neurotubule-dependent transport*. This fast transport along the neurotubules is generated by the motor proteins *kinesin* and *dynein*. Linked with ATP they act as motors (**Fig. 2.5**). They are responsible for generating the forces for the organelle movements that underlie axonal transport along the neurotubules. ATP is obligatory as it furnishes the energy for the fast transport in either direction. These proteins and ATP seem to provide a mechanistic basis for microtubules-associated movement.

The following is a current scheme for the role of these motor (motility) proteins in fast transport (**Fig. 2.5**). Both anterograde motor kinesin and retrograde dynein attach to appropriate binding sites on the precursors or organelle to be transported. The organelle is conveyed by anterograde transport along the "rail" of the track on the neurotubule by the "motors" of kinesin and powered by ATP on the organelle toward the plus (+) or axon terminal end of the neurotubule. During this phase the dynein is transported in an inactive form. Then the kinesin is transported back in an inactive form to the cell body for recycling. The retrograde motor dynein, after being transported in an inactive form to the terminal, is activated and becomes the motor to organelles that are destined to be transported along the rails of the track on the neurotubules toward their minus (−) or cell body ends. Each neurotubule contain several tracks along which different particles move. On a single neurotubule (1) a vesicle can pass another vesicle moving in the same direction on a separate track or (2) two vesicles can move bidirectionally in opposite directions simultaneously on separate tracks of the same neurotubule. In addition, a vesicle can shift from one tubule to another tubule.

The slow axonal transport is an anterograde transport involved with the movement of soluble enzymes and the components of the cytoskeleton and plasma membrane. Proteins and other substances are conveyed to renew and maintain the axoplasm (cytosol) of mature neurons and to supply the axoplasm for axon and dendrite growth of developing and regenerating neurons. The protein dynamin has been suggested to be the motor protein with a role in slow transport.

Conceptually, axonal transport is an expression of the unity of the neuron in that, through transport, a continuous communication is maintained between the cell body (trophic center) and its processes. By this means, the cell body is kept informed of the metabolic needs and condition of its most distal parts. Through axonal uptake of extracellular substances, such as nerve growth factor (see later) followed by retrograde transport, the cell body can sample the extracellular environment. However, retrograde transport has its debit side, in that through its mechanism neurotropic viruses such as rabies, herpes simplex, and poliomyelitis are conveyed to the CNS. Defects in microtubules may be involved in some human neurologic disorders.

Dendrites and Axons

Dendrites contain the same cytoplasmic organelles (e.g., Nissl bodies and mitochondria) as the cell body. They are true extensions of the cell body. The axon is specialized for transmission of coded information as all-or-none action potentials. It arises from the *axon hillock* of the cell body at a site called the *initial segment* (**Figs. 2.1, 2.4**). It extends from less than a millimeter to as much as 1 meter before arborizing into *terminal branches*. The axon hillock, initial segment, and the axon lack Nissl bodies. The branches of an axon may have two types of *boutons*. Each ends as a *terminal bouton* (bouton terminaux or end-foot) that forms a synapse with the dendrite, cell body or axon of another neuron (**Fig. 2.9**). Along some branches are thickenings called *boutons en passage*, which form synapses with another neuron or smooth muscle fiber (**Fig. 2.3**). The dendrites of many neurons are studded with tiny protuberances called *spines* (e.g., pyramidal neurons of the cerebral cortex **Figs. 25.1, 25.2**). These dendritic spines increase the surface area of the membrane of the receptive segment of the neuron (Chap. 3). On them are located over 90% of all the excitatory synapses in the central nervous system. Because of their widespread occurrence on neurons of the cortical areas of the cerebrum they are thought to be involved in learning and memory (Chap. 25).

Axons and dendrites are often called *nerve fibers*. The *neuropil* is a collective term for a meshwork of axons, dendrites, and neuroglia fibers within the central nervous system.

Synapse

The *synapse* is the site of contact of one neuron with another (Figs. 2.1, 2.3, and 2.4). A submicroscopic space, the synaptic cleft, which is about 200 Å, exists between the bouton of one neuron and the cell body of another neuron (*axosomatic synapse*), between a bouton and a dendrite (*axodendritic synapse*), and between a bouton and an axon (*axoaxonic synapse*). In addition, *dendrodendritic synapses* (between two dendrites) have been noted (e.g., in olfactory bulb and retina). The axon of one neuron may terminate in only a few synapses, or up to many thousands of synapses. The dendrite-cell body complex may receive synaptic contacts from many different neurons (up to well over 15,000 synapses). The termination of a nerve fiber in a muscle cell (neuromuscular junction) or a glandular cell (neuroglandular junction) is basically similar to the synapse between two neurons. The synapse of each axon terminal of a motoneuron on a voluntary muscle cell is called a *motor end plate* (Figs. 2.1, 2.4, 8.1, and 8.2).

The cell membrane of the axon at the synapse is the *presynaptic membrane*, and the cell membrane of dendrite-cell body complex, muscle, or glandular cell is the *postsynaptic membrane*. The *subsynaptic membrane* is that region of the postsynaptic membrane that is juxtaposed against the presynaptic membrane at the synapse. A concentration of mitochondria and *presynaptic vesicles* is present in the cytoplasm of the bouton; none are present in the cytoplasm adjacent to the subsynaptic membrane. Most neurons contain at least two distinct types of vesicles: (1) small vesicles 50 nm in diameter and (2) large vesicles from 70 to 200 nm in diameter. The vesicles contain the precursors of the active neurotransmitter agents (Chaps. 3 and 15).

TROPHIC EFFECTS AND NERVE GROWTH FACTOR (NGF)

Trophic is a term implying certain long-term effects exerted through specific chemical substances (*trophic factors*) passing from one cell (or tissue) to affect another cell (or tissue). Trophic interactions associated with the nervous system are expressed in one of two ways: (1) the nervous system can exert trophic influences on other cells or (2) neurons may be the recipients of trophic factors from non-neural sources. These neurotrophic chemical agents initiate or control molecular modifications in the other cells and are responsible for various aspects of the formation and maintenance of the structural, chemical, and functional integrity of the target cells. Of the numerous potential trophic factors, one, the *nerve growth factor (NGF)*, was characterized by Levi-Montalcini and Cohen, for which they received the 1986 Nobel Prize. Trophic actions may occur at any time from early embryonic life through adulthood, with a progressive reduction with age without ever being totally lost.

The "*trophic action*" of neurons on a peripheral structure is illustrated by the role of the "taste nerves" upon the taste buds. Not only do the gustatory nerve fibers convey taste information from the taste buds, but also they have a critical role in maintaining the taste buds. Following the transection of the gustatory nerve fibers, the taste buds degenerate. When the nerve fibers regenerate, the taste buds reform. Presumably, only gustatory neurons contain the essential trophic factor, because only taste fibers are capable of inducing the taste buds to reappear.

The *nerve growth factor (NGF)* is a diffusible protein that is essential for the survival of two types of neurons, namely, sympathetic neurons (Chap. 19) and sensory neurons, both derived from the neural crest (Chap. 6). Neurotrophic agents are synthesized in the target region and act via specific membrane-bound receptors. Other trophic factors that exert trophic influences on other neurons remain to be discovered. NGF has an essential role in the differentiation and the maintenance of the viability of these neurons, even in preventing cell death. NGF reaches its target neurons by being taken up by the axon terminals, where it has certain local effects. Some is carried by retrograde axonal transport to the cell body, where it exerts its broad effects on neuronal growth and maintenance. This is expressed in the concept that NGF acts as a trophic messenger conveying information from the periphery to and through the axon to the trophic segment of the neuron, thereby preserving the integrity of the neuron. NGF's local effects are demonstrated by its ability to stimulate and to direct the outgrowth and regeneration of axonal fibers and in stabilization of synapses of the sensory and sympathetic neurons and even in the survival of neurons. Evidence for several other neurotrophic factors have now been established, namely *brain-derived neurotrophic factor (BDNF)* from the brain itself, neurotrophin 3 (NT3), and ciliary neurotrophic factor (CNF). The trophic proteins are closely related chemically. Each supports the growth and survival of distinct groups of neurons. Many questions remain concerning these factors and their mode of action.

STRUCTURE OF PERIPHERAL NERVES AND GANGLIA

The *peripheral nerves* are the cranial and spinal nerves including their branches. The peripheral ganglia are collections of cell bodies associated with the peripheral nerves. Each nerve consists of three basic tissue elements: (1) axons (nerve fibers of neurons); (2) Schwann (neurolemma) cells and myelin sheath (interstitial element); and (3) endoneurium, perineurium, and epineurium (connective tissue elements). A peripheral ganglion consists of the same three elements: (1) cell bodies and nerve fibers (of the neurons), (2) inner satellite cells (interstitial element), and (3) outer satellite cells (connective tissue elements).

A peripheral nerve with its numerous nerve fibers is comparable to a telephone cable. The axons are analogous to the wires and the Schwann cells and the endoneurium to the insulation encapsulating each wire. Groups of insulated nerve fibers are bound together into fascicles by the perineurium. In turn, groups of fascicles are bound together by the epineurium.

Each of these layers is continuous with its counterpart in most peripheral ganglia. The connective tissue elements contain the blood vessels that nourish the neurons; they are also essential for the strength and flexibility exhibited by nerves. The flattened cells of the perineurium form a sheath that acts as a physiological barrier preventing substances from reaching the fascicles of axons. This is a means of maintaining an optimal environment for axonal activity. The numerous generally longitudinal organized collagen fibers are oriented to resist the stretching of axons. Impulse conduction is altered in slightly stretched axons.

The myelin sheath is a structure composed of many concentric layers of the plasma membrane of Schwann cells (neurolemma) in the PNS (and of oligodendroglia in the CNS) surrounding an axis cylinder (axon). The sheath resembles the layers of a jelly roll (**Fig. 2.6**).

The myelin sheath is interrupted at regular intervals by the *nodes of Ranvier* (**Figs. 2.1, 2.4**). The interval between adjacent nodes is an internode. Each internode is ensheathed by one Schwann cell. The length of an internode is roughly proportional to the diameter of the fiber (including myelin sheath); the thicker the fiber, the longer its internode. In addition, the diameter of a fiber and the length of an internode are directly related to the speed of conduction of the nerve impulse—*the greater the diameter of a fiber, the faster the speed of conduction.* Three features of the nodes are important: (1) nerve fibers branch at a node, (2) a high concentration of mitochondria in the axis cylinder at these sites indicates a local high level of metabolic activity, and (3) extracellular fluids are close to the axis cylinder at each node. Nerve fibers are bound as fascicles by connective tissue. Nearly all nerve fibers over 2 μm in diameter are myelinated and those under 2 μm are unmyelinated.

Adjacent to the outer surface of each Schwann cell is a basal lamina, which is synthesized by the Schwann cells. It is a homogeneous layer composed of such proteins as type IV collagen and laminin. The glial cells and neurons of the CNS are not associated with a basal lamina. This layer may have a critical role in the regeneration of peripheral nerve fibers (see later).

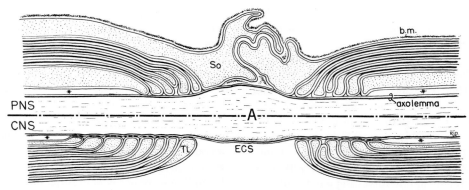

Figure 2.6: Regions of the nodes of Ranvier in the peripheral nervous system (PNS) compared with those in the central nervous system (CNS). In the PNS the Schwann (neurolemma) cell has an outer collar (So) of cytoplasm which loosely interdigitates in the nodal region with the outer collar of the adjacent Schwann cell. In the CNS the axis cylinder (A) in the nodal region is exposed directly with the extracellular space (ECS). In both the PNS and CNS the compact-layered myelin surrounding the axis cylinder forms terminal loops (TL), which are in close apposition to the axolemma; this apposition may form a "seal" preventing ready movement of materials between the periaxonal space (*) and the nodal region. The Schwann cell is covered by a basement lamina (b.m.). (Courtesy of Dr. R.P. Bunge and the American Physiological Society.)

Whereas a myelinated nerve fiber is ensheathed in its private layer of Schwann cells (**Fig. 2.6**), a group of *unmyelinated fibers* share a common Schwann cell (neurolemma) (**Fig. 2.7**). As many as 20 or more unmyelinated fibers may share one Schwann cell. These fibers are separated from one another, for each is embedded in a private trough of the surface of a Schwann cell's plasma membrane. The axons of the olfactory nerve present an unusual arrangement. Up to two dozen or more axons are grouped into clusters of several fine fibers enclosed in troughs of a Schwann cell (**Fig. 2.7**).

NEUROGLIA (GLIA)

The *neuroglia (glia)* are the non-neural cells of the CNS. Depending on the region, they outnumber the neurons from 5 to over 50 times and comprise about 40% of the total CNS volume. Their main functions are to support, to nurture,

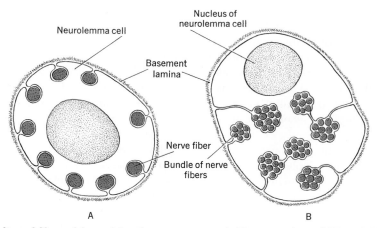

Figure 2.7: Unmyelinated fibers of the peripheral nervous system. **A.** Nine unmyelinated fibers enclosed in individual troughs of a Schwann (neurolemma) cell. **B.** Clusters of groups of fine fibers enclosed in troughs of neurolemma cells in the olfactory nerve. (After Dr. R.P. Bunge.)

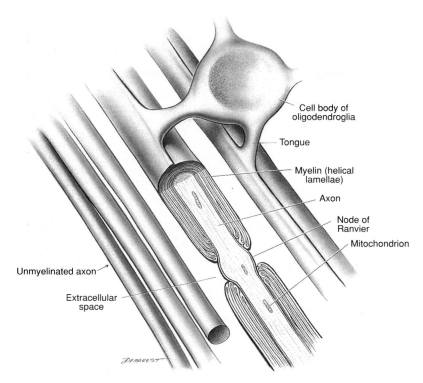

Cell body of
oligodendroglia

Tongue

Myelin (helical
lamellae)

Axon

Node of
Ranvier

Mitochondrion

Unmyelinated axon

Extracellular
space

Figure 2.8: Relation of oligodendroglia to the axons of the central nervous system, as reconstructed from electron micrographs. The three unmyelinated axons on the left are naked. The two myelinated axons of the right share one oligodendroglia cell. The myelin sheaths of each of the myelinated fibers are continuous through the protoplasmic tongue with the glial cell body. The glial tongue spreads out as a ridge, which extends throughout the entire length of an internode. The loop of the cell membrane at the ridge makes the site where the membrane is doubled (myelin unit of two plasma cell membranes) and is continuous as a laminated myelin sheath. (Adapted from Drs. M. Bunge, R. Bunge, and H. Ris.)

and to maintain a relatively constant environment (milieu) for the neurons.

The *oligodendrocytes (oligodendroglia)* of the CNS are the equivalent of the neurolemma cells of the PNS (**Figs. 2.1, 2.8**). Every oligodendrocyte has several processes, each of which forms the myelin sheath of an internode of a different nerve fiber. Thus, each oligodendrocyte forms the internodes of several nerve fibers (**Fig. 2.8**). Myelination of axons commences prenatally. Many pathways in the human nervous system are not fully myelinated until 2 years after birth.

The cell bodies of *astrocytes (astroglia)* have sheet-like processes that extend out among the neurons (**Fig. 2.9**). These processes extend to the (1) basement membrane of the capillaries, (2) cell bodies and dendrites of the neurons to envelop the synapses and thereby insulate each synapse from another, and (3) to the pia mater to form the pia-glial membrane adjacent to the subarachnoid space (**Fig. 5.5**). These cells act to store and to transfer metabolites from the capillaries to the neurons. They can act as a potassium sink taking up excess extracellular potassium and other substances such as neurotransmitters from the extracellular space which accumulated following intense neuronal activity. In essence, astrocytes have critical roles in maintaining and regulating the homeostatic composition of the extracellular fluid essential for the normal functioning of the neurons of the brain and spinal cord.

The *macroglia (oligodendroglia and astroglia)* act to maintain a homeostatic environment for the neurons. In the labyrinth of

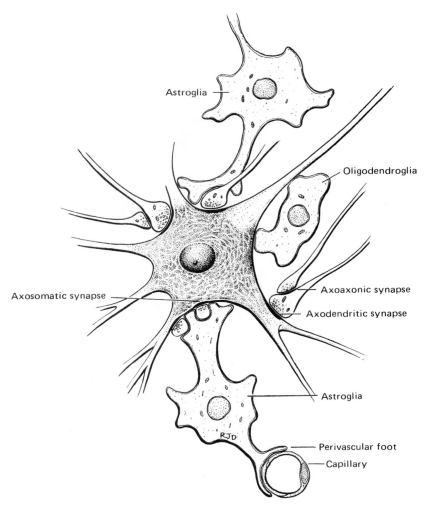

Figure 2.9: Relation of a neuron, astroglia, oligodendroglia, and nerve terminals. Note axosomatic synapse, axodendritic synapse, and axoaxonic synapse. Astroglia have processes extending to a capillary (Fig. 5.4) and to neurons.

glia and their processes distributed throughout the CNS, the neurons, including their processes, are encapsulated and isolated from each other, except at synapses. Glial cells react to the injury of neurons and they can form permanent scars or plaques by a process known as *gliosis*.

The *microglia* are small cells with relatively small nuclei that comprise 10% or more of all glial cells. They contain lysosomes and vesicles characteristic of macrophages and only sparse ER and a few cytoskeletal fibers. Existing in both a resting form and as activated macrophage-like cells, they are found in the CNS as parenchymal microglia, the choroid plexus, the circumventricular organs (Chap. 15) and as perivascular cells. The resting microglia are presumed to be activated by local factors to become the macrophage-like cells of the CNS. They remove the debris of cells that die during normal development of the nervous system. Following injuries such as a stab wound or inflammation, microglia are transformed as both their nucleus and cytoplasm enlarge; they become mobile and became filled with phagocytosed debris, like tissue macrophages.

The *ependymal cells* are the glial cells that line the ventricular cavities and the choroid plexuses. They are involved in the production of cerebrospinal fluid (Chap. 5).

NERVE REGENERATION

The trauma inflicted on an injured neuron acts as a potent stimulus that sets in motion a series of events directed to preserve the neuron and to regenerate its processes (Fig. 2.10).

Axon Reaction

Following the transection of an axon, the neuron responds through a series of events, known as the *axon reaction*. These include changes in the (1) cell body and (2) nerve fibers both proximal and distal to the transection.

The cell body swells and the nucleus becomes eccentrically located. There is an increase and redistribution of the ribosomes (RNA) such that they are concentrated. This activity, near the plasma membrane, resulting

in a relative lack of staining in the central part of the soma, known as *chromatolysis*, is indicative of an enhanced synthesis of proteins prior to their distribution to the regenerating axon by axonal transport.

The severed ends of axis cylinders of the proximal stump from the cell body side of the transection site are sealed by newly formed plasma membrane within a day. During the weeks following the trauma, the myelin sheaths and axis cylinders of nerve fibers in the distal stump break up. The fragmented products are phagocytized by microglia and removed. The neurolemma (Schwann) cells of the distal stump divide by mitosis and form continuous cords (tubes or columns of Schwann). Each cord is surrounded by a basal lamina and each extends distally to the location of the original nerve terminal. This applies to both myelinated and unmyelinated fibers.

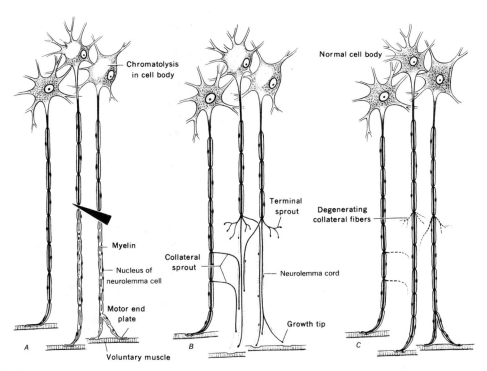

Figure 2.10: Degeneration and regeneration of peripheral somatic motor nerve fibers. **A.** Several days after transection (at the wedge). Note the chromatolysis and eccentric nuclei, increase in number of neurolemma cells, and fragmentation of myelin sheaths. **B.** Several weeks later, the neurolemma cord receives regenerating axis cylinders from the transected fibers and collateral branches from the adjacent normal fiber. **C.** Several months later, collateral branches of axis cylinders that failed to innervate motor end plates degenerate. The regenerated portions of the fibers contain more internodes than before: hence they conduct nerve impulses more slowly.

Regeneration in the Peripheral Nervous System

Each axis cylinder in the proximal stump elongates, grows out of the stump, and branches into many sprouts which spread randomly across the gap between the stumps. Many of the sprouts cross the gap and contact neurolemma cords to which they may be presumably attracted by chemical substances such as neurotrophic factors located in the basal laminae (Chap. 6). The sprouts from each axis cylinder may enter many different cords and, in turn, each cord may receive and act as a guide for the growth cones of the sprouts from many different axons. In a crushed nerve it is likely that each regenerating axon extends into and remains within its parent cord. Each branch elongates within the cleft between the basal lamina and the neurolemma cells at from 1 to 3 mm per day. Remyelination of the regenerating branches commences after 1 week. In a sense, the growth of the branches and remyelination recapitulate early development. The basal lamina is a critical element as it contains such neurotrophic factors as the glycoproteins laminin, fibronectin, and tenascin. These proteins, especially laminin, are apparently effective substrates for the attraction and guidance for axonal outgrowth. The axons that enter the appropriate cords and then terminate in a suitable matched terminal can form functionally effective connections—motor fibers to reconstituted motor end plates and sensory fibers to reconstituted sensory endings. Those axons that do not reach appropriate terminals will eventually degenerate (**Fig. 2.10**). Suggestions are made that trophic and related factors, such as NGF, and nerve cell adhesion molecules, such as NCAM (Chap. 6) may also have roles such as guidance cues during regeneration. The internodal distances between nodes of Ranvier are shorter following regeneration. This may account for slower conduction velocities of regenerated nerves. Those regenerating axons that do not enter a stump may grow locally and form a *neuroma*. The resulting tender mass, when irritated, can evoke severe pain, called *causalgia*, which is perceived as coming from the original region supplied by the nerve (see Phantom limb, Chap. 9).

Regeneration in the Central Nervous System

An injury to the brain and spinal cord can be severe and irreversible. The exceptions include the successful axonal regeneration of hypothalamic neurosecretory neurons to the hypophysis (Chap. 21) and certain neurons containing such amines as dopamine, norepinephrine, and serotonin (Chap. 15). In general, the damaged axons can generate some short branches, which then abort. Axonal regeneration of CNS neurons can be demonstrated to occur experimentally into transplanted grafts of peripheral nerves.

Some current suggestions explain, in part, why the growth of neurites (term used to designate either an axon or a dendrite when it is not possible to establish whether a growing nerve fiber is one or the other) can occur in the PNS throughout life, but in the CNS only during development and not in the adult.

During early development the extracellular matrix of both the CNS and PNS contains laminin and fibronectin, the glycoproteins that promote axon growth. These glycoproteins are present in the mature PNS, but are virtually absent in the mature CNS. Thus, the mature CNS lacks these proteins which may be essential for axonal growth. In addition, the oligodendroglia in the region of the injured CNS synthesize glycoproteins that actively suppress neurite outgrowth. These inhibitory glycoproteins are absent in Schwann cells during regeneration in the PNS. Thus, the combination of the absence of these growth promoting glycoproteins and the presence of the growth inhibitory glycoproteins in the CNS of the adult may explain, in part, this loss of the capacity of CNS axons to regenerate. The glial scar forms by astrocytes in the vicinity of the injury act as a physical obstruction to neurite regeneration.

Experimental evidence indicates that the axons of mature CNS neurons will regenerate if the severed proximal ends of these axons are brought into contact with the Schwann cords of a peripheral nerve. Subsequently, these axons will acquire myelin sheaths and be able to function by conducting nerve impulses. This indicates that the axons of the CNS of adults have the potential to regenerate, remyelinate, and function. This also demonstrates that Schwann cells play a critical role and do substantially influence regeneration of the axons of both the PNS and CNS, probably through the production and release of trophic factors (Chap. 6). It is thought that the oligodendrocytes of the CNS do not have this factor or do not release it. Some evidence suggests that the oligodendrocytes do have a membrane-bound inhibitor on their surface and their myelin sheaths have a factor that inhibits the regeneration of axons. If such a substance can be suppressed, then the regeneration of CNS axons could be enhanced. This inhibitor is said to be present in these glial cells in mammals, birds, and reptiles, animals in which CNS axons do not regenerate, but absent in oligodendrocytes of fish and amphibians, animals in which CNS axons can regenerate and function.

Some current research is directed to the possibility that the NGFs may have therapeutic roles for the restoration of malfunctioning neurons in such neurodegenerative diseases as amyotrophic lateral sclerosis (Chap. 12) and Parkinson's disease (Chap. 24). This is consistent with the concept of the critical roles of NGFs in neuronal survival and functioning. In addition, during embryological and fetal development, the NGFs are associated with establishing the basic network of the nervous system (Chap. 6). This includes guiding the neuroblasts, including their dendrites and axons, in establishing the neuronal network and synaptic connections, resulting in the organization of the connectivity of the nervus system. After having carried out these roles, the NGFs are inhibited during and following the perinatal period. In their place, other NGFs become operative during infancy and childhood. These new NGFs are presumed to be involved in maintenance functions and subtle adjustments occurring throughout postnatal life. An obstacle to evaluating the therapeutic value is the inability to deliver the NGFs to the neurons via the vascular system. Because the NGFs are large protein molecules, they are unable to penetrate the blood brain barrier.

PLASTICITY AND AXONAL SPROUTING

The neurons of the mammalian CNS possess the capacity to generate new branches (*axonal sprouting*), to form new synapses (*synaptic replacement*), and thus to renew the neuronal circuits. The expression of this potential, known as *neuronal plasticity*, is maximal during development, but it is retained in part in the adult CNS. In the mature brain, neuronal plasticity is manifest as a response to such changes as hormonal levels, learning new skills, response to changes in the environment, and injury. This indicates that, although the cell body of each neuron is a relatively fixed component within each processing center, the synaptic connections it makes with other neurons are modifiable throughout life. In this respect, the CNS is not a static, "hard-wired" organ but rather a sensitive organ capable of limited change induced by natural stimuli. Neuronal plasticity is, in essence, the capability of synaptic connections of a neuron to be replaced, to be increased or decreased in quantity, and to modify functional activity. Presumably, this plasticity is influenced by chemical factors (such as NGF) released by the target cells. This plasticity may be involved in part in the functional recovery occurring following small lesions in the brain.

SUGGESTED READINGS

Altman J. Microglia emerge from the fog. *Trends Neurosci.* 1994;17:47–49.

Edelman G. Cell adhesion molecules in the regulation of animal form and tissue pattern. *Annu Rev Cell Biol.* 1986;2:81–116.

Fawcett D, Raviola E. *Bloom and Fawcett, A Textbook of Histology.* 12th ed. New York, NY: Chapman & Hall; 1994.

Jones E. The nervous tissue. In: Weiss L, ed. *Cell and Tissue Biology: A Textbook of Histology.* 6th ed. Baltimore, Md: Urban & Schwarzenberg; 1988:277–352.

Kimelberg H, Norenberg M. Astrocytes. *Sci Am.* 1989;260(4):66–76.

Levi-Montalcini R. The nerve growth factor 35 years later. *Science.* 1987;237:1154–1162.

Levitan I, Kaczmarek L. *The Neuron: Cell and Molecular Biology.* New York, NY: Oxford University Press; 1991.

Murphy S. *Astrocytes: Pharmacology and Function.* New York, NY: Academic Press; 1993.

Peters A, Palay S, Webster H. *The Fine Structure of the Nervous System. The Neurons and Their Supporting Cells.* 3rd ed. New York, NY: Oxford University Press; 1990.

Robinson P, Liu J-P, Powell K, Fykse E, Südhof T. Phosphorylation of dynamin I and synaptic-vesicle recycling. *Trends Neurosci.* 1994;17:348–353.

Schwartz J. The transport of substances in nerve cells. *Sci Am.* 1980;242(4):152–171.

Shepherd G, ed. *The Synaptic Organization of the Brain.* 3rd ed. New York, NY: Oxford University Press; 1990.

Thoenen H, Kreutzberg G, eds. The role of fast transport in the nervous system. *Neurosci Res Prog Bull.* 1982;20:1–138.

Resting potential

Nernst equation

Excitability of the neuron

Generator (receptive and synaptic) potentials and action potentials

Structural and functional organization of the neuron

Receptive segment and the receptor potentials

Initial segment and the integrated potential

Conductile segment and the action potential

Transmissive segment (synaptic or effector segment)

Synapses and chemical transmission in the central nervous system

Second messenger system

Electric (electronic) synapse

Neuron as an integrator

Presynaptic inhibition and presynaptic facilitation

Anatomy of a first-order neuron

Some general concepts associated with coding and processing in the nervous system

Some general concepts associated with neuronal processing

Each neuron is said to possess "in miniature the integrative capacity of the entire nervous system." Neurons can transform information and, in addition, transmit it to other neurons. In most neurons the dendrite-cell body unit is specialized as a receptor and integrator of synaptic input from other neurons, while the axon is specialized to convey coded information from the dendrite-cell body unit to the synaptic junctions, where transformation functions take place with other neurons or effectors (muscles and glands). To serve these tasks, the neuron is organized into (1) a receptive segment (dendrites and cell body), (2) an initial segment, (3) a conductile segment (axon), and (4) an effector segment (synapse) (Fig. 3.1).

Information about the external world and the organism's internal environment is conveyed to the CNS by neurons of the peripheral nervous system called *first-order neurons*. The peripheral processes of these neurons terminate in the retina, cochlea, vestibular end organs, skin, muscles, joints, and internal viscera (e.g., stomach), while their central processes terminate within the CNS. The structural and functional features of a typical first-order neuron, in relation to the receptor, conductile and effector segments, are described later in the chapter. Before then, the resting membrane potential and excitability of the neuron, which are essential to its function, will be examined.

RESTING POTENTIAL

The resting neuron is a charged cell that is not conducting a nerve impulse. Critical in main-

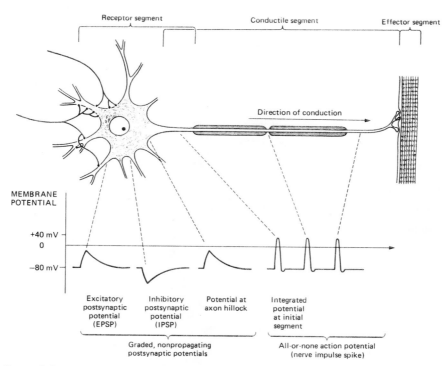

Figure 3.1: Types of electric potential changes recorded across the plasma membrane at various sites of a motoneuron. On the surface of the dendrites and cell body are excitatory and inhibitory synapses, which, when stimulated, produce local, graded, nonpropagating potentials. These are exhibited as an excitatory or depolarizing postsynaptic potential (EPSP) and an inhibitory or hyperpolarizing postsynaptic potential (IPSP). These local potentials are summated at the axon hillock and, if adequate, may trigger an integrated potential at the initial segment and an all-or-none action potential, which is conducted along the axon to the motor endplate. (Adapted from Gray's Anatomy, WB Saunders.)

taining this charged state, or *resting potential*, is the plasma membrane, which acts as a thin boundary between two fluids. One is the extracellular (interstitial) fluid outside the neuron. The other is the intracellular fluid (neuroplasm) inside the neuron (**Fig. 3.2**). The electric charge across the plasma membrane results from a thin mist of positive and negative ions, unequally distributed across the membrane. These are (1) sodium (Na^+) and chloride (Cl^-) ions that are in higher concentration in the interstitial fluid and (2) potassium (K^+) and protein (organic) ions that are in higher concentration in the neuroplasm. A tendency exists for the Na^+, K^+, and Cl^- ions to diffuse across the membrane from regions of high to low concentration (along concentration gradients), through Na^+, K^+, and Cl^- channels, respectively. The passage of ions across the membrane is known as *conductance*. Thus, the semipermeable plasma membrane is selectively permeable

through non-gated open channels (Chap. 2) to Na^+, K^+, and Cl^- ions and impermeable to large protein ions. These channels, which are always open, are important in determining the resting potential. The ionic concentrations on either side of the membrane are produced and maintained by a system of membrane pumps (**Fig. 2.2**) called the *sodium (or sodium-potassium) pump* requiring metabolic energy released by adenosine triphosphate (ATP). The sodium-potassium exchange pump is an integral membrane protein that utilizes ATP as an energy source for its role in *active transport*. This transport is an energy dependent process in which the movement of Na^+ ions and K^+ is "uphill" against a concentration gradient. The activity of the pump results in the passage of 3 Na^+ ions out of, and 2 K^+ ions into, the neuron. The consequence is the restoration of a concentration of K^+, that is 30 or more times higher within the neuroplasm than the interstitial fluid,

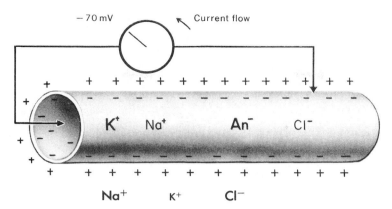

Figure 3.2: Resting potential. The intracellular neuroplasm potential of the normal nerve fiber "at rest" is negative to the extracellular potential. Sodium (Na$^+$) and chloride (Cl$^-$) ions are in high concentration in the extracellular fluid, and the potassium (K$^+$) ions and protein (An$^-$) are in high concentrations in the neuroplasm. The potential across the plasma membrane is -60 to -70 mV.

and in a concentration of Na$^+$ that is 10 times and Cl$^-$ that is 14 times higher in the interstitial fluid than in the neuroplasm. Most neurons do not have a Cl$^-$ pump; hence Cl$^-$ ions diffuse passively across the membrane. These are the ionic concentrations responsible for establishing an electric potential across the membrane. This potential difference across the membrane, known as the *resting potential*, is about -60 to -70 mV (millivolts) with an excess of negative charge inside the neuron (**Fig. 3.2**).

The resting potential is in a steady state (*dynamic equilibrium*) requiring metabolic energy to maintain the ionic gradients across the membrane. When the neuron is "at rest," its membrane potential is the result of a balance (involving Na$^+$ and K$^+$ ions) between the active fluxes (movements) of ions metabolically driven by *pumps* and the passive fluxes caused by *diffusion*. The active fluxes result from the pump extruding three Na$^+$ ions for every two K$^+$ ions it brings into the neuron. The passive fluxes of ions take place through nongated channels. The outward flux of positive charges by the pump tends to hyperpolarize the membrane. The greater the hyperpolarization, the greater the inward electrochemical force driving Na$^+$ into the neuron, and the smaller the force driving K$^+$ out. The steady state for the neuron is attained when the resting potential is reached at the point when the net passive inward current (movement of electrical charge) through the ion

channels exactly counterbalances the active outward current driven by the pump. The steady state is not basically due to *passive diffusion*, which is the diffusion of a solute down a concentration gradient without the expenditure of energy (**Figs. 3.2 and 3.3**).

NERNST EQUATION

The *Nernst equation* is fundamental to the nature of electrical potentials of all cells, including neurons. It is derived from basic thermodynamic principles. From this equation, the magnitude of the membrane potential at which ions (e.g., K$^+$) are in equilibrium across a membrane can be calculated. The Nernst equation is:

$$E = 2.3 \frac{RT}{F} \log \frac{C_o}{C_i}$$

in which:

E = the difference in the electrical potential between inside and outside the neuron—called Nernst potential

R = universal gas constant,

T = absolute temperature,

F = electric charge per gram equivalent of univalent ions (Faraday's constant),

C$_i$ = concentration of ions inside the membrane, and

C$_o$ = concentration of ions outside the membrane.

The following summary is based on the classic studies on the giant squid axon by Hodgkin and Huxley of England. The resting potential of -70 mV is primarily due to (1) the much greater concentration of K^+ ions inside than outside the neuron and (2) the passive movement of K^+ ions that diffuse freely through permanently open channels in the membrane. Both of these points have been established experimentally. In addition, only open channels, without gates, are involved in creating resting potentials (gated channels remain closed; see subsequent discussion regarding gates and gating). Thus, the concentrations of ions on either side of the membrane result from the opposite actions of the diffusion forces (flow of K^+ ions out of cell to regions of low concentration) and the electric forces (negative charge on the organic molecules inside the neurons that attract the positive charge of K^+ ions). The diffusion of the Na^+ and Cl^- ions contributes only slightly to the resting potential (see later). The distribution of the ions is maintained at a steady state by the sodium-potassium pump that drives the Na^+ out of, and the K^+ into, the neuron. Actually, the pump is a self-regulating system; the more the sodium accumulates inside the neuron, the more active the pump becomes. *When the known concentrations of K^+ ions inside and outside the squid giant axon are applied to the Nernst equation, a resting (Nernst) potential of -75 mV is obtained. This potential, predicted by the Nernst equation, differs slightly but importantly from the actual resting potential of -70 mV recorded by microelectrode studies of the squid axon. This slight discrepancy is explained by the fact that Cl^- and Na^+ make small contributions.* Sodium does not have a major role, because application of the Nernst equation to the known Na^+ concentrations on either side of the membrane yields a potential of $+50$ mV. The explanation is that Na^+ is kept out of the neuron because only a few open sodium channels exist in the resting membrane. Practically all sodium channels are gated.

The Nernst equation expresses a significant relationship that defines the equilibrium potential inside the cell for the K^+ ion in terms of its concentration on both sides of the plasma membrane. This relation between K^+ concentration and membrane potential is not quite per-

fect, because Cl^- and Na^+ do make small contributions. A more exact relation is expressed by the *Goldman-Hodgkin-Katz equation* which takes into account the actual permeability for several ions. On the basis of actual ionic concentrations and ionic permeabilities, calculations using the latter equation agree with the measurements of these values in living cells (see more comprehensive references for detailed accounts).

EXCITABILITY OF THE NEURON

Excitability is a property that enables a neuron to respond to a stimulus and to transmit information in the form of electrical signals. The flow of information within a neuron and between neurons is conveyed by both electrical and chemical signals. The electrical signals —called receptor potentials, synaptic potentials, and action potentials—are all produced by temporary changes in the current flow in and out of the neuron. These changes are deviations away from the normal value of the resting membrane potential. The current flow into and out of the neuron is controlled by ion channels within the plasma membrane. The channels possess three features: (1) they conduct ions across the plasma membrane at rapid rates up to 100,000,000 ions per second, (2) channels can recognize specific ions and be selective as to the ion or ions that can pass through, and (3) open and close the channels in response to specific electrical, chemical, and mechanical stimuli. Each neuron is presumed to have over 20 different types of channels with thousands of copies of each channel. The flux (movement of ions) through the ion channels is passive requiring no expenditure of metabolic energy. The direction of the flux is determined by the electrochemical driving force across the plasma membrane.

The primary role of ion channels in neurons is to mediate rapid signaling. These channels, called *gated channels*, have a molecular "cap" or *gate*, which opens briefly to permit an ion species to pass before the gate closes to the passage of more ions (**Fig. 3.4**). They open and close in response to various stimuli. There are (1) *ligand-gated channels* (e.g., *transmitter-gated* and *hormone-gated channels*), (2) *volt-*

age-gated channels, and (3) *modality-gated channels*. Ligands are specific chemical agents to which the channels respond by opening or closing. Gating is the process by which a channel is opened or closed during activity. The ligand-gated channels have gates that respond to specific chemical agents. The voltage-gated channels have gates that are activated to open or to close when the potential across the membrane changes. The modality gated channels respond to specific modalities involving mechanical forces (e.g., touch, pressure, or stretch). Each channel consists of several plasma membrane-spanning polypeptide subunits (proteins) arranged around a central pore. Each of these classes of channels belong to a different gene family. Each member of each family shares common similar structural and biochemical features, which presumably have evolved as the products of a common ancestral gene of that family. The channels of the voltage-gated gene family are selective for Na^+, K^+, and Ca^{++} ions. The channels for the transmitter-gated channels respond to acetylcholine, gamma amino butyric acid (GABA), and glycine. In the future, other families will be identified when the genes for other ion channels have been sequenced.

Most gated-channels are closed with the membrane at rest. They open when activated following with the binding of a ligand (ligand gating), a change in the membrane potential (voltage gating), or the stretch of the membrane (modality gating). In the transmitter-gated channel, the transmitter binds to a specific site on the external face of a channel that activates it to open briefly.

The energy to open the channels is derived (1) from the binding of the transmitter to the receptor protein in the ligand-gated channels, (2) from the changes in the membrane voltage in the voltage-gated channels, and (3) presumably from the mechanical forces resulting from cytoskeletal interaction at the modality-gated channels.

There are two types of membrane responses: by becoming (1) *hyperpolarized* or (2) *depolarized*. During *hyperpolarization*, the membrane becomes more negative on its inside with respect to its outside (i.e., it may go from -70 mV to -80 mV; **Fig. 3.1**). During *depolariza-*

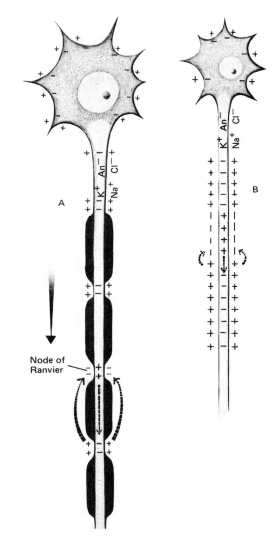

Figure 3.3: A neuron with a myelinated axon (**A**) and a neuron with an unmyelinated axon (**B**) showing the charges on the cell membrane and the location of certain ions in each neuron "at rest" and at active sites (one in each neuron) during conduction of an all-or-none action potential. The minus ($-$) signs within the neurons signify intraneuronal negativity with respect to the positivity ($+$) within the extracellular fluid outside the neurons. The two large arrows indicate the direction in which the nerve impulses are propagated. The arrows within the axons indicate the direction of the flow of current. Na^+ = sodium; K^+ = potassium; Cl^- = chloride; An^- ions = protein.

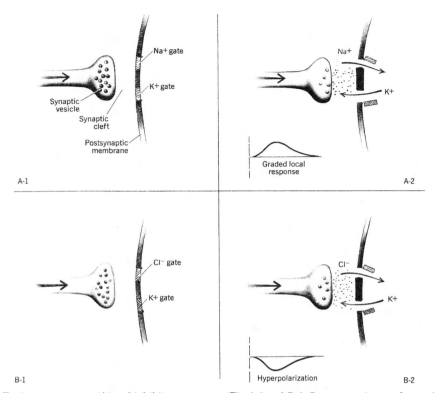

Figure 3.4: Excitatory synapses (**A**) and inhibitory synapses (**B**). *A-1* and *B-1*, Synapses prior to release of neurotransmitter. *A-2*, Excitatory postsynaptic response (EPSP) following release of neurotransmitter with Na$^+$ ion inrush through Na$^+$ gate and K$^+$ ion outrush through K$^+$ gate. *B-2*, Inhibitory postsynaptic response (IPSP) following release of neurotransmitter with Cl$^-$ ion inrush through Cl$^+$ gate and K$^+$ ion outrush through K$^+$ gate.

tion, the membrane becomes less negative on its inside with respect to its outside and even may reverse the polarity with its inside becoming positive with respect to the outside (**Figs. 3.1, 3.3 to 3.5**); this is still called depolarization because the membrane potential is less negative than the resting potential (i.e., from −70 mV to 0 to +40 mV; **Fig. 3.1**).

GENERATOR (RECEPTIVE AND SYNAPTIC) POTENTIALS AND ACTION POTENTIALS

Neurons are specialized to convey and to encode information employing electric signals generated and conducted along their cell membranes. These signals are expressed as *voltage changes* of the underlying basic resting potentials. Voltage changes that occur at the sites where neurons are stimulated are called *genera-*

tor potentials. These potentials can lead to the generation of *action potentials (nerve impulses or spikes)*, which transmit information for substantial distances along an axon. Receptor and synaptic potentials are essentially similar to each other because both have roles in the processing leading to generation of an action potential; they are called *generator potentials*. Sensory stimuli from the environment (both inside and outside the body) stimulate the receptors to produce *receptor potentials*. Information that passes from one neuron to another at synapses can produce *synaptic potentials* on the postsynaptic neuron. The activity of both receptor and synaptic potentials can result in the generation of action potentials, which can, in turn, stimulate other neurons to generate synaptic potentials. Effectors, such as muscles and glands, are activated by synaptic potentials which can influence the contraction of a muscle or the secretion of a gland (see later).

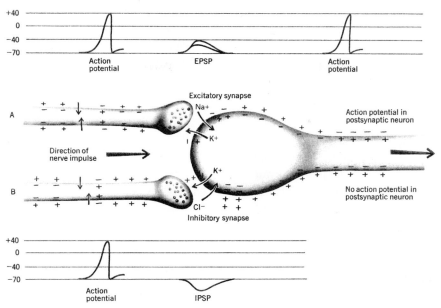

Figure 3.5: Sequences in excitatory (**A**) and inhibitory (**B**) transmission from presynaptic neurons (left) across synapses to postsynaptic neuron (right). **A**. The action potential conducted along the presynaptic axon to an excitatory synapse produces an EPSP, which, in turn, can contribute to the generation of an action potential in the postsynaptic neuron. **B**. The action potential conducted along the presynaptic axon to an inhibitory synapse produces an IPSP, which, in turn, suppresses the generation of an action potential in the postsynaptic neuron.

Generator potentials differ from action potentials in the means by which they code information. In essence, the generator potentials code information by amplitude modulation (an AM system), and the action potential code by frequency modulation (an FM system). The generator potentials code by response amplitude: that is, weak stimuli evoke small potentials (small voltage changes) and, in contrast, strong stimuli evoke large potentials (greater voltage changes). These different responses to the intensity of the stimuli are said to be *graded responses*. A small depolarization (small voltage change), called an *excitatory postsynaptic potential (EPSP)*, occurs at the postsynaptic membrane of an excitatory synapse. A small hyperpolarization, called an *inhibitory postsynaptic potential (IPSP)*, occurs at the postsynaptic membrane of an inhibitory synapse (Fig. 3.5).

In contrast, action potentials code by response frequency. That is, weak stimuli evoke the generation of only a few action potentials per unit time and strong stimuli evoke the generation of many action potentials per unit time.

The following outline the responses of generator potentials as contrasted with those of action potentials. More details will be discussed later.

Generator Potentials

1. Graded Response: the amplitudes of the responses are graded with respect to the intensity of the stimulus—the stronger the stimulus the larger the membrane potential.
2. Maintenance of Response: the membrane potentials may last as long as the stimulus is sustained.
3. Threshold for Response: there is no discrete threshold. Small potentials may be evoked with the weakest stimulus. For example, one quantum of light or the transmitter from one synaptic vesicle will elicit a weak receptor (rod or cone of retina) or synaptic potential (postsynaptic membrane).
4. Summation of Responses: the potentials will sum when the stimuli are presented close together.
5. Response Remains Local: potentials will spread passively from the stimulus site (site of generation)—they are largest at the stim-

ulus site and become progressively smaller away from that site.

Action Potentials

1. All-or-None Response: regardless of the strength of the stimulus, the potentials are all the same size (about 100 millivolts or 0.1 volts).
2. Transient Response: the potentials are of constant duration (about 1.5 milliseconds).
3. Threshold for Response: for their generation, action potentials respond to substantial change in the membrane potential (up to 15 millivolts).
4. Refractory Responses: a refractory period of about 1.5 milliseconds follows every action potential. During this period another action potential cannot be generated, regardless of the strength of the stimulus.

5. Propagation of Response: potentials are actively regenerated and propagated along the length of an axon. A potential at the beginning of an axon (site of stimulation) is of the same strength as at the axon terminal. Thus the *neural code* for the message conveyed by an axon is the frequency (number of action potentials per unit time) and the pattern of these potentials.

STRUCTURAL AND FUNCTIONAL ORGANIZATION OF THE NEURON

A typical neuron may be conceived of as a cell with (1) a receptive segment, (2) an initial segment, (3) a conductile segment, (4) a transmissive segment, and (5) a trophic segment (Figs.

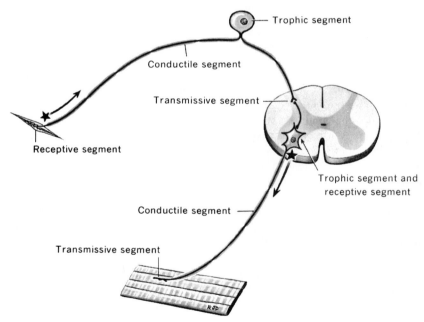

Figure 3.6: A structural and functional schema of a neuron. A neuron may be parceled into segments other than the classical dendrite, cell body, axon, and nerve endings. The sensory neuron may be parceled as follows: the receptive segment, which conducts with decrement, is the nerve ending; the initial segment (star) is the nodal site where the decremental conduction becomes the nondecremental (all-or-none) conduction of the conductile segment; the conductile segment, which conducts without decrement (all-or-none), extends from the initial segment to the synaptic endings within the spinal cord; and the terminal (transmissive) segment includes the synaptic endings. In this neuron, the cell body is located within the conductile segment. The motoneuron may be subdivided as follows: the receptive segment includes the dendrites and cell body; the initial segment (star) is located just distal to the cell body; the conductile segment to the motor endplates; and the terminal segment is located within the motor endplates. In this neuron the cell body is located within the receptive segment. The cell body is the trophic segment, which is the metabolic center of the neuron.

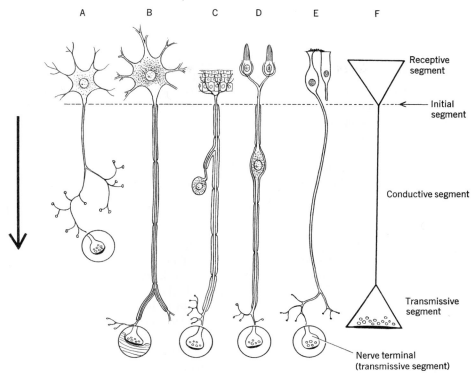

Figure 3.7: Structural and functional organization of representative neurons. Most neurons are composed of a receptive segment, an initial segment, a conductile segment, and a transmissive segment. The transmissive segment of each neuron is encircled. An arrow indicates the normal direction of conduction of the nerve impulse. A = Interneuron, B = Lower motoneuron, C = Sensory neuron with cell body in cranial or spinal ganglion, D = Neuron of vestibulocochlear nerve, E = Neuron of olfactory nerve, and F = Functional organization of neuron. Note that the cell body (trophic segment) may be located within the receptive segment (A, B, and E) or within the conductile segment (C and D). The receptive segment of the vestibulocochlear nerve is associated with a hair cell. (Adapted from Bodian.)

3.1 and 3.6). Each of these segments can be defined by functional criteria.

The *receptive segment* is the portion that senses, receives, and integrates information from numerous synapses for neural processing. It is specialized for the reception of stimuli (input), which results in the generation of local potentials. Each *local potential* generated at a synapse is the product of a transient shift of the membrane potential in the immediate vicinity of the synapse of the receptive segment. The membrane may respond by either hyperpolarizing or depolarizing. This occurs because of local alterations in the permeability to certain ions (i.e., Na^+, K^+, and Cl^-). In those neurons in which the dendrites and cell body comprise the receptive segment, the local potential is called the *synaptic (postsynaptic) potential* or *chemical potential* (see local potential later). The channels involved in generating these potentials are chemically (transmitter) gated. In sensory neurons of the peripheral nerves, the receptive segment is located in sensory receptors in the body (i.e., touch receptors). This segment contains modality specific gated Na^+ and K^+ channels. In these neurons, the local potential is called the *receptor* or *generator potential* (see Anatomy of a First-Order Neuron, p. 52).

The *initial segment* is the *junctional* or *trigger zone* between the receptive zone and conductile zone. It is the locale where the collective effects of the receptive zone generate an *integrated (integral) potential*, which is able to trigger the generation of an *action potential* of the conductile segment **(Fig. 3.1)**.

The *conductile segment* is specialized for the

conduction of neural information from the receptive segment to the transmissive synaptic segment. To perform this role, the conductile segment conveys all-or-none *action potentials* (nerve impulses). This segment contains voltage-gated Na^+ and K^+ channels.

The *transmissive segment* contains the presynaptic membrane and the synaptic vesicles. The action potentials arriving from the conductile segment activate, through voltage-gated channels, the release of the chemical neurotransmitter, which, in turn, influences the receptor sites of the postsynaptic cell.

The *trophic segment* is the cell body, that is the metabolic center essential for the viability of the neuron. In most neurons, the trophic center is usually located within the receptive segment. In the sensory neurons of the peripheral nerves, the cell body is located within the conductile segment (**Figs. 3.6 and 3.7**).

RECEPTIVE SEGMENT AND THE RECEPTOR POTENTIALS

In most neurons, the receptive segment consists of the *dendrite-cell body* unit. In the sensory neurons of the peripheral nerves, it is the nerve terminals distal to the first node of Ranvier.

Dendrite-Cell Body Unit

The cell membrane of the dendrite-cell body unit is a postsynaptic membrane, also known as the *receptor membrane*, because its permeability channels are responsive to the *transmitters (neurotransmitters)* released by the presynaptic neuron. Thus, its channels are transmitter-gated (chemically-gated). In addition, each of these channels is permeable to both Na^+ and K^+ ions or to both K^+ and Cl^- ions. When stimulated, this membrane propagates its response, called a *receptor potential or synaptic potential*, which is a graded response. Each graded response propagates a potential along the cell membrane for a short distance and lasts for only 1 or 2 milliseconds, but is not sufficient to generate an action potential (**Figs. 2.1 and 3.1**). Successive stimuli, when timed close together, can add on and enhance or facilitate the previous graded response. When a synaptic potential

is increased in size, it is said to be *facilitated*. Action potentials are not generated across the membrane of the dendrites and cell body because these membranes do not contain voltage sensitive Na^+ and K^+ channels. In contrast, action potentials are usually generated in most neurons in the region of the initial segment because of the high concentration of voltage sensitive Na^+ and K^+ channels in the membrane at this site.

Excitation of the receptor membrane is explained as the response to a transmitter that partially depolarizes the postsynaptic membrane. Such a response is a graded response known as an excitatory postsynaptic potential (EPSP) (**Figs. 3.1, 3.4, and 3.5**). It, like the action potential noted later, is associated with Na^+ inrush into the segment and K^+ outrush through the same chemically-gated channels driven by molecular pumps (**Fig. 3.4**). A single EPSP does not lower the membrane potential sufficiently to generate an action potential (**Fig. 3.5**). However, many EPSPs, generated collectively, can, by facilitation, become strong enough to lower the membrane potential of the initial segment sufficiently to generate an action potential (nerve impulse). The transmitter eliciting EPSPs opens channels that allow both Na^+ and K^+ to cross the plasma membrane.

Whereas an EPSP brings a neuron to a state closer to its generating potential in which it is more likely to generate an action potential, an *inhibitory postsynaptic potential (IPSP)* creates a state in which the neuron is prevented from firing. Inhibition is the response of the postsynaptic membrane to a transmitter by hyperpolarizing the receptor membrane, i.e., to increase the potential to, for example, -80 mV (**Fig. 3.1**). The inhibitory response is associated with Cl^- inrush and K^+ outrush through the channels of the postsynaptic membrane (**Figs. 3.4 and 3.5**). The transmitter eliciting IPSP's opens channels that allow both Cl^- and K^+ to cross the plasma membrane. The major inhibitory transmitters are GABA and glycine. The postsynaptic receptors for these transmitters are associated with channels permeable to Cl^- ions. The resulting influx of Cl^- ions into the neuron hyperpolarizes the membrane and produces IPSPs.

In a sense, EPSPs oppose IPSPs. A neuron

may have numerous excitatory postsynaptic channels as well as numerous inhibitory postsynaptic transmitter-gated channels. Both types are able to alter the ionic permeability of the receptor membrane. The integration of such synaptic activity is the function of the dendrites and cell body of a neuron (see later). In essence, the receptive segment integrates synaptic inputs, which, if they summate sufficient excitatory activity to reach the initial segment, can trigger an action potential in the axon (**Fig. 3.1**).

In general, excitatory synapses, evoking EPSPs, are found in greater numbers in the dendrites, while inhibitory synapses are found in greater numbers in the cell body. This is a functionally desirable distribution. The EPSPs can summate to excite the neuron, while the IPSPs, by being located closer to the initial segment, can effectively control and modulate the quantity of excitatory influences arriving at the initial segment to trigger the generation of an action potential. The nozzle of a hose is analogous to the role of the inhibitory synapses: the set of the nozzle (degree of inhibition) regulates the amount of water (summated EPSPs) ejected by the hose.

Receptive Segment of Peripheral Sensory Neurons

The sensory or afferent neurons conveying information from the external and internal environment via the peripheral nerves to the CNS have a special structural organization. The peripheral sensory endings of these fibers—many of which are associated with specialized sensory receptors such as rods and cones of the retina, spiral organ of Corti of the ear, and neuromuscular spindles within muscles—have a short receptive segment (**Figs. 3.6 and 3.7**). Its plasma membrane contains modality-specific gated Na^+ and K^+ channels. They produce graded potentials that are called *receptor* or *generator potentials*. Pressure in touch receptors, stretch in muscle spindle sensory endings and light in retinal rods and cones open these channels. When the generator potentials reach the first node of Ranvier, which is the initial segment, an integrated potential is generated.

INITIAL SEGMENT AND THE INTEGRATED POTENTIAL

The *initial segment* of an axon of most neurons or the *first node of Ranvier* of peripheral sensory neurons (**Fig. 3.6**) is a specialized segment of a neuron where an *integrated potential* is generated. In essence, this segment is the integrative region where the (algebraic) summation of the EPSPs and IPSPs of the receptive (synaptic) segment are recorded and integrated. It is called the *trigger zone* or *spike generating zone* because it can trigger the generation of the spike of the action potential (AP) of the axon. This occurs because it is the site of the lowest threshold of each neuron—roughly about -45 mV. When this threshold is reached, the newly generated integrated potential of this segment orchestrates and initiates the generation of the spike. This integrated potential will spark the firing of an AP only if the excitation exceeds the inhibition by a critical minimum at the trigger zone. If the membrane potential falls below the spike-firing threshold, no more action potentials are generated.

Each receptor transfers the stimulus energy into the electrochemical energy of the neuron, and thus establishes a common language for all the sensory systems.

CONDUCTILE SEGMENT AND THE ACTION POTENTIAL

The *conductile segment* is the segment specialized to convey an *action potential (AP, nerve impulse)*, which is a rapidly propagated traveling wave of electrical excitation advancing without decrement in an all-or-none fashion along the axon's plasma membrane. Because of the sharp inflection recorded on the oscilloscope, it is also called a *spike* (**Fig. 3.1**). All-or-none refers to the fact that an impulse travels either as a full-blown spike or not at all. The *integrated potential* of the initial segment activates the voltage-gated channels of the conductile segment. This alters the permeability of the cell membrane. When the stimulus to the axon lowers the resting potential to a critical voltage level, usually about 10 to 15 mV lower than the resting potential, an explosive event occurs with the opening of the voltage-gated channels of the conductile segment. The result is the AP, which is an expression of the sudden depolarization. This is due to changes in conductance associated with the opening of the voltage-gated Na^+ and K^+ channels. For a few milliseconds a polarity reversal occurs from the resting potential of -60 to -70 mV to the AP of $+30$ mV with an excess of negative charge outside the neuron. The axis cylinder gains Na^+ and loses K^+ ions during the passage of the AP. At each patch along the axon, the voltage-gated Na^+ channels are activated first and then followed by the opening of the voltage-gated K^+ channels (Fig. 3.3). The conductance of the Na^+ and K^+ ion channels presumably occurs through separate and independent channels. Through these independent channels, the AP is propagated sequentially along the nerve fiber at essentially a constant velocity. As soon as the AP passes by each patch along the nerve fiber, the K^+ conductance is increased by the opening of the voltage-gated K^+ channels and thus the cell membrane returns to its resting level. The repolarization of the membrane occurs when the K^+ conductance restores internal negativity.

The following is a rough approximation. The assumptions that the membrane potential (1) is due solely to K^+, leads to a value near that of the resting potential and (2) is due solely to Na^+, leads to a value near that of the action potential. These assumptions are essentially correct because K^+ is primarily responsible for the resting potential and Na^+ is primarily responsible for the action potential.

In summary, the AP is produced by the movement of ions across the plasma membrane through voltage-gated channels. The movement only occurs after the channels are open, which results in changes in the distribution of charges on either side of the membrane. The influx of Na^+ ions reverses the resting charge distribution. This is followed by an influx of K^+ ions which repolarizes the membrane by restoring the initial charge distribution.

Unmyelinated Fibers

In an unmyelinated fiber, the AP is propagated sequentially along all parts of the cell membrane of the axon. Each depolarized patch on the membrane produces a flow of current (AP) that triggers events to depolarize the adjacent patch that, in turn, depolarizes the resting membrane further ahead (Fig. 3.3B). The AP travels along the cell membrane as a chain reaction at a constant speed. It regenerates itself from point to point along the axon without loss of amplitude, i.e., it propagates via voltage-gated channels without decrement. The smooth progression of the AP is characteristic of unmyelinated fibers (Fig. 3.3).

Myelinated Fibers and Saltatory Conduction

The AP in a myelinated nerve fiber is propagated by discontinuous spread or saltatory (hop or jump) conduction, in which the AP hops along the nerve fiber from node of Ranvier to node of Ranvier (Fig. 3.3A). The current spreads only from an active depolarized node to an inactive polarized node by activating its voltage sensitive Na^+ and K^+ channels. These channels are highly concentrated in the axis cylinders exposed at the nodes. The myelinated internodes act as passive conductors. Myelinated fibers are fast conductors of the action potentials. The speed of conduction of the AP is related to the thickness of the myelin sheaths and the length of the internodes of a nerve fiber. The thicker the myelin sheath and the longer the internodes, the faster an axon conducts an action potential. The myelin improves the signaling (conductile) efficiency of the axon.

TRANSMISSIVE SEGMENT (SYNAPTIC OR EFFECTOR SEGMENT)

The *transmissive* or *synaptic segment* is that portion (or portions) of a neuron through which it exerts its influence on another neuron, muscle, or gland cell. Anatomically this is the presynaptic portion of a synapse comprising the presynaptic membrane and vesicles containing neurotransmitters or their precursors. Physiologically, the arrival of an action potential in the transmissive segment activates the voltage-gated calcium channels in the presynaptic membrane to trigger the inward passage of Ca^{++} ions. This is the critical final step for the release of neurotransmitter into the synaptic cleft. These voltage-gated Ca^{++} channels control what is essentially the secretory function of a neuron, which is, in essence, a secretory cell.

The synapse acts as a one-way valve permitting the action potential of a neuron to exert its influence through the release of neurotransmitters across the synaptic cleft of the receptive segment of the postsynaptic neuron. An exception is the axoaxonic synapse (Fig. 2.9), in which the synapse is between two transmissive segments (discussed later in connection with presynaptic inhibition and excitation).

Synapse at Motor End-Plate (Neuromuscular Junction)

The synapse at the motor end-plate between an axon terminal and voluntary muscle is a well-documented example of interaction at a synapse (Fig. 3.8). Acetylcholine (ACh) is the transmitter at this synapse. The ACh is released into the synaptic cleft from a vesicle as a quantum of ACh with each quantum containing about 6,000 to 10,000 ACh molecules. The release is continuous with a quantum resulting in the slight activity known as miniature end-plate po-

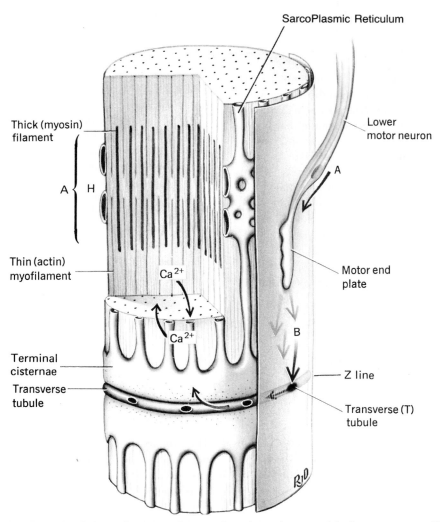

Figure 3.8: Neuromuscular linkage. Sequence of events from the action potential of a motor nerve (**A**), to motor endplate, to action potential of muscle cell membrane (**B**), to T tubule and to sarcoplasmic cisternae. The release and uptake of calcium ions are involved with excitation-contraction (EC) coupling.

tentials (MEPPs), that do not produce an action potential (AP) in the postsynaptic membrane (sarcolemma of muscle fiber). Each AP releases from 100 to 200 quanta. A more active synaptic transmission commences with the depolarization of the membrane by the arrival of the action potential (AP) at the presynaptic terminal. Upon depolarization, the voltage-sensitive Ca^{++} channels open, resulting in the influx of Ca^{++} ions into the terminal. The Ca^{++} facilitates the binding and confluence of many synaptic vesicles to the presynaptic membrane. Following the arrival of volleys of APs and the increase in the influx of Ca^{++} ions into the nerve terminal, there is a 100,000 times surge in ACh molecules as numerous quanta are released by exocytosis into the synaptic cleft. Following exocytosis the vesicle membrane is recycled (Fig. 3.9).

The ACh molecules activate an estimated 20 to 40 million receptor sites on the sarcolemma of the motor end-plate. This results in end plate potentials (EPPs) in the membrane that depolarize the sarcolemma adjacent to the neuromuscular junction (NMJ). This activates its voltage-sensitive Na^+ and K^+ channels of the sarcolemma to generate action potentials. The AP is conducted rapidly along the muscle surface and to the interior of the muscle fiber via the membrane of the many transverse tubules (T-tubules) (Fig. 3.8). The AP stimulates the release of Ca^{++} ions from the sarcoplasmic reticulum (SR) of the muscle to initiate the contraction of the muscle fiber as a unit (known as excitation-contraction or EC coupling). The relaxation of the muscle fiber is associated with the return of the Ca^{++} ions to the sarcoplasmic reticulum. The basal lamina of the muscle in the end-plate is filled with the enzyme acetylcholinesterase, which inactivates the excess ACh. This enzyme serves two purposes, it (1) permits only a small proportion of ACh released to stimulate receptors and their channels on the sarcolemma of the end plate and (2) creates breakdown products, such as choline, which is taken up by the nerve terminals and utilized in the resynthesis of ACh (Fig. 3.9).

In brief, the neurotransmitter precursor is synthesized within a neuron, stored and packaged in a vesicle within the nerve terminal, and the activated form is released by exocytosis from the vesicle into the synaptic cleft.

Neither Na^+ influx nor K^+ efflux is required for synaptic transmission. Only Ca^{++} ions which enter the neuron through voltage-dependent Ca^{++} channels in the presynaptic ending are essential. Ca^{++} ions are the intraneuronal messengers. They serve as the only link to transduce depolarization into all the nonelectrical activities regulated by excitation. Without Ca^{++} channels, the neurons and, as a consequence, the nervous system, would have no outputs. In essence, synaptic delay, i.e., the time interval between the arrival of the action potential at the transmissive segment and the release of neurotransmitter, is an expression of the time it takes for the Ca^{++} ions to diffuse to the site of action within the terminal and the release of transmitter from the synaptic vesicles. At the neuromuscular junction, the normal synaptic potential of -70 mV at the postsynaptic membrane results from the release of about 150 quanta of acetylcholine.

In the innervated muscle fiber, the channels capable of responding to acetylcholine are restricted to the region of the neuromuscular junction. Following the denervation of a muscle fiber, the fiber becomes sensitive to acetylcholine over its entire surface. In response to denervation, the fiber synthesizes new ACh-sensitive channels and inserts them into its plasma membrane. In a sense, this is a reversion to its early development when newly differentiated muscle fibers have ACh-sensitive channels scattered over their entire surface. Upon reinnervation, the membrane's ACh sensitivity becomes restricted to the region of the NMJ.

SYNAPSES AND CHEMICAL TRANSMISSION IN THE CENTRAL NERVOUS SYSTEM

The primary means of communication between neurons is via chemical transmission at synapses (Fig. 3.9). Within the CNS, this process consists of four steps. They are similar in principle to those at the neuromuscular junction, which is actually a synapse between a neuron and a muscle fiber. These steps are (1) synthesis of the transmitter, (2) storage and release of the

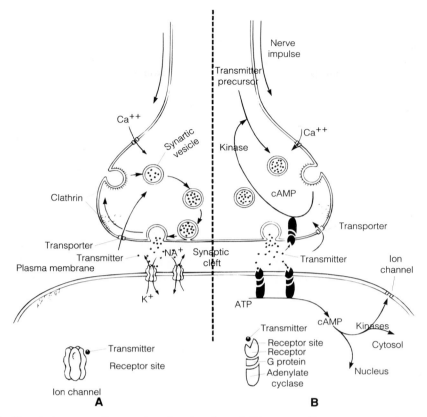

Figure 3.9: A. Chemical synapse-direct gating of an ion channel. In nerve endings, neurotransmitters are packaged in synaptic vesicles and released by exocytosis. Empty synaptic vesicles are rapidly recycled for re-use by endocytosis. The action potential conveyed by the axon depolarizes the nerve terminal to trigger an influx of Ca^{++} ions through voltage-gated channels. This activates synaptic vesicles to fuse with the presynaptic membrane and to release transmitter molecules into the synaptic cleft by exocytosis. These transmitters diffuse across the cleft and bind to specific receptor sites on the postsynaptic membrane. Each receptor controls an ion channel (selective to specific ions) by direct gating of the ion channels. *The direct gating of an ion channel is mediated by a transmitter receptor that is a part of the ion channel.* The resulting ion flux alters the voltage of the postsynaptic membrane. This can either depolarize the membrane to generate excitatory postsynaptic potentials (EPSPs) or hyperpolarize the membrane to generate inhibitory postsynaptic potentials (IPSPs). Transmitter molecules then uncouple from the receptor sites, and thus their role in the synaptic response is consummated. The transmitter (or its breakdown product) can be conveyed through a membrane *transporter* into the axon terminal to be recycled. The vesicle membrane is also recycled—the protein *clathrin* becomes transiently associated with the vesicle membrane to assist its being incorporated into a new vesicle by endocytosis. A critical means for sustaining the vesicle population at the endings in the presence of active transmitter release is by the rapid recycling of synaptic vesicles. The entire process, from the activation of the exocytosed synaptic vesicle for recycling until the vesicle with transmitter is competent to exocytose again, can presumably occur in less than 3 minutes. This insures the maintenance of the population of about 200 vesicles in a single nerve ending. (Refer to text). **B.** Chemical synapse—indirect gating of an ion channel via a second messenger. The neuromodulator (transmitter) released from a synaptic vesicle into the synaptic cleft binds with a receptor on the postsynaptic membrane. The receptor activates a G-protein and an intracellular enzyme such as adenylate cyclase. This enzyme converts adenosine triphosphate (ATP) to the second messenger cyclic adenosine monophosphate (cAMP). In turn cAMP activates other enzymes, called kinases (cAMP-dependent kinases), and phosphorylates ion channels to modulate their function (also to influence activity in the nucleus and the cytosol). Second messengers frequently act through protein phosphorylation to open and close ion channels. *The indirect gating of an ion channel is mediated by a second messenger that couples to the receptor of an ion channel.* Neuromodulators can also bind with autoreceptors located on the presynaptic terminal membrane. These receptors activate the second messenger system in the axonal terminal to modulate transmitter release. Neurotransmitter transporters are glycoproteins in the cell membrane that are active in reuptake systems conveying neurotransmitters from the synaptic cleft to the axon terminal for recycling. (Refer to text).

transmitter, (3) interaction of transmitter with receptors, and (4) removal and recycling of synaptic vesicles and transmitters (**Fig. 3.9**).

For signaling, the nervous system utilizes two classes of neurotransmitters which are contained within vesicles located in the synaptic terminals. There are (A) small molecule transmitters and (B) neuroactive peptides (Chap. 15). The *small molecule transmitters* include (a) acetylcholine; (b) the four amino acids—glutamate, aspartate, GABA, and glycine; and (c) the four monoamines comprising the catecholamines—dopamine, norepinephrine and epinephrine, and the indolamine—serotonin. The *neuroactive peptides* include at least 50 different pharmacologically active peptides such as the hypothalamic peptide *somatostatin*, the pituitary peptide *vasopressin*, the digestive system peptide *substance P* and such peptides as *enkephalins*.

Synthesis of the Transmitters

The transmitters are synthesized within the presynaptic neuron. The small molecule transmitters are generated in all regions of the neuron including the nerve terminals. Its macromolecular components are synthesized in the cell body and rapidly delivered by fast transport to the nerve terminal. Some are derived from released transmitters in the synaptic cleft and recycled back into the terminal. The neuropeptides are generated in the cell body (see later for more details).

Storage and Release of the Transmitters

Once formed these transmitters are immediately sequestered within the vesicles and tethered to the cytoskeleton in the reserve pool (storage or cytoskeletal anchored compartment) of the nerve terminal. If left free in the cytoplasm, the transmitter is vulnerable to intracellular digestion. Vesicle stores constitute a reserve of transmitters, protected from intracellular enzymes. Thus, only an appropriate level of transmitter is available within the cytoplasm. The small transmitters are stored in *small, clear vesicles* of about 50 nm in diameter. Vesicles are then transported to *docking sites* near the sites of release, called *active zones*, where they are docked to *fusion pore complexes* in the presynaptic

plasma membrane. The entry of calcium into the nerve terminal through voltage-gated channels triggers the opening of the fusion pore complex and transmitter release into the synaptic cleft. The calcium also mobilizes cytoskeletally anchored vesicles and makes them available for docking with the fusion pore complex.

In contrast to small molecule vesicle transmitters, the precursors of the neuroactive peptides are synthesized and packaged into secretory granules and synaptic vesicles in the cell body. They are then transported by fast transport via neurotubules to the terminal. In this respect, they are unlike the small-molecule transmitters. The neuropeptides are stored in large (with an electron dense core) vesicles of about 120 nm in diameter.

A *transmitter* is a substance that is released at a synapse by a neuron and affects another neuron or effector cell (muscle fiber or glandular cell) in a specific manner. A mature neuron makes use of the same transmitter (or transmitters) at all of its synapses. A small molecule transmitter and a neuroactive peptide transmitter can coexist in the same mature neuron. The corelease of several transmitters from the presynaptic neuron and the presence of appropriate receptors on the postsynaptic neuron is one expression of the combination of diverse information transfer.

Interaction of Transmitter with Receptors

The released transmitters diffuse quickly across the synaptic cleft, bind to specific receptor proteins on the postsynaptic membrane and *initiate* changes in the membrane. There are two general groups of transmitters: *neurotransmitters* and *neuromodulators*. Neurotransmitters are substances that act directly on the postsynaptic membrane channels and, by altering their permeability, allow ions to pass through the channel mediated by the transmitter receptor that is an integral part of the channel. The neurotransmitters include acetylcholine and the amino acids glutamate, aspartate, GABA, and glycine. They are involved with the generation of fast EPSPs and IPSPs. These local potentials commence within a fraction of a millisecond after the release of the transmitter and seldom persist longer than 100 milliseconds. Glutamate and aspartate are excitatory neurotransmitters and GABA and glycine are inhibitory neurotransmitters. Depending upon the nature of the receptor, acetylcholine can act either as an excitatory or inhibitory transmitter.

Some substances released at synapses modify or modulate neural activity rather than initiate it. These transmitters are known as *neuromodulators*. Their responses are of slow onset that last for seconds or even for minutes, hours, or longer. They operate in the postsynaptic neuron through other molecules called *second messengers* (see later). These long-term changes may be involved with such phenomena as memory and learning. The neuromodulators include the monoamines dopamine, norepinephrine, epinephrine and serotonin, and the neuroactive peptides. Of the many neuropeptides in the brain, most act as neuromodulators.

The receptor protein to which the transmitter binds determines whether the response to the transmitter will act as neurotransmitter to a neuromodulator. A substance such as acetylcholine can, depending on the specific receptors, act as both (see Second Messenger System).

Removal and Recycling of the Synaptic Vesicles and Transmitters

Vesicle Membrane

In order to release its transmitters into the synaptic cleft, a vesicle containing the transmitters initially fuses with the presynaptic membrane. Following the release by a process known as *exocytosis*, the vesicle membrane becomes incorporated in the presynaptic membrane and coated on its inner surface by a dense layer of the protein *clathrin*. A coated "pothole" is then retrieved as a vesicle by the reverse process of *endocytosis* (**Fig. 3.9**). The budding off of the new vesicle, which is energetically unfavorable, is aided by the clathrin, which remains as a temporary coat around the vesicle. After being pinched off from the plasma membrane, the clathrin-coated vesicles are enzymatically uncoated within a few seconds. Most of the recycled membranes form intermediary structures called *cisterna* before forming vesicles that become filled with newly synthesized or reuptaken transmitters. Thus, the vesicle membrane and

transmitters are recycled. Some exocytosed vesicle membranes may be returned by retrograde transport to the cell body to be degraded by lysosomes.

Removal and Reuptake of Transmitters

Following their release from the nerve terminals, most transmitters are rapidly removed from the synaptic cleft by a sodium-dependent cotransport reuptake system into the axon terminal (or into glial cells). By cotransporting the transmitter with sodium, the energy stored in the transmembrane electrochemical gradients can be used to drive the transmitter back into the axon terminal through the *glycoprotein transporters* in the plasma membrane (**Fig. 3.9**). Once within the axon terminal, the transmitter is incorporated into a new synaptic vesicle. Such neuroactive transmitters as serotonin, glutamate, aspartate, glycine, GABA, and the catecholamines dopamine and norepinephrine are taken up by the transmembrane transporters, each of which is linked to a specific transmitter. Transporters are implicated as sites for drug action. Drugs that block neurotransmitter reuptake exert powerful physiologic effects. The action of many antidepressant drugs, such as Prozac, results from the blocking of the serotonin transporter. Thereby, the amount of serotonin in the synaptic cleft is increased (Chap. 15).

The neurotransmitter acetylcholine (ACh) released from cholinergic endings (e.g., motor end plate) is not taken up into the axon terminal as ACh. Rather, it is degraded into choline and acetate by the enzyme acetylcholinesterase located in the basal membrane of the synaptic cleft (**Fig. 2.4**). The choline is taken up into the axon terminal to be used in the synthesis of new ACh. The choline is combined with *acetyl coenzyme A* (an activated form of acetate) by the enzyme *choline acetyltransferase*, as the catalyst, to become ACh, which is then concentrated in new synaptic vesicles.

Activity at the Synapse

Following release, the neurotransmitter molecules diffuse across the synaptic cleft, resulting in a *synaptic delay* of about 1 millisecond. Depending on the chemical structure of the transmitter and of the receptor sites on the postsynaptic membrane, the resulting permeability changes at the receptor channels lead either to excitation or inhibition. The response of the postsynaptic membrane (excitation or inhibition) cannot be attributed exclusively to the transmitter, because the properties of the receptor are also critical. The stimulation of the excitatory receptors results in excitatory responses on the postsynaptic membrane, while the stimulation of the inhibitory receptors results in inhibitory responses. For example, the transmitter acetylcholine stimulates excitatory activity in voluntary muscle and inhibitory activity in cardiac muscle. Neurons exert either excitatory or inhibitory influences. Presumably, they are never ambivalent. As a rule, such transmitters as glutamate, aspartate, and acetylcholine produce excitatory responses, and such transmitters as glycine and GABA produce inhibitory responses.

Hormones and drugs may also bind to receptor sites of the plasma membrane. The molecules of neurotransmitters, hormones, or drugs do not just bind to their receptors; each is in a process of binding and unbinding that results in a state of dynamic equilibrium. In this continuous process, each molecule-receptor combination has its own dynamic steady state and rate of binding and unbinding between free and bound molecules and between free and bound receptors. In addition, molecular pumps act quickly to remove transmitters from the receptor sites.

In summary, two physiologic events occur at a synapse between a transmissive segment and a receptive segment: (1) the nerve impulse by depolarizing the presynaptic membrane brings about Ca^{++} entry followed by transmitter release into the synaptic cleft and (2) there is a response at the postsynaptic membrane initiated by the transmitter-receptor protein interaction followed by the generation of a graded potential. These two events can be broken down into eight steps: (1) the arrival of the nerve impulse results in presynaptic depolarization, which (2) triggers the opening of calcium channels with the inrush of Ca^{++} ions through the presynaptic membrane, which (3) triggers transmitter release from presynaptic vesicles followed by (4) diffusion of transmitter across the synaptic cleft and (5) the binding of the

transmitter to the receptor sites on the postsynaptic membrane, after which there are (6) molecular events in the postsynaptic membrane resulting in (7) the opening of ion channels and (8) the generation of graded postsynaptic potentials. Each of the receptor sites is a complex of proteins with an active binding portion facing the synaptic cleft and channel through the postsynaptic membrane. In effect, the transmitter binds to the receptive site and opens the channel through which the ions flow.

SECOND MESSENGER SYSTEM

The neurotransmitters have been called the *first messenger system* utilizing a *first messenger*. The first messenger is a neurotransmitter, released by a presynaptic neuron, that interacts with a specific postsynaptic receptor protein associated with an ionic channel. The latter protein directly influences the channel (Fig. 3.9). This entire sequence is fast; it takes place within a millisecond. These receptors have been recently designated as Class I (fast) receptors (Chap. 15).

Another type of synaptic activity is the *second messenger system* utilizing a *second messenger*. The sequence in this system is relatively slow: it lasts from a few milliseconds to seconds and even minutes. The first messenger, a neuromodulator (or hormone), is released by the presynaptic neuron and then binds to a specific postsynaptic receptor protein to produce a single graded response. Following the binding, in one family, the receptor contacts and activates a G-protein which is attached to the inner surface of the plasma membrane (named after a family of membrane proteins that bind to guanine nucleotide-binding protein, G-protein). The activated G-protein functions as an intermediary between the receptor in the plasma membrane and an effector intracellular enzyme, such as adenylate cyclase (Fig. 3.9). In turn, this effector enzyme converts ATP into cyclic adenosine monophosphate, (cAMP), which acts as a diffusible *second messenger* or *intracellular signaling molecule*. This messenger triggers a cascade of molecular reactions that alters the biochemical state within the neuron. Receptor proteins activated by neuromodulators commonly are linked to G-proteins or receptor kinases. Depending on the neuromodulator, G-proteins may increase or decrease activity of enzymes that produce second messengers such as adenylate cyclase which produces cAMP. The cAMP activates other enzymes, namely protein kinases, which add phosphate groups (through the process called phosphorylation) to molecules, thus activating them. Phosphorylation is a common mechanism for regulating biochemical reactions. Receptor, G-proteins, second messengers and protein kinases interact through subtle and highly integrated biochemical reactions that operate throughout the neuron—including the nucleus (gene expression can be altered), in the cytosol (protein synthesis can be modified) and in the plasma membrane (channel activity can be modulated). The second messengers may be conceived as acting directly on the channels or more commonly as acting through the kinases. The latter can modulate channel activity by phosphorylating either the channel protein or a regulatory protein that also acts on the channel. These receptors have recently been designated as Class 2 (slow) receptors (Chap. 15).

Neuromodulators can exert presynaptic as well as postsynaptic effects. Presynaptic terminals may have their own receptors, called *autoreceptors* (Fig. 3.9). Autoreceptors are presynaptic receptors that are able to recognize, and to bind with, the neuron's own transmitter. In the figure, the autoreceptor is activated to instigate a cAMP cascade which modulates the synthesis of neuroactive agents in the terminal. The neuromodulator released by the presynaptic terminal can regulate, through a feedback sequence, the formation of neuroactive substances.

Several second messenger systems, as well as variations within each of these systems, are known to exist in neurons. More systems remain to be uncovered. Complexity of these systems results from the myriad of linkages involving different types of receptors, G-proteins, second messengers, and protein kinases. A current estimate suggests that neurons have 100 or more receptors that communicate through 20 or so G-proteins. The G-proteins are considered to be a key component within the plasma membrane

of the complex processing messenger network within the neuron.

ELECTRIC (ELECTRONIC) SYNAPSE

Another type of synapse, the electric (electronic) synapse, is relatively infrequent in the mammalian nervous system. In these synapses there is cytoplasmic continuity between two adjacent neurons through 1.5 nm channels. Because of this continuity, ions can flow between cells at these junctions; these low-resistance *"gap junctions"* result in *"electrically coupled"* neurons. In these synapses, no transmitter is involved. There is essentially no synaptic delay, because the electrical activity readily spreads from neuron to neuron. Because these synapses cannot be modulated, they are not compatible with most neural functions. However, these are found occasionally where activity must be tightly synchronized. For example, they occur in the neural circuits involved with stereotypic saccadic eye movements (Chap. 16), and also in the junctions (nexus) between smooth muscle cells involved in peristalsis of the gut, and between cardiac muscle fibers (intercalated disks) in synchronizing the heart beat (Fig. 2.3).

Because the current can flow across gap junctions in either direction (bidirectionally), it may be difficult to decide which is the presynaptic and which is the postsynaptic side of the junction. They can be either, especially when the electric synapse adjoins two dendrites, two cell bodies, or two axons. Some evidence suggests that, at some gap junctions, there is only a unidirectional transport of ions.

NEURON AS AN INTEGRATOR

Each neuron is an integrator of stimuli (neurotransmitters) streaming into its dendritic field and onto its cell body. Some of the receptive patches (subsynaptic membranes) on the dendrites and cell body are excitatory, others inhibitory. In addition, as will be described, presynaptic inhibitory activity may indirectly affect some excitatory receptive sites. At any one moment, a neuron may receive hundreds or even thousands of stimuli on its excitatory and inhibitory membrane patches.

Most neurons are under constant *synaptic bombardment*. In this battleground of activity, the neuron reacts and may respond. If the summation of the EPSPs exceeds the summation of the IPSPs, the initial segment of the axon may be excited to initiate the production of an action potential in the axon (Figs. 3.4 and 3.5). If the algebraic summation of these potentials (EPSPs and IPSPs) is not sufficient to stimulate the initial segment, an action potential is not generated in the axon. The depolarization of the initial segment to the critical voltage is a prerequisite to the generation of an action potential. Thus, each dendrite-cell body complex of a neuron is a *miniature integration center*; it will respond with an action potential according to the net effect of the excitatory and inhibitory synaptic activity on the receptive membrane of the neuron. The axon is the vehicle for signaling coded information, via action potentials, from the dendrite-cell body complex to other neurons or effectors (muscles or gland cells).

Each postsynaptic membrane of the signaled neurons and effectors contains hundreds or even thousands of receptor sites. Each receptor site, which is composed of macromolecular proteins acting as specialized decoders, responds to a given stimulus in its own, probably predetermined way. For example, acetylcholine is an excitatory agent at a motor end-plate (contraction of voluntary muscle) and an inhibitory agent at the synapses of the vagus nerve with heart tissue (decrease in heart rate).

A neuron may in turn be influenced by its own activity through a *negative feedback loop* involving an interneuron (Fig. 3.10). Such an interneuron, called a *Renshaw cell*, is intercalated between an axon collateral branch of a lower motoneuron of the spinal cord and the dendrite-cell body region of the same motoneuron and other motoneurons. The axon collateral terminates at an excitatory synapse on the Renshaw cell; the axons of this cell have, in turn, inhibitory synaptic connections with the parent lower motoneuron (Chap. 10).

Neurons in the CNS may be classified into two major types: (1) projection neurons and (2) local circuit neurons. Projection neurons have long axons coursing from one region of the central nervous system to another. Local circuit neurons have axons passing and interacting with neurons in the immediate vicinity.

PRESYNAPTIC INHIBITION AND PRESYNAPTIC FACILITATION

Presynaptic Inhibition is the phenomenon that occurs when a presynaptic neuron (neuron A) exerts inhibitory influences through transmitters at an axoaxonic synapse with the axon terminal of a postsynaptic neuron (neuron B) (Fig. 3.10). In turn, this presynaptic inhibition of neuron B depresses the release of excitatory transmitter at the synapse of neuron B with neuron C. In the figure, note that the axon terminal of neuron A synapses with the axon terminal of axon B. When terminal B is stimulated alone, EPSPs are evoked in the postsynaptic neuron C. When terminal A is stimulated alone, no response occurs in the terminal B. When A and B are stimulated simultaneously, the generation of EPSPs in the postsynaptic neuron C is decreased.

The explanation for this phenomenon involves the Cl^-, K^+, and Ca^{++} channels on terminal B. The release of inhibitory transmitter from terminal A opens Cl^- and K^+ channels on terminal B. In turn, this reduces the influx of Ca^{++} through the voltage-gated channels on terminal A. This reduction of Ca^{++} influx depresses the release or excitatory transmitter by terminal B at its synapse with the postsynaptic neuron C.

Presynaptic Facilitation (Presynaptic Excitation) is the phenomena that occurs when a presynaptic neuron (A) exerts excitatory influences through transmitters at an axoaxonic synapse upon the axon terminal of a postsynaptic neuron (B). The presynaptic release of the transmitter is presumed to close the K^+ channels, resulting in a prolongation of the action potential (because of a slower repolarization phase). This acts to increase calcium influx into the postsynaptic axon terminal (neuron B), and thereby enhances excitatory transmitter release by neuron B at its synapse with the postsynaptic neuron C.

The mediation of presynaptic inhibition and presynaptic facilitation through axoaxonic syn-

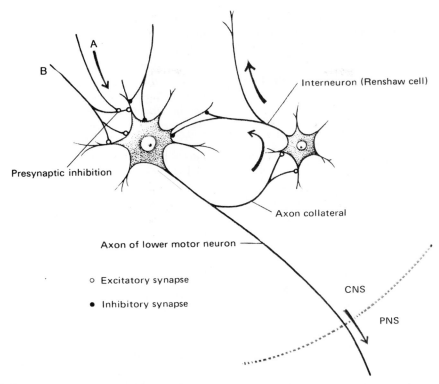

Figure 3.10: The neuron as an integrator. The interrupted line represents the boundary between the central nervous system and the peripheral nervous system. Arrows indicate the direction in which nerve impulses are propagated. Neurons from many sources in the brain, spinal cord, and body convey influences to each lower motor neuron (see Chap. 10), which in turn innervates some voluntary muscle fibers. The axon collateral of the lower motoneuron excites the interneuron (Renshaw cell), which feeds back inhibitory influences to the lower motoneuron. (See text for significance of presynaptic inhibition at axoaxonic synapse of synapse of neurons A and B.)

apses contributes to the elegant neural processing that takes place in the central nervous system. Of significance is that, axoaxonic synapses can control and alter the Ca^{++} influx into the axon terminals. As a consequence, presynaptic activity makes it possible to influence selectively the signal transmission from one neuron to another, without affecting the general excitability of the postsynaptic neuron and thus, its responsiveness to other synaptic inputs.

Importance of Inhibition

Inhibition is a most significant neural activity. It is as important as excitation. The inhibitory neurons and their neural circuits act as governors that prevent, shape, and control the excitatory neurons and their neural circuits from firing to excess. In a simplistic explanation, imagine

the consequences of excitatory influences without braking (as the brakes in a car) to keep these influences from getting out of hand. Inhibitory influences function to channel and to modulate the effects of excitation and to direct activity to attain a desired end. In learning the intricate movements of writing, a child initially has control difficulties because, in part, too many unnecessary movements are made. During the learning process these movements are gradually eliminated through inhibition. The desired excitatory channels are sustained to produce the focal movements. In this case, the inhibition of the nonessential movements is significant to the learning process. The inhibitory circuits prevent an excess of neural firing and, in addition, time the specific responsiveness of the excitatory networks. This also applies to neural networks (pathways) that convey and interpret information about the external and internal world. Inhibition, including lateral inhibition, is presumably involved to shape the excitatory activity in the neural pathways that form the basis of the experience of sensation and feeling (sentience) as distinguished from perception and thought.

Channels—Precis on Neuronal Signals

The control of the flow of ions across the channels of the cell membranes of neurons is the basis for electrical signals utilized by the nervous system. These channels possess two significant properties. (1) They are *ion-specific* as expressed in the independent control of a variety of channels that allow for the flow of different ions (estimates suggest that there are over 75 distinct types of channels). (2) They are *regulated* in expressing their roles by being either in an open state or in a closed state. The balance between these two states can be regulated by external ligands (e.g., cAMP), voltage, and mechanical stimuli (e.g., stretch and vibrations).

Numerous combinations of the many types of channels are used by neurons to create a variety of signals in different neurons and in various sites of the same neuron. This is accomplished by the use of the many types of channels and by their distribution and numbers on the cell membrane. These electrical signals are the substrates for the intricacy and flexibility expressed by the neuronal components that are essential for the subtlety and plasticity embedded in the tapestry or signal systems of our brain.

ANATOMY OF A FIRST-ORDER NEURON

The sensory or afferent neurons conveying information from the external and internal environment via the peripheral nerves to the CNS have a different structural organization from other neurons (Figs. 3.6, 3.7, 7.2, and 8.3).

Most of the first-order neurons, called *unipolar* or *pseudounipolar neurons*, are present in all spinal nerves and most cranial nerves. The first-order sensory neurons of the olfactory, optic, and vestibulocochlear systems are *bipolar neurons* (e.g., cochlear nerve, Fig. 16.5). A unipo-

lar neuron has only one process (which, in turn, divides into two processes) extending from the cell body; the distal process extends to the sensory nerve ending and the proximal process extends to the central nervous system. A bipolar neuron has two processes extending from the cell body: one process to the nerve endings and the other to the CNS.

The peripheral sensory endings of these fibers—many of which are associated with specialized sensory receptors such as rods and cones in the retina, organ of Corti in the ear, and muscle spindles within muscles—compose the receptive segment of the neurons; this portion propagates by graded potentials (generator potential) for a short distance. Except for the receptive portion, the rest of the process (or processes) propagates action potentials by all-or-none conduction, either as myelinated or unmyelinated fibers, which terminate as axodendritic and axosomatic synaptic junctions within the CNS (Fig. 3.6). The initial segment is located at the junction of the receptive segment and the conductile segment.

The cell bodies of the first-order neurons are located in the dorsal root ganglia of the spinal nerves (Fig. 7.2) and the sensory ganglia of the cranial nerves (Fig. 14.2). The bipolar cells in the nasal mucosa (olfactory system) and in the retina (visual system) (Fig. 19.2) are also first-order neurons.

SOME GENERAL CONCEPTS ASSOCIATED WITH CODING AND PROCESSING IN THE NERVOUS SYSTEM

Neural Signals: Label Line Codes and Pattern Codes

The body responds to external and internal environmental stimuli through receptors that are associated with modalities of the sensory systems. The recognized receptors are mechanoreceptors, nociceptors, thermoreceptors, photoreceptors, and chemoreceptors. The modalities comprise general somatic senses, balance, audition, vision, taste, and smell. Most sensory receptors are sensitive to specific stimulus energies, called receptor specificity, that results in generating a neural signal as a *labeled line code* in a first order neuron. The code of specific modalities associated with, for example, touch (Chap. 10) are conveyed via specific lines through series of neurons and neural centers of the central nervous system where they are processed to evoke the perception of the sensation. Each sensory receptor responds in a specific manner when it is adequately stimulated, regardless of the stimulus. Whether activated by a natural or an artificial (e.g., electrical) stimulus, the same sensation is elicited. Chemoreceptors lack the specificity of responding to a single stimulus signal and thus, do not project their information on labeled lines. Rather, the modalities associated with taste and smell use a *pattern code* signal in which several receptors are activated. The resulting discharge pattern of signals formed by a group of neurons is the basis for the perception of a flavor or odor sensation.

Transformation of the Neural Signals at Processing Centers of Pathways

Neural processing occurs within the neural centers (laminae, nuclei, and cortices) of each pathway system. Neurons within these centers process the patterns of incoming signals and transform them so that the relay neurons project a different pattern of signals to other centers. *Each center performs a transformation function.* Each center consists of (1) relay neurons whose axons project to other centers, (2) interneurons with processes located wholly within the center, and (3) axons of neurons from other sources.

Processing Within the Nervous System

The ascending (and descending) pathways function both as processors and as transmitters of coded information. The processing within a center of the pathways is information-linked, not energy-linked. For example, stimulation of the optic system evokes sensations related to vision, regardless of whether the stimulus is light, an electrical shock, or a blow to the eye.

The sensory input to the relay neurons within a center are examples of convergence (input of axons from many neurons to one relay neuron) and divergence (input of an axon to more than one relay neuron). These inputs form a basis for

some of the complexities of interactions among neurons. The numerous signals arriving at each processing center and interaction with the local interneurons act to bias, enhance, or dampen signals and their transmission. In effect, each center acts as an editor. A major role in the processing is performed by the local inhibitory interneurons in (1) feedback inhibition, (2) feed-forward inhibition, and (3) reflected inhibition (Fig. 3.11)

Feedback (or Recurrent) Inhibition

In feedback inhibition, the most actively firing relay neurons, utilizing inhibitory interneurons, depresses the activity of the adjacent, less actively firing relay neurons (Fig. 3.11). Thus, the more active neurons enhance and amplify the contrast between the actively firing relay neurons and their less active neighboring neurons. This leads to a selective emphasis of one stimulus over another. Stated otherwise, the signal is enhanced and the adjacent noise of the less active neurons suppressed. It is called feedback or recurrent inhibition because the recurrent collateral branches of the axon of the relay neuron feedback to excite the inhibitory interneurons to inhibit the adjacent relay neurons.

Feed-forward (or Reciprocal) Inhibition

In feed-forward inhibition, the activity of one or more neurons inhibit another neuron or group of neurons (Fig. 3.11). This acts in what is called the *singleness of action* in which only a limited number of competing responses are expressed, while the others are suppressed. The feed-forward neuronal circuits consist of the branches of the axons of relay neurons entering a nucleus and terminating by synapsing with local circuit interneurons. In turn, these neurons exert inhibitory influences upon relay neurons via either presynaptic or postsynaptic inhibition. *Presynaptic inhibition* occurs when the axons entering a relay nucleus synapse with excitatory local circuit interneurons that, in turn, synapse with the terminals of neighboring entering axons. *Postsynaptic inhibition* occurs when the axons entering the nucleus synapse with local interneurons that, in turn, synapse with the cell bodies of adjacent relay neurons. A *feed-forward inhibitory circuit* is characterized by having one or more inhibitory

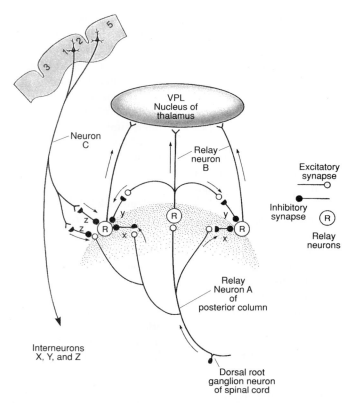

Figure 3.11: Diagram illustrating three types of neural processing involving inhibition. The neurons represent relay (R) neurons and local inhibitory neurons (X, Y, and Z) associated with the nuclei gracilis and cuneatus of the posterior column-medial lemniscus pathway (Chap. 10). The relay neurons (R) project to the ventral posterior lateral nucleus (VPL) of the thalamus. (1) Feed-Forward Inhibition. Relay neuron A of a dorsal root ganglion has an axon that ascends to and diverges within the nuclei gracilis and cuneatus into branches that have excitatory synapses with several neurons (shaded area). These feed-forward to excite the relay neurons (R) and, in addition local inhibitory interneurons (X). The latter inhibit adjacent relay neurons. (2) Feedback Inhibition. Relay neuron (B) has recurrent branches that feedback to excite local inhibitory interneurons (Y). The latter inhibit the adjacent relay neurons. (3) Reflected Inhibition. Neurons (C) of the somatic sensory areas 3, 1, 2, and 5 of the cerebral cortex (C) have long axons that excite local inhibitory interneurons (Z). The latter modulate the relay neurons by both presynaptic and postsynaptic inhibition. (Adapted from Kandel, Schwartz, and Jessell).

interneurons within the circuit. These interneurons convey influences in a *forward direction* toward the more distal levels of the pathway. Because these inhibitory circuits utilize ascending or afferent relay neurons, their activity is referred to as *afferent inhibition.*

Feed-forward inhibition is utilized by the influences of muscle spindles in the stretch reflex (Chap. 8). The afferent fibers from neuromuscular spindles excite inhibitory interneurons that exert inhibitory influences upon the alpha motor neurons innervating voluntary muscles.

An expression of feed-forward inhibition is known as *lateral* or *surround* inhibition. This

physiologic activity is utilized by all sensory systems in processing neural information. For example, to discriminate between two points close together (two-point discrimination, Chap. 10), the two label lines for the two points are each maintained in order for the perception to occur. Each label line enhances its signal and suppresses the surrounding relay neurons in order to maintain its identity. *Inhibitory interneurons* interact with adjacent relay neurons with the result that the *signal-to-noise* is enhanced. In effect, the excitatory neurons of the circuit or pathway convey the signal and also stimulate the inhibitory interneurons in adjacent (lateral) locales to suppress the circuits conveying the noise within the sensory pathway. This emphasis on the signal and suppression of the noise is also known as the *focusing effect* or *sharpening effect*. For example, background noise such as potential sound generated by blood flow through the inner ear is not normally heard because it is filtered out by lateral inhibition within the auditory pathways and the neural activity associated with the sound to be heard is increased. In the visual system, inhibitory interneurons have a role in enhancing information to heighten the contrast, to make borders and contours more pronounced to the viewer, and to the generation of the center-surround receptor fields (Chap. 19).

Reflected (or Distal) Inhibition (or Excitation)

This type of feedback involves descending centrifugal fibers (reflected descending fibers) from the rostrally located cerebral cortex and brainstem nuclei to the more caudally located nuclei of the ascending pathways (Fig. 3.11). Some influences may be projected from the brainstem and spinal cord via fibers known as efferents to some sensory receptors. These descending fibers generally form excitatory synapses with inhibitory interneurons. Cortical and brainstem neurons can regulate, through inhibition, the information flow into the relay nuclei. This so-called distal inhibition can express itself by exciting interneurons that modulate the relay neurons through both inhibitory presynaptic and postsynaptic synapses. By this means, the higher centers of the brain can control the sensory input from the peripheral receptors to the relay nuclei (Chap. 10). Efferent neurons, with their cell bodies in the brainstem and spinal cord, that send axons to sensory receptors may facilitate or inhibit and thus alter the receptivity of the receptors. The gamma efferent fibers to the neuromuscular spindles (Chap. 8) and the cochlear efferent fibers to the organ of Corti (Chap. 16) are examples of such feedback neurons.

SOME GENERAL CONCEPTS ASSOCIATED WITH NEURONAL PROCESSING

Processing consists of a series of actions or operations directed to some end. In the nervous sys-

tem, neuronal processing occurs through interactions among complexes of neurons in a center (processing center). Following processing, the neural information is relayed to other centers. Sequences of processing centers may be organized as sensory pathways, motor pathways, or as feedback circuits. For example, touching a hot object can evoke several reactions including the perceptions of pain and heat. The hot object stimulates pain and heat receptors in the skin and, in response, nerve impulses are conveyed to centers in the spinal cord. Following neuronal processing in the spinal cord, the neural information can be distributed to other centers. (1) Some information is relayed to motor centers in the spinal cord, which results in the stimulation of muscles to withdraw the hand. (2) Other information can be relayed through a sequence of centers (pain pathway) for further processing. The higher centers of the pain pathway are involved in the awareness of pain and in the appreciation of such qualities as the intensity and location of the pain.

Serial Processing

In *serial processing*, neurons are arranged with connections in a sequential order; e.g., a neuron (or group of neurons) has synaptic connections with another neuron (or group of neurons) which has, in turn, connections with another neuron, muscle, or glandular cell. Such a serial sequence occurs in the knee-jerk reflex in which each sensory neuron from a muscle spindle receptor has synaptic connections in the spinal cord with motor neurons innervating and stimulating muscle fibers to contract (Fig. 8.1).

Parallel Processing

In *parallel processing*, each receptor in a constellation of receptors may have synaptic connections with different sequences of neurons, often called *channels*. These channels act to process and convey neural information in parallel sequences. At some center or centers, these channels are integrated with each other and with other channels. Actually, the receptors in the head and body send impulses simultaneously by many parallel channels through the central nervous system. These signals may be processed in parallel and then compared (comparator mechanisms); their "significance" is relayed to other centers. In a broader context, parallel processing is a phylogenetically evolved specialization of the organism to facilitate more subtle interpretations of environmental stimuli and to integrate appropriate responses to the complex demands of the environment.

Hierarchical Organization

A *hierarchy* is a systematic organization whose members or levels can be assigned to specific ranks in relation to each other. Many functional pathways and systems of the nervous system are hierarchically organized with each successive level in the sequence processing at a more complex level. For example, the retina of the eye is so structured, with the photoreceptors (rods and cones) responding to light, followed by a more advanced level of processing by the bipolar cells and, in turn, followed by a still more advanced level of processing by the retinal ganglion cells (Chap. 19).

Modulation

Modulation is an expression of the neuronal process by which the nervous system regulates and alters the resting or base level of excitability and responsiveness of a neuron or a neuronal circuit. Modulatory influences can raise the base level of excitability and thus make the input more effective, or lower the base level and make the input less effective. Certain therapeutic drugs are known to raise (augment or potentiate) this base level. An example of modulation is expressed in the variations in our attentiveness following stimulations during different stages and phases of sleep, drowsiness, boredom, and alertness. Modulation is conceived as the ability of neurons and neuronal circuits to alter their electrical properties as a response to intracellular or extracellular events resulting from synaptic or hormonal stimulation. Recent studies have demonstrated that neurotransmitters may alter the properties of the postsynaptic membrane over a somewhat longer time span than the well-known simple depolarization or hyperpolarization of brief duration on the postsynaptic membrane. These differences in the time span have their role in modulation. Modulation may be short-term as in motivational states or long-term as in learning. Modulation changes the degree, quality, and even speed of responsiveness to stimulation within the sensory, motor, and highest integrative centers and systems of the nervous system.

SUGGESTED READINGS

Alberts B, Bray D, Lewis J, Raff M, Roberts K, Watson J. *Molecular Biology of the Cell*. 3rd ed. New York, NY: Garland; 1994.

Barde Y-A. What, if anything, is a neurotrophic factor? *Trends Neurosci*. 1988;11:343–346.

Black I. *Information in the Brain. A Molecular Perspective*. Cambridge, Mass: MIT Press; 1994.

Catteral W. Structure and function of voltage and ion channels. *Science*. 1988;242:50–61.

Chesselet M. Presynaptic regulation of neurotransmitter release in the brain. *Neuroscience*. 1984; 12:347–375.

Conneally P. *Molecular Basis of Neurology*. Boston, Mass: Blackwell Scientific Publications; 1992.

Corey D, Roper D, eds. *Sensory Transduction*. New York, NY: Rockefeller University Press; 1992.

Dowling J. *Neurons and Networks: An Introduction to Neuroscience*. Cambridge, Mass: Harvard University Press; 1993.

Eccles J. The synapse: from electrical to chemical transmission. *Ann Rev Neurosci*. 1982;5: 325–339.

Emson P, ed. *Chemical Neuroanatomy*. New York, NY: Raven Press; 1983.

Gardner D, ed. *The Neurobiology of Neural Networks*. Cambridge, Mass: MIT Press; 1993.

Guyton A. *Basic Neuroscience: Anatomy and Physiology*. 2nd ed. Philadelphia, Pa: WB Saunders Co; 1991.

Hall Z. *An Introduction to Molecular Neurobiology*. Sunderland, Mass: Sinauer; 1992.

Hille B. *Ionic Channels of Excitable Membranes*. Sunderland, Mass: Sinauer; 1992.

Iversen L. Neuropeptides—what next? *Trends Neurosci*. 1983;6:293–294.

Kaczmarek L, Levitans I, eds. *Neuromodulation. The Biochemical Control of Neuronal Excitability*. New York, NY: Oxford University Press; 1986.

Laufenburger D, Linderman J. *Receptors—Models for Binding, Trafficking, and Signaling*. New York, NY: Oxford University Press; 1993.

Lentz T. Cellular membrane reutilization and synaptic vesicle recycling. *Trends Neurosci*. 1983;6: 48–53.

Linder M, Gilman A. G proteins. *Sci Am.* 1992; 267(1):56–65.

Llinás R. Calcium in synaptic transmission. *Sci Am.* 1982;247(4):56–65.

Nicholls J, Martin A, Wallace B. *From Neuron to Brain.* 3rd ed. Sunderland, Mass: Sinauer; 1992.

Schwartz J, Kandel E. Modulation of synaptic transmission: second messenger systems. In: Kandel, E, Schwartz J, Jessell T, eds. *Essentials of Neural Science and Behavior.* Norwalk, Conn: Appleton & Lange; 1995:243–267.

Shepherd G. *Neurobiology.* 3rd ed. New York, NY: Oxford University Press; 1994.

Siegel G, Agranoff B, Albers R, Molinoff P, eds. *Basic Neurochemistry: Molecular, Cellular, and Medical Aspects.* 5th ed. New York, NY: Raven Press; 1994.

Stein R. *Nerve and Muscle: Membranes, Cells and Systems.* New York, NY: Plenum; 1980.

Zimmermann H. *Synaptic Transmission, Cellular and Molecular Basis.* New York, NY: Oxford University Press; 1994.

Blood Circulation

4

Arterial supply
Venous drainage
Functional considerations
Blood-brain barrier

A copious blood supply is required to sustain the ever-active brain, which gets about one-fifth of the blood pumped by the heart and consumes about 20% of the oxygen utilized by the body. Roughly 800 mL of blood flows through the brain each minute, with 75 mL present in the brain at any moment. Each day the brain utilizes about 400 kilocalories, or about one fifth of a 2,000-kilocalorie diet. It takes about 7 seconds for a drop of blood to flow through the brain from the internal carotid artery to the internal jugular vein. The necessity for this continuous flow is because the brain stores only minute amounts of glucose and oxygen and derives its energy almost exclusively from the aerobic metabolism of glucose delivered by the blood. Paradoxically, this blood circulation is the minimum required; consciousness is lost if the blood supply is cut off for less than 10 seconds. The demand for blood is the same whether one is resting, sleeping, thinking, or exercising.

Neurons differ from cells of other organs in their requirements for oxygen. Deprived of oxygen, neurons almost always die within a few minutes. Neurons cannot build an oxygen debt, as can muscle cells and other body cells; that is, they cannot survive anaerobically. This constraint has enormous medical implications. When the oxygen supply is cut off following a heart attack or suffocation, the brain dies first. Only if oxygen is restored to the brain in a few minutes will the brain retain its functional viability.

Blood is supplied to the brain by the internal carotid arteries and the vertebral arteries. It is drained from the brain largely by the internal jugular veins.

ARTERIAL SUPPLY

The arterial blood supply to the brain is derived from two pairs of trunk arteries: (1) the vertebral arteries and (2) the internal carotid arteries.

Vertebral

Vertebral arteries enter the cranial cavity through the foramen magnum and become located on the anterolateral aspect of the medulla (Fig. 4.1). They unite at the pontomedullary junction to form the *basilar artery*, which continues to the midbrain level, where it bifurcates to form the paired *posterior cerebral arteries*. The branches of the vertebral and basilar arteries supply the medulla, pons, cerebellum, midbrain, and caudal diencephalon. Each posterior cerebral artery supplies part of the caudal diencephalon and the medial aspect (and adjacent lateral aspect) of the occipital lobe including the primary visual cortex (area 17) and the inferior posterior temporal lobe. The branches of the vertebral and basilar arteries that supply the medial aspect of the brainstem adjacent to the midsagittal plane are called *paramedian arteries (anterior spinal artery, paramedian branches of the basilar artery)*; those that supply the anterolateral aspect of the brainstem are called *short circumferential arteries (branches of the vertebral artery, short pontine circumferential*

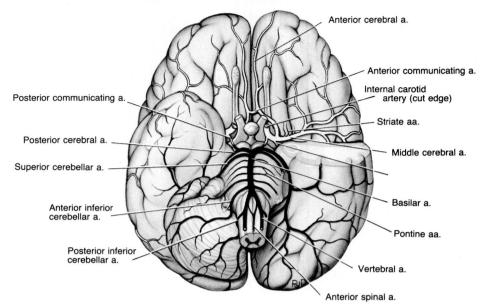

Figure 4.1: Major arterial supply to the brain. The vertebral-basilar-posterior cerebral arterial tree is indicated as solid black vessels and the paired middle and anterior cerebral tree is indicated as white vessels. Note the circle of Willis, which comprises the single anterior communicating artery and the paired anterior cerebral, internal carotid, posterior communicating, and posterior cerebral arteries. The last paired arteries are formed by the bifurcation of the basilar artery. The circle of Willis is located beneath the hypothalamus and surrounds the stalk of the hypophysis and optic chiasm.

branches of the basilar artery); and those that supply the posterolateral and posterior aspect of the brainstem and cerebellum **(Figs. 17.1 and 17.2)** are the *long circumferential branches (posterior spinal artery, posterior inferior cerebellar artery, anterior inferior cerebellar artery, superior cerebellar artery).*

Internal Carotid

Each internal carotid artery passes through the cavernous sinus as the S-shaped carotid siphon and then divides, level with and lateral to the optic chiasma, into two terminal branches: (1) the *anterior cerebral artery*, which supplies the orbital and medial aspect of the frontal lobe and medial aspect of the parietal lobe and (2) the *middle cerebral artery*, which passes laterally through the lateral fissure between the temporal lobe and insula and divides into a number of branches supplying the lateral portions of the orbital gyri and the frontal, parietal, and temporal lobes **(Fig. 4.2)**. The peripheral branches of the middle cerebral arteries anastomose on

the lateral surface of the cerebrum with the peripheral branches of the anterior and posterior cerebral arteries. Branches of the middle cerebral artery and the choroidal arteries penetrate the cerebrum to supply the basal ganglia, most of the diencephalon, internal capsule, and adjacent structures; these central or ganglionic branches (e.g., striate arteries) and the choroidal arteries are variable in their extent and in their anastomotic connections. Other branches of the internal carotid arteries include the *ophthalmic artery* (to the orbit), the *anterior choroidal artery* (to the arc structures adjacent to the choroidal fissure; Chap. 5), and the *posterior communicating artery* (joins posterior cerebral artery).

Circle of Willis

Although the *vertebral-basilar arterial tree* and the *internal carotid arterial tree* are essentially independent, there are some anastomotic connections between the two systems (e.g., between the terminal branches of posterior cerebral ar-

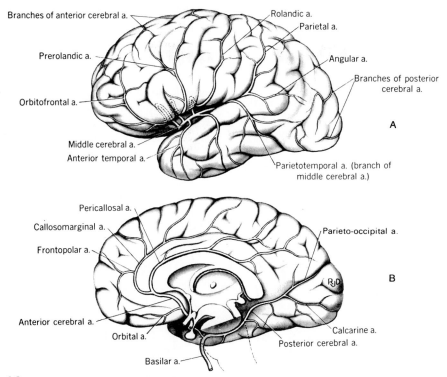

Figure 4.2: Distribution of the arteries on the surface of the brain. **A.** Lateral surface. **B.** Medial surface.

teries and those of the anterior and middle cerebral arteries). The *cerebral arterial circle of Willis* (Fig. 4.1) is an arterial ring in which the two systems are connected by the small posterior communicating arteries. The circle is completed by the anterior communicating artery which connects the two anterior cerebral arteries. There is actually little exchange of blood through these communicating arteries; the circle of Willis may act as a safety valve when differential pressures are present among these arteries.

The arteries meeting at the cerebral arterial circle of Willis form branches comparable to those of the basilar artery. Thus, (1) the anterior, middle, and posterior cerebral arteries are actually long circumferential arteries; (2) the subbranches (e.g., striate arteries, Fig. 4.1) of these three major cerebral arteries close to the circle of Willis are short circumferential branches; and (3) the small medial arteries from the circle of Willis are paramedian branches.

Anastomotic connections within the vertebral and internal carotid systems are extensive

in the brain. Those that occur among the large branches of the superficial arteries on the surface are usually physiologically effective, so that occlusion need not result in impairment of blood supply to the neural tissues. Rich anastomoses do exist among the capillary beds of adjacent arteries within the substance of the brain, but sudden occlusions of these arteries most often are followed by neural damage. The anastomotic connections may not be sufficient to allow adequate blood to reach the deprived region rapidly enough to meet its high metabolic requirements.

VENOUS DRAINAGE

The veins draining the brainstem and cerebellum roughly follow the arteries to these structures. On the other hand, the veins draining the cerebrum do not usually form patterns which parallel its arterial trees. In general, the venous trees in this region have short stocky branches that come off at right angles, resembling the silhouette of an oak tree.

Dural Sinuses

Venous anastomoses are extensive and effective between the deep veins within the brain and the superficial surface veins **(Fig. 4.3)**. The veins of the brain drain into superficial venous plexuses and the dural sinuses. The *dural (venous) sinuses* are valveless channels located between two layers of the dura mater. Most venous blood ultimately drains into the *internal jugular veins* at the base of the skull.

The blood from the cortex on the upper, lateral, and medial aspects of the cerebrum drains into the *superior sagittal (dural) sinus* to the occipital region. From there it flows to the *transverse (lateral)* and *sigmoid sinuses* into the *internal jugular vein*. All dural sinuses receive blood from veins in the immediate vicinity.

The deep cerebral drainage is to the region of the *foramina of Monro* where the paired internal cerebral veins (posterior to the choroid plexus

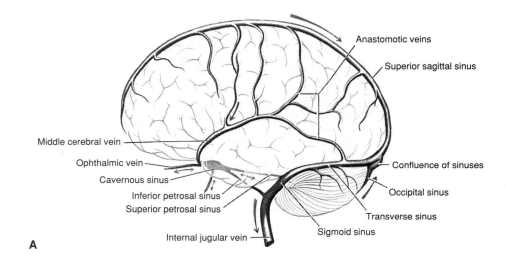

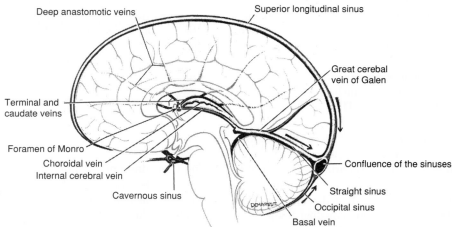

Figure 4.3: Venous drainage from the brain. **A.** Lateral view of the brain. * = Location of emissary veins. **B.** Medial view of the brain.

of the third ventricle) extend to the region of the pineal body. There they join to form the *great vein of Galen*. Blood then flows, successively, through the *straight sinus* (located along the midline within the tentorium, which is dura mater lying between cerebellum and occipital lobe), *transverse sinus*, and *sigmoid sinus* before draining into the *internal jugular vein* (**Fig. 5.1**).

Some blood from the base of the cerebrum drains into the *superior* and *inferior petrosal sinuses* and then flows into either the *sigmoid sinus*, or the *cavernous sinus* in the region of the hypothalamus (on the sides of the sphenoid bone). The cavernous sinus is connected via the superior petrosal sinus with the transverse sinus, via the inferior petrosal sinus with the jugular vein, and via the basilar venous plexus with the venous plexus of the vertebral canal (**Fig. 4.3**).

Emissary Veins

Some dural sinuses connect with the veins superficial to the skull by *emissary veins*. These veins act as pressure valves when intracranial pressure is raised and are also routes for the spread of infection into the brain case (infection in the nose may spread via an emissary vein high in the nose into the meninges and may result in meningitis). The cavernous sinus is connected with emissary veins, including the ophthalmic vein, which extends into the orbit.

FUNCTIONAL CONSIDERATIONS

The mean blood flow in the normal brain is 50 mL per 100 g of brain tissue per minute. It takes about 7 seconds for a drop of blood to flow through the brain. At any given moment, however, the flow through a specific region may be greater, the same, or less than the mean flow through the CNS. The brain is similar to other tissues of the body where the amount of blood flow varies with the level of metabolic and functional activity. For example, dynamic voluntary movements of the hand are associated with an increase in the blood flow within the cerebral cortical motor areas associated with hand movements and with sensory areas receiving signals

from skin, joints, and muscles associated with these movements (Chap. 25).

Anastomotic connections within the vertebral and internal carotid arterial systems form extensive patterns of collateral circulation in the brain. A sudden deprivation of the blood supply to a region of the brain may, if the vascular insufficiency lasts for more than a few minutes, result in the necrosis (infarct) of brain tissue. The inadequate oxygen and glucose supply at the lesion (*infarct*) site is the essential cause of a "stroke" (sudden appearance of focal neurologic deficits). This may result from the sudden occlusion by a *thrombus* (blood clot formed within the blood vessel), or an *embolism* (a portion of clot transported along in the blood stream) to the occlusion site, or the rupture of an artery often due to arteriosclerosis or hypertension; this is called a *cerebrovascular accident (CVA)*. A stroke is often preceded by a significant warning sign, known as a *ministroke* or *transient ischemic attack (TIA)*. These temporary spells are due to impaired neural function caused by a brief but definite reduction in blood flow to the brain. Depending on the location that is deprived of oxygen and glucose, the symptoms may include difficulty in talking, temporary weakness or paralysis on one side, dizziness, blurred vision, loss of hearing, et cetera.

Interconnections among the large branches of the superficial arteries are usually physiologically effective, so that an occlusion of one need not result in a marked impairment of the blood supply to the neural tissues. For example, following an occlusion within the circle of Willis, or its proximal branches, the collateral circulation is often adequate, especially if the involved artery becomes occluded slowly before the stroke. In contrast, anastomoses among the distal arterial branches of the circle of Willis are variable; consequently, the collateral circulation may not be adequate, and occlusion of a vessel may result in an infarct. Rich anastomoses exist among the capillary beds of adjacent arteries within the substance of the brain, but an occlusion of the supplying arteries is often followed by neural damage causing symptoms and signs correlated with the site (Chaps. 17 and 25). This occurs because the anastomotic connections are not sufficiently rich to allow adequate blood flow to reach the deprived areas rapidly enough to meet the high metabolic requirements.

An occlusion of the *anterior cerebral artery* results in a lesion of the paracentral lobule that has the general sensory and motor cortical areas for the contralateral lower extremity (Chap. 25). A lesion in this area results in contralateral paresis as a motor sign and diminished sensitivity (hypoaesthesia) of the general senses in this extremity (Chap. 12). Blockage of the *calcarine branch of the posterior cerebral artery* (supplies the primary visual cortex of one side) results in a contralateral hemianopsia (Chap. 19). Occlusion of small branches of the *posterior cerebral artery* (supplies the posterior thalamus and adjacent tissues) produces the *thalamic syndrome* (Chap. 23). Strokes following the rupture and bleeding of the *striate arteries*, branches of the *middle cerebral artery* (supply portions of the internal capsule and adjacent structures), result in signs that include an upper motoneuron paralysis of the face and upper and lower limbs on the opposite side as well as sensory disturbances (Chaps. 12 and 25). Signs associated with vascular lesions of branches of the *vertebral artery* supplying the brain stem are outlined in Chapter 17.

Although collateral circulation provides certain regions of the CNS with a margin of safety during arterial occlusion, the anastomotic network also allows for a degree of vulnerability. With a reduction in the systemic blood pressure, a region supplied by an anastomotic network is susceptible to ischemia; such an anastomosis occurs at the terminal ends of two or more arterial trees, a border region where perfusion pressure is lowest. These border regions, which are supplied by major arteries, are called *border zones* or *watershed zones*. An infarction occurring in such a region is called a *border zone* or *watershed zone infarct*.

BLOOD-BRAIN BARRIER

The selective restriction of blood-borne substances from entering the CNS is called the *blood-brain barrier* (BBB). This BBB is associated with the capillary endothelial cells. They act more like secretory cells, that mediate the diffusion of substances from the blood directly

into the interstitial fluid. Adjacent endothelial cells are attached to each other by impermeable tight junctions to form a physical barrier. The astrocytes have foot processes that encapsulate the capillaries (Figs. 2.9 and 5.4). In addition, the high concentrations of mitochondria within the endothelial cells are indicative of high oxidative metabolic activity associated with active transport systems. These features explain why large molecules such as serum proteins and penicillin do not pass through the normal brain capillaries and also why small molecules pass through the barrier more rapidly than medium sized molecules. Lipid solubility does enhance the passage of substances through the barrier; such lipid-soluble chemicals as oxygen, carbon dioxide, and some drugs pass through the barrier into the brain rapidly. Many essential substances, such as glucose, amino acids, lactate, ribonucleosides, and several vitamins penetrate the barrier by being conveyed by facilitated diffusion (carrier-mediated transport) systems. In this form of transport, the solute (e.g., glucose) combines with a specific membrane carrier on one side of the membrane which then "shuttles" across the membrane to release the solute on the other side. Facilitated diffusion is not energy dependent; it usually occurs "downhill," i.e., down a concentration gradient. The transport systems that move molecules rapidly without consuming energy, act bidirectionally by conveying certain chemical substances from the brain and CSF to the blood and vice versa, thereby influencing the passage of substances to and from the brain and blood plasma. Facilitated diffusion is ideal for transporting glucose and critical nutrients that must be supplied into the brain continuously and in large amounts. Should the brain be inadequately supplied with glucose or oxygen, loss of consciousness, and even death can occur within minutes.

The astrocytes have processes with end-feet that cover most of the surface of the brain capillaries. Their other processes are in contact with neurons and with the pia-glial membrane (Fig. 5.5). It is probable that the astrocytes have a transport function transferring metabolites bidirectionally between the capillaries (endothelial cells) and the neurons. In addition, the astrocytes may (1) take up from the extracellular fluid the excess extracellular potassium ions generated during intense neuronal activity and (2) regulate the extracellular concentrations of neurotransmitters by an uptake process and store them.

Another permeability barrier, called the *blood-cerebrospinal fluid barrier*, is present between the capillaries of the choroid plexus and the cerebrospinal fluid (Chap. 5).

Homeostasis of the neuronal environment is vital for the normal functioning of each neuron. In turn, these barriers are essential for the preservation of the homeostasis by maintaining the ionic constancy of the interstitial fluid (fluid surrounding the glial cells, neurons, and capillaries), by promoting the entry of required substances, by preventing entrance of unwanted substances, and by removing unwanted substances. Following infection, stroke, tumors,

and trauma, the blood-brain barrier may be breached.

SUGGESTED READING

Duvernoy H. *Human Brainstem Vessels.* New York, NY: Springer-Verlag; 1977.

Fisher C. The anatomy and pathology of the cerebral vasculature. In: Meyer J, ed. *Modern Concepts of Cerebrovascular Disease.* New York, NY: Spectrum Publications; 1975:1–41.

Netter F. *Atlas of Human Anatomy.* West Caldwell, NJ: Ciba-Geigy; 1989: plates 130–141.

Osborn A. *An Introduction to Cerebral Angiography.* Philadelphia, Pa: JB Lippincott Co; 1980.

Purves M. *The Physiology of the Cerebral Circulation.* Cambridge, NY: Cambridge University Press; 1972.

Stephens R, Stelweall D. *Arteries and Veins of the Human Brain.* Springfield, Ill: Charles C Thomas; 1969.

Meninges, Ventricles, and Cerebrospinal Fluid

5

Meninges

Ventricles

Fluid environment of the brain

Circumventricular (periventricular) organs

Imaging of the brain and its arteries

Hydrocephalus

Clinical aspects of cerebrospinal fluid

The meninges are the three layers of connective tissue that surround and protect the soft brain and spinal cord. Cerebrospinal fluid (CSF) passes between two of the layers of the meninges and thus slowly circulates over the entire perimeter of the central nervous system. The CSF also flows through the ventricles, which are the cavities within the brain derived from the central canal of the embryonic neural tube.

MENINGES

Each of the meningeal layers—pia mater, arachnoid, and dura mater—is a separate, continuous sheet: thin strands of connective tissue called *trabeculae* extend from the arachnoid to the pia mater (Fig. 5.1).

The *pia mater* is intimately attached to the brain and spinal cord, dipping into every sulcus and fissure. It is a vascular layer containing blood vessels whose branches nourish the neural tissue.

The *arachnoid* is a thin, avascular, delicate layer, which does not follow each indentation of the brain, but rather skips from crest to crest. The *subarachnoid space*, between the pia mater and the arachnoid, contains CSF and large blood vessels. In several places the subarachnoid space is enlarged into *cisterns* (Fig. 5.1). The *cisterna magna (cerebellomedullary cistern)* is located dorsal to the medulla and inferior to the cerebellum. The *pontine* and *interpeduncular cisterns* are located on the anterior brainstem, and the *superior cistern* is located posterior to the midbrain. The *spinal (lumbar) cistern* is located caudal to the spinal cord (lumbar-2 to sacral-2 vertebral levels).

The major branches of the circle of Willis traverse the large cisterns at the base of the brain. The pulsations of these arteries are transmitted through the CSF within the subarachnoid space.

In the head, the tough nonstretchable *dura mater* consists of two layers—the *outer and inner dura mater*. The skull and dura mater form an inelastic envelope enclosing the CNS, CSF, and blood vessels. This inelasticity permits but a slight increase in the cranial contents; the concept that the volume of the intracranial contents cannot change is the basis of the Monro-Kellie doctrine (see below under "CSF Pressure"). The *outer dura mater* is actually the periosteum of the skull. The *inner dura mater* is a thick membrane which extends (1) between the two cerebral hemispheres in the midsagittal

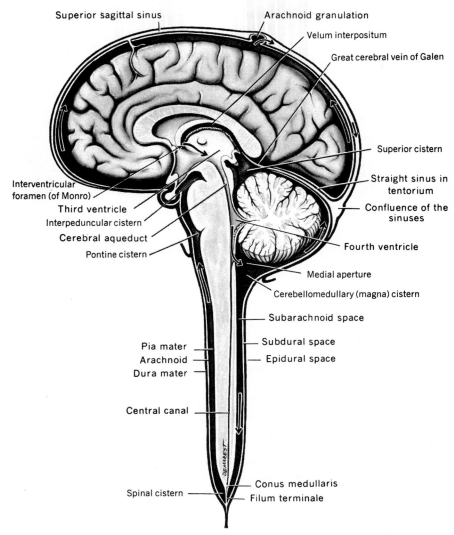

Figure 5.1: Midsagittal view of the meninges, ventricles, subarachnoid spaces, and cisternae. Arrows indicate the normal direction of flow of the cerebrospinal fluid.

plane as the *falx cerebri* and (2) between the occipital lobes and the cerebellum as the *tentorium cerebelli*. The *subdural space* is the potential thin space located between the inner dura mater and the arachnoid. The film of fluid in the subdural space is not CSF (Chap. 7).

The dura mater is also called the *pachymeninx* and the arachnoid and pia mater comprise the *leptomeninges.*

In head injuries, bleeding may occur into the subarachnoid space (*subarachnoid hemorrhage*), into the subdural space (*subdural hemorrhage*), and between the outer dura mater and the skull (*extradural hemorrhage*). An extradural hemorrhage may result from the bleeding of meningeal vessels after a fracture of the skull. A subdural hemorrhage may be caused by the tearing of veins crossing the subdural space, which may follow after the sudden movement of the cerebral hemispheres relative to the dura and skull. A subarachnoid hemorrhage may result from the rupture of an aneurysm in a branch of the internal carotid or vertebral arteries; the presence of bloodstained CSF obtained from a lumbar puncture into the lumbar cistern is confirmatory.

VENTRICLES

The *ventricular system* is a series of cavities within the brain, lined by ependyma, and filled with CSF. The ependyma is a simple cuboidal epithelial layer of glial cells. Each cerebral hemisphere contains a *lateral ventricle*, each of which is continuous through one of the paired interventricular *foramina of Monro* with the *third ventricle* of the diencephalon (**Figs. 5.2 and 5.3**). The third ventricle is continuous with the tubelike *cerebral aqueduct of Sylvius* (iter) of the midbrain, and the latter with the *fourth ventricle* of the pons and medulla. The fourth ventricle, in turn, is continuous with the central canal that extends from the caudal medulla to the lower end of the spinal cord where it terminates without outlet. It has a small bore and is, for the most part, occluded. Each lateral ventricle is subdivided into four parts: anterior horn in the frontal lobe (rostral to foramen of Monro), body in the parietal lobe, inferior horn in the temporal lobe, and occipital horn in the occipital lobe.

Each ventricle contains a *tela choroidea*, which is a thin sheet of ependyma appended directly to the pia mater. Thus, each tela is actually the site where the lining of each ventricle (structure within the brain) is in contact with the pia mater (structure on the outer surface of the brain). The *choroid plexus* is that portion of the tela choroidea composed of a rich vascular network functionally integrated with the adjoining specialized ependyma (see later). The choroid plexus of each lateral ventricle is located in the body and inferior horn; it is continuous through a foramen of Monro with the unpaired choroid plexus of the roof of the third ventricle (**Fig. 5.2**). The choroid plexus of the fourth ventricle is located in the roof of the medulla, in which there are three foramina through which CSF escapes from the fourth ventricle into the cisterna magna of the subarachnoid space. The two lateral openings are the *lateral apertures* (*foramina of Luschka*) and the medial opening is the *medial aperture* (*foramen of Magendie*) (**Fig. 5.3**).

FLUID ENVIRONMENT OF THE BRAIN

The brain and spinal cord can only function in a chemically stable homeostatic fluid environ-

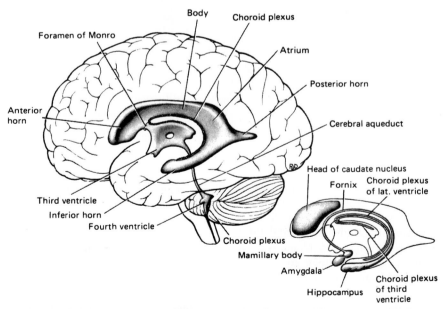

Figure 5.2: Lateral view of the ventricles of the brain. Note in the small drawing that the choroid plexus of the lateral ventricle, the hippocampus-fornix complex, and the caudate nucleus, follow the curvature of the lateral ventricle. The caudate nucleus is cut off just behind its head in this view.

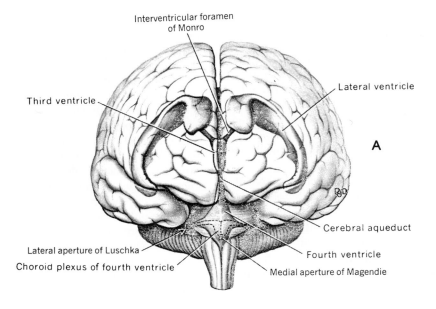

Interventricular foramen
of Monro

Third ventricle

Lateral ventricle

A

Cerebral aqueduct

Lateral aperture of Luschka

Fourth ventricle

Choroid plexus of fourth ventricle

Medial aperture of Magendie

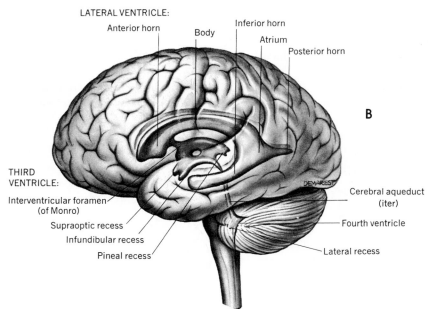

LATERAL VENTRICLE:

Anterior horn   Body   Inferior horn

Atrium

Posterior horn

B

THIRD
VENTRICLE:

Interventricular foramen
(of Monro)

Supraoptic recess

Infundibular recess

Pineal recess

Cerebral aqueduct
(iter)

Fourth ventricle

Lateral recess

Figure 5.3: Frontal (**A**) and lateral (**B**) views of the ventricles of the brain.

ment. This comprises (1) the interstitial fluid bathing the neurons, glia, and blood vessels within the central nervous system; and (2) the CSF. These two fluids are essentially similar in composition.

The extracellular fluid occupies a space of about 15 to 20% of the volume of the brain. This interstitial space is greater in the gray mat-

ter than in the white matter. The former has a higher water content than the latter. This fluid joins the choroid plexus produced CSF within the subarachnoid space. This CSF is constantly being renewed by production and reabsorption so that the total volume is replaced several times a day.

Two structures have critical roles in the for-

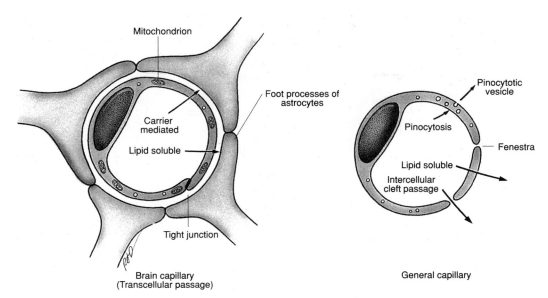

Figure 5.4: Ultrastructural features of capillary endothelial cells of the brain as compared with those of other capillaries of the body. **A.** *Brain capillary.* The endothelial cells of the brain capillaries constitute the blood-brain barrier. The transendothelial passage from the blood to the brain is essentially restricted to lipid soluble substances and by carrier mediated transport. Features of capillaries contributing to this selective barrier are the numerous mitochondria and the tight junctions between their cell membranes. The energy supplied by the mitochondria is utilized to transport nutrients into the brain. The scattered few pinocytotic vesicles contribute minimally. The foot processes of the astrocytes almost completely surround the brain capillary. **B.** *General capillary.* The unselective capillary endothelial lining of other organs differs by being characterized with numerous pinocytotic vesicles, absence of tight junctions, presence of fenestra, and having few mitochondria. (Adapted from Fishman.)

mation and maintenance of this environment: (1) the brain capillaries and (2) choroid plexuses. They act as selective barriers and major transfer sites of certain substances that constitute these fluids.

The cerebral capillaries form the so-called blood-brain barrier between the blood and the interstitial fluid. The capillaries and the ependymal epithelial cells of the choroid plexus form the blood-CSF barrier between the blood and CSF (Figs. 5.4 and 5.5). In addition, the arachnoid is essentially impermeable to water-soluble substances and its role is largely passive.

Cerebrospinal Fluid

The *Cerebrospinal Fluid (CSF)* is a crystal clear, colorless solution that looks like water and is found in the ventricular system and the subarachnoid space. It consists of water, small amounts of protein, gases in solution (oxygen and carbon dioxide), sodium, potassium, mag-

nesium and chloride ions, glucose and a few white cells (mostly lymphocytes).

The CSF, formed primarily by a combination of capillary filtration and active epithelial secretion, serves two major functional roles. (1) *Physical Support.* By acting as a "water jacket" surrounding the brain and by providing buoyancy for it, the CSF protects, supports and keeps the brain afloat in a sea of fluid. (2) *Homeostasis.* The CSF of the ventricles and the subarachnoid space comprises a pool to which some of the endogenous water-soluble products, including unwanted substances, drain by diffusion from extracellular fluids of the brain to the ventricles and subarachnoid space. Other products of brain metabolism are removed to the blood flowing through the capillaries. The CSF and capillaries act as substitutes for the lack of a lymphatic system in the brain and spinal cord. The CSF along with extracellular fluids surrounding the neurons are the "expressions" of state of chemical equilibrium of the neural environ-

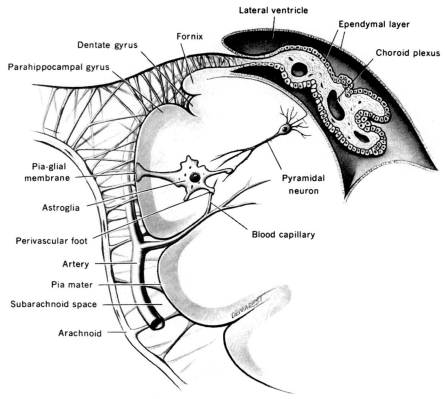

Figure 5.5: Relations of the leptomeninges, subarachnoid, choroid plexus, ventricle, astroglia, and neurons of the central nervous system. The subarachnoid space is located between the arachnoid and pia mater. The choroid plexus is composed of an ependymal layer and a highly vascularized connective tissue core. Subarachnoid blood vessels and subarachnoid space are continuous with the core of the choroid plexus. The astrocyte has several processes: one extends to a blood capillary and terminates as a perivascular foot; another process extends to and contacts the pyramidal neuron; and another extends to the pia mater. The pia mater and arachnoid make up the leptomeninges. The dura mater is called the pachymeninx.

ment, called *homeostasis*, essential for the normal functioning of the central nervous system.

The brain and spinal cord actually float in the CSF; the 1,400 g brain has a net weight of about 25 g while suspended in the CSF (reduces brain weight 60-fold). The brain is "shock mounted" in the CSF and thus is able to withstand the stress during sudden movements of the head. When the CSF is removed, the patient suffers intense pain and headaches with each movement of the head. The headaches are due to the irritated nerve endings in the meninges and intracranial blood vessels. They persist for a time until the CSF is naturally replaced. The volume of CSF in an adult is about 150 ml (60 ml in the ventricles and 90 ml in the subarachnoid space, including the lumbar cistern; Chap.

7). The choroid plexuses can form sufficient CSF to replace the total volume of CSF every 3 or 4 hours.

The interstitial fluid within the brain is readily exchanged with CSF. As the CSF flows through the ventricles and the subarachnoid space around the spinal cord and brain, the exchange between the two fluids occurs (1) at the leaky spaces (gap junctions; Fig. 5.6) of the ependymal layer within the ventricles and (2) at the perivascular spaces on the pial surface of the CNS.

Choroid Plexus and the Blood-CSF Barrier

The choroid plexus comprises a single row of choroidal epithelium, arranged as villi around

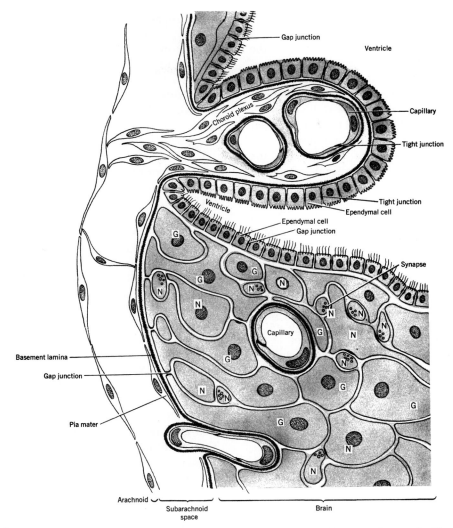

Figure 5.6: Ultrastructural features in the brain, choroid plexus, pia-arachnoid layer, and ventricle. The continuous extracellular space is located among the glia (G), neurons or their processes (N), and the capillary. The basement lamina (also surrounds capillary) is a porous structure. Note tight junctions between capillary endothelial cells and choroid plexus ependymal cells and gap junctions between pial cells and ependymal cells lining ventricle.

a core of blood vessels derived from the pia mater and connective tissue (**Figs. 5.5 and 5.6**). The choroidal epithelium is continuous with the ependyma of the ventricles (**Fig. 5.6**). The extensive vascular network of the plexus is an expression of its active metabolic activity. The ventricular surface of each choroidal cell has a brush border comprised of microvilli, which is a feature of epithelial cells noted for fluid transport. These cells contain many oxidative enzymes, which are indicative of their role in the active transport of electrolytes and other

solutes. Tight junctions join adjacent endothelial cells of the brain and the choroid plexus, adjacent choroidal epithelial cells and adjacent cells of the arachnoid membrane. These tight junctions are a barrier to the passage of macromolecules (1) from the blood to the ventricular CSF (CSF secretion) and (2) from the CSF to the capillary blood (absorption by the choroid plexus). The mechanism of CSF secretion and absorption from the CSF may be summarized as follows. The hydrostatic pressure within the choroidal capillaries initiates the passage of water and ions across the endothelial cells to the interstitial connective tissue and then to the choroidal epithelium. The completion of the transfer to the CSF takes two routes: (1) *transcellular movement* through the epithelial choroidal cells and across the plasma membrane into the ventricular cavity and (2) *paracellular movement* across the tight junction to the ventricular cavity. Both of these transfers are thought to be dependent upon ion pumps. The details of the means for the transfer of molecules from the ventricular CSF to the capillaries has not been fully resolved.

Most of the CSF is being continuously secreted by the choroid plexuses of the four ventricles where the *blood-CSF barrier* is located. Impermeable *tight junctions* join the endothelial cells and also the cuboidal ependymal cells of the choroid plexus (Fig. 5.6). These junctional barriers prevent the serum proteins from entering the CNS and inhibit the free diffusion of water-soluble molecules. The formation of the CSF by the choroid plexus involves capillary filtration and active secretion transport by the ependymal cells. Flow of molecules across the cells of the choroid plexus occurs via active transport (energy required), facilitated diffusion (no energy required), and facilitated exchanges of ions (e.g. sodium, potassium, and chloride ions). Although the CSF is characterized as a cell-free, low protein ultrafiltrate of blood and that the CSF and blood plasma are in osmotic equilibrium, some small but significant differences do exist between the two fluids. As compared to the blood plasma, CSF contains less potassium, bicarbonate, calcium and glucose, and more magnesium and chloride; its pH is lower.

The choroid plexus acts as a *"kidney" of the brain* that maintains the chemical stability of the CSF in a similar fashion as the kidney maintains the chemical stability of the blood. A key difference in this comparison is that the kidney removes waste products from the blood, whereas the choroid plexus pumps some "waste products" (by-products of metabolic activity) from the CNS into the blood.

These barriers consist of permeability barriers that comprise systems whose primary roles are to preserve *homeostasis* in the central nervous system. They facilitate the entry of essential substances and metabolites and they block the entry or facilitate the removal of toxic substances and unnecessary metabolites. In many neurologic diseases, the blood-brain barrier breaks down and does not function as usual with some substances normally excluded passing through the barrier. This occurs in some infections, strokes, brain tumors and trauma.

Flow of CSF

After its formation at the choroid plexuses and in the ventricular surfaces, there is a bulk flow of CSF through the ventricular system, the subarachnoid spaces and cisterns surrounding the CNS before entering the blood systemic circulation. The CSF travels from the lateral ventricles through the foramina of Monro into the third ventricle, through the narrow cerebral aqueduct into the fourth ventricle, through the paired apertures of Luschka and the median aperture of Magendie within the tela choroidea in the roof of the fourth ventricle into the cisterna magna, and then slowly circulates rostrally through the subarachnoid space to the region of the superior sagittal venous sinus at the top of the skull. Most of the CSF enters the blood by *bulk flow* through narrow channels in the *arachnoid villi* (pacchionian granulations) by giant vacuole transport. These villi are grossly visible spongelike herniations of the arachnoid that penetrate into the lumen of the superior sagittal sinus. CSF extends into and fills the tubular extensions of the arachnoid and subarachnoid space that form the sleeves around the roots of the spinal nerves (Fig. 5.7). Some CSF is absorbed by these numerous microscopically visible arachnoid villi associated with spinal veins of the spinal roots.

CSF Pressure

The CSF pressure is lower than blood pressure. In the individual lying on his side, the pressure varies from 60 to 180 mm of water throughout the subarachnoid space. In the seated subject, the pressure may rise to between 200 and 300 mm of water in the lumbar cistern, reach zero in the cisterna magna, and go below atmospheric pressure in the ventricles. Fluctuations in the pressure occur in response to phases of the heartbeat and the respiratory cycle. These shifts occur because the rigid box of dura and skull does not yield, so that the intracranial pressure

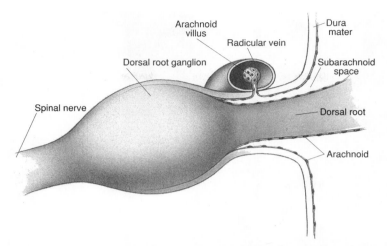

Figure 5.7: Dorsal view of a dorsal root ganglion and dorsal root illustrating an *arachnoid villus* adjacent to a dorsal root (spinal cord to the right of figure). The arachnoid, cerebrospinal fluid (CSF), and subarachnoid space of the spinal canal extend as sleeves that surround the ganglion and roots of each spinal nerve. The arachnoid of this sleeve protrudes into a spinal root (radicular) vein to form an arachnoid villus from which some CSF can pass into a vein. (Adapted from Fishman.)

changes if additions or subtractions to the intracranial contents occur (*Monro-Kellie doctrine*).

An obstruction to the normal passage of CSF results in a backup of CSF and an increase in intracranial pressure. Because the CSF extends to the optic disk (optic nerve head, blind spot) of the subarachnoid space within the dural sleeve along the optic nerve, an elevated CSF pressure results in dilated retinal veins and forward thrust of the optic disk beyond the level of the retina. This *papilledema*, or so-called "*choked disk*," can be observed during an inspection of the fundus of the eye with an ophthalmoscope. A persistent papilledema may result in damaged optic nerve fibers.

CIRCUMVENTRICULAR (PERIVENTRICULAR) ORGANS

Adjacent to the median ventricular cavities (third ventricle, cerebral aqueduct, and fourth ventricle) are several specialized regions of ependymal origin called *circumventricular organs* (**Fig. 21.5**). The common vascular, ependymal, and neural organization of these structures differs from that found in typical brain tissue. They are referred to as "being in the

brain, but not of it" in part because their capillaries are lined by fenestrated endothelial cells—indicative of a defective blood brain barrier to macromolecules. In humans, these anatomically well-defined organs include (1) *the median eminence of the tuber cinereum* (hypothalamus), the *neurohypophysis* and the *pineal body*, all of which have a role in neuroendocrine regulation (Chap. 21), and the (2) *subcommissural organ, organum vasculosum of the lamina terminalis, subfornical organ*, and *area postrema* (Chap. 21).

IMAGING OF THE BRAIN AND ITS ARTERIES

Angiography

Angiography (arteriography) is the method by which blood vessels—usually arteries—are visualized radiographically following the injection of a nontoxic radiopaque substance into an artery. In cerebral angiography, the sites for the injection of such substances are generally the internal carotid or the vertebral arteries. Injections into the former outline the anterior and middle cerebral arteries, while injections into

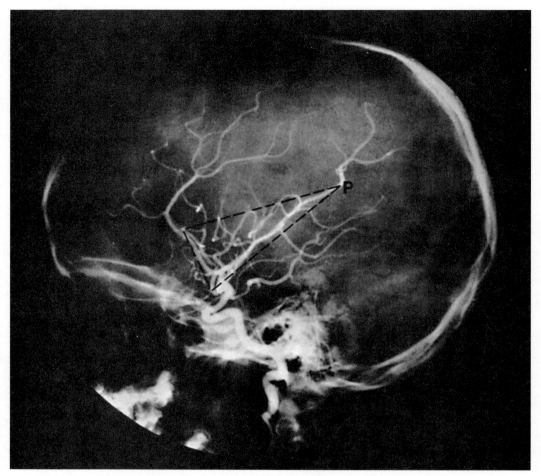

Figure 5.8: Cerebral angiogram demonstrating the internal carotid artery and middle cerebral artery and some of its branches (Figs. 4.1, 4.2). The 5 to 8 branches of the middle cerebral artery are framed in the Sylvian triangle. The Sylvian point (P) is the posterior point of the triangle. The inferior margin of the triangle is formed by the lower branches of the artery. The superior margin is a line formed by the superior margin of the insula. This is the line where the arterial branches reverse their course; they pass from the vertically oriented insula and continue laterally and downward until they emerge from the lateral (Sylvian) sulcus (Fig. 4.2). The anterior margin is formed by the most rostrally located branch. The *Sylvian triangle* is a useful triangle for the interpretation of angiograms. (Courtesy of Juan Taveras, MD, and the late John Wood, MD. *Diagnostic Neuroradiology.* Baltimore: Williams & Wilkins; 1976.)

the latter outline the basilar artery and its major branches, including the posterior cerebral arteries (**Fig. 5.8**). Angiography is used to outline aneurysms and anomalous arrangements of certain arteries. By changes in the usual arterial patterns, the sites of edema, hemorrhage, or tumors may be pinpointed.

Tomographic Methods

Three noninvasive and nondestructive techniques, *computerized tomography (CT)*, *mag-*

netic resonance imaging (MRI), and *positron emission tomography (PET)*, are available for producing high resolution images of the regional anatomy of the living brain and spinal cord without the use of a contrast substance. One method, PET, is valuable for identifying certain ongoing metabolic processes *in vivo*.

Computerized tomography (CT) (**Fig. 5.9**), also called *computerized axial tomography (CAT) scanning*, produces images of cranial contents and the internal anatomy of the brain

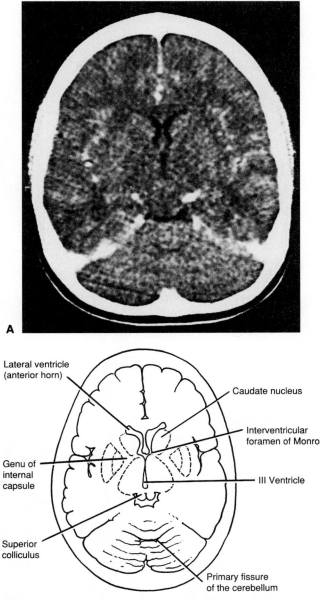

Figure 5.9: A. Computerized axial tomography (CT) image of a horizontal scan of the cerebrum. **B.** Diagram illustrating some major structures in A (Refer to Figure 1.8). (Courtesy of Sadek K. Hilal, MD, Department of Radiology, Columbia-Presbyterian Medical Center, New York.)

as a series of adjacent slices with a remarkable degree of accuracy and detail. This method, based on x-ray transmission, is widely used for the clinical evaluation of disease and lesions, and has reduced the need for invasive procedures such as cerebral angiography and pneumoencephalography. Emissions from an x-ray source are collimated to define a beam that passes through a single plane to a detector. With the aid of a computer, information from many scan "slices" are used to build an image revealing, for example, differences between gray and white matter, an outline of the ventricular system and brain surface convolutions. A CT scan

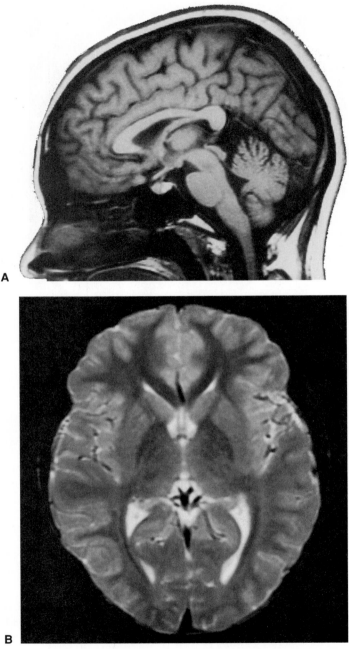

Figure 5.10: **A**. Magnetic resonance image (MRI) scan of the median sagittal section of the brain and part of the head illustrating the cerebral hemisphere, cerebellum, and brainstem. Refer to Figure 1.5 for structures visible on the scan. **B**. MRI scan of a horizontal (axial) section through the cerebrum in a plane A—A of Figure 5.10 E. Refer to Figure 1.8 for some structures visible on the scan. **C**. MRI scan of a coronal section through the cerebral hemispheres an diencephalon in a plane B—B of Figure 5.10 E. Refer to Figure 5.10 D for some structures visible on the scan. **D**. Diagram illustrating the structures visible in the MRI scan in Figure 5.10 C. **E**. Diagram illustrating the planes of (1) the horizontal section A—A of the MRI scan in Figure 10.5 B and (2) the coronal section B—B of the MRI scan in Figure 10.5 C. (Courtesy of Alan J. Silver, MD, Department of Radiology, Columbia-Presbyterian Medical Center, New York.)

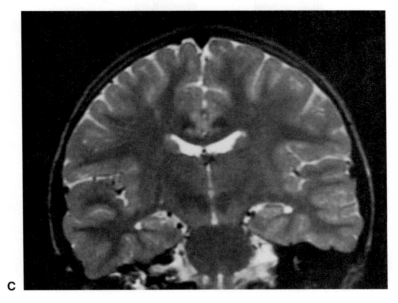

C

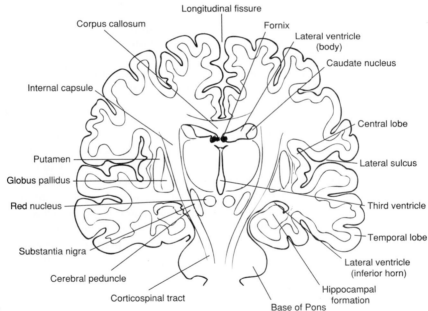

D

Figure 5.10: *(continued).*

does not give any indications of metabolic processes.

Magnetic resonance imaging (MRI) **(Fig. 5.10 A-E)**, also called *nuclear magnetic resonance (NMR)*, is based upon the principle that certain atomic nuclei in the living organism will emit radio signals when placed in a strong magnetic field and stimulated by radio frequency

waves (RF). Instead of x-rays, they will re-emit some absorbed energy in the form of radio signals (known as nuclear magnetic resonance). Biologically important nuclei of atoms that are MRI sensitive are hydrogen, carbon, sodium, phosphorus, and potassium. An MR image is superior to that of CT because of its ability to enhance the contrast between white and gray

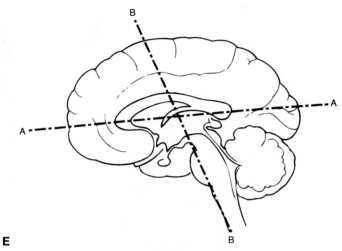

Figure 5.10: *(continued)*.

matter. In fact, the MR image has a similar quality in anatomic detail to that visualized in the classic fixed and stained sections of the brain. When placed in a magnetic field, the protons of the patient become oriented in a certain direction. This orientation is then disturbed as the RF current is briefly passed through the selected region. With stoppage of the RF current, the protons re-orient to the magnetic field and emit signals that produce the image. Phosphorus is present in the high energy phosphates adenosine triphosphate (ATP) and phosphocreatine. The scan with these elements enables the clinician to determine if ischemia is present, how widespread it is, and to evaluate the efficacy of prescribed drugs in reducing the oxygen-deprived areas.

Positron emission tomography (PET) (**Fig. 25.8**) combines CT with radioisotope scanning. Although its resolution is relatively poor as compared to CT and MRI, PET is most valuable because its images reflect functional activity. This method utilizes an on site cyclotron-produced positron-emitting (positive charged electrons) chemicals such as carbon, hydrogen, nitrogen, fluorine, and oxygen, which are converted into positron emitters. Having the cyclotron near the PET scanner is important because these isotopes decay rapidly and immediately need to be delivered and then given to the patient. When these elements are synthesized into such compounds as glucose and then injected

intravenously, the radioactive compound is taken up by the brain. There, via the collision of positrons with electrons, the degradation of the radioactive substances takes place. The resulting emission of gamma rays is detected by photo multiplier tubes. The tomographic image of the sites of the metabolic activity is constructed by computer processing. It partially fulfills the need for quantitative regional metabolic, biochemical and hemodynamic measurements in the human brain in vivo. These include cerebral blood flow and volume; oxygen utilization; glucose metabolic activity; and localization of neurotransmitter sites in the CNS. For example, it is possible to distinguish those areas of the brain permanently damaged from those just rendered nonfunctional by a severe reduction in oxygen supply following a stroke.

Pneumoencephalography

The ventricles and the subarachnoid space, when they contain air, can be visualized on an x-ray plate. This is accomplished after some CSF is withdrawn and replaced by air, which acts as a contrast medium. The air is introduced by passing a needle either directly into the ventricle or between the lower two lumbar vertebrae (*spinal tap*) into the lumbar cistern (caudal to the spinal cord). The air in the lumbar region can ascend and outline the subarachnoid space of the spinal and cranial cavities (by *pneumoen-*

cephalography); it can also pass through the foramina of Magendie and Luschka to outline the entire ventricular system (in a ventriculogram) by serial radiograms (x-rays), taken as the subject is slowly rotated through 360 degrees in a special apparatus. Access to the lateral ventricles is usually made by drilling trephine holes through the parietal bones. Hollow needles are passed through these holes and the brain into the lateral ventricles, permitting air to be introduced.

Myelography

Myelography is a method utilizing x-rays to outline the spinal cord, nerve roots, and bony margins of the vertebral canal. Iodinated contrast material that is radiopaque to x-rays is introduced into the subarachnoid space of a patient lying on a tilt table. The radiopaque material can be made to move up and down the subarachnoid space by tilting the table, can be visualized fluoroscopically, and can be radiographed to reveal the contours of structures within the vertebral canal.

HYDROCEPHALUS

An increase in the volume of CSF within the skull is known as hydrocephalus. Several types exist. In *compensating hydrocephalus*, there is no increase in pressure; this usually occurs when cerebral atrophy associated with a primary CNS disease is compensated for with an increase in CSF volume. In *obstructive hydrocephalus* and *communicating hydrocephalus*, there is both an increase in volume and in pressure of the CSF. Obstructive hydrocephalus occurs when there is an obstruction to the flow of CSF within the ventricles, cerebral aqueduct, or the apertures in the roof of the fourth ventricle. The blockage results in an increase in the volume of CSF above the obstruction, which may be caused by a tumor, developmental anomaly, or some inflammatory process. In communicating hydrocephalus, the ventricular CSF can readily flow into the subarachnoid space; the hydrocephalus results either from an obstruction to its flow within the subarachnoid space or from an alteration in the rate of formation and absorption of the CSF.

CLINICAL ASPECTS OF CEREBROSPINAL FLUID

The CSF is used for diagnostic testing. Samples of CSF for examination are usually obtained by a *lumbar puncture (spinal tap)* into the *spinal cistern*; this is done by inserting a long needle in the midline between the spines of vertebrae L3 and L4, or L4 and L5, with the patient lying curled up on one side. There is no risk to injuring the spinal cord, which terminates above these levels. The nerve roots of the cauda equina are usually deflected by the needle and thus rarely injured. With the relaxed patient lying sideways, the normal pressure ranges from 65 to 195 mm water. The pulsations of the cerebral arteries are registered as small oscillations on the manometer. Compression on the internal jugular veins draining blood from the brain results in a brisk rise in the CSF pressure. A lumbar puncture is contraindicated in the presence of an elevated intracranial pressure or an obstruction in the subarachnoid space. In such cases, removal of CSF from lumbar cistern would lower pressure below the blockage with several possible results: herniation of (1) the uncus of temporal lobe through the tentorium or (2) the cerebellar tonsils into the foramen magnum. The former, through pressure on the midbrain, can result in coma and the latter, through pressure on the medulla, can cause death from malfunctioning of the cardiac and respiratory centers.

The removed CSF is examined for the presence of cells (lymphocytes and erythrocytes), plasma protein, gamma globulins, and glucose. Special tests are carried out for specific diseases.

SUGGESTED READING

Bradbury M. The structure and function of the blood-brain barrier. *Federation Proceedings.* 1984;43: 186–190.

Davson H. Formation and drainage of the cerebrospinal fluid. In: Shapiro K, Marmarou A, Portnoy H, eds. *Hydrocephalus.* New York, NY: Raven Press; 1984:1–40.

Davson H, Kealey W, Segal M. *Physiology and Path-*

ophysiology of the Cerebrospinal Fluid. Edinburgh: Churchill Livingstone; 1987.

Fishman R. *Cerebrospinal Fluid in Diseases of the Nervous System.* 2nd ed. Philadelphia, Pa: WB Saunders; 1992.

Goldstein G, Betz A. The blood-brain barrier. *Sci Am.* 1986;255(3):74–83.

McCulloch J. Perivascular nerve fibres and the cerebral circulation. *Trends Neurosci.* 1984;7: 135–138.

Netter F. *Atlas of Human Anatomy.* West Caldwell, NJ: Ciba-Geigy; 1989: plates 94–98.

Osborn A. *Introduction to Cerebral Angiography.* Hagerstown, Md: Harper & Row; 1980.

Raichle M. Positron emission tomography. *Annu Rev Neurosci.* 1983;6:249–267.

Risau W, Wolburg H. Development of the blood-brain barrier. *Trends Neurosci.* 1990;13: 174–184.

Sochurek H. Medicine's new image (computed tomography, magnetic resonance imaging, and positron emission tomography). *National Geographic.* 1987;171:2–41.

Sokoloff L, ed. Brain Imaging and Brain Function. In: Research publication of the Association for Research in Nervous and Mental Diseases. New York, NY: Raven Press; 1985:63:1–290.

Walz W. Role of glial cells in the regulation of the brain ion microenvironment. *Prog Neurobiol.* 1989;33:309–333.

Wilson M. *The Anatomic Foundation of Neuroradiology of the Brain.* 2nd ed. Boston, Mass: Little Brown & Co; 1972.

Development and Growth of the
Nervous System
6

Origin of the nervous system

Differentiation of neurons and glial cells

Neuron: early development through maturity

Development of the cerebellum

Neural specificity and plasticity

Intraneuronal transport of signals

Reciprocal Schwann cell-axon interactions

Apoptosis or naturally occurring neuronal death

Aging of the brain during postnatal life

Spinal cord and peripheral nervous system

Brain

Critical periods: effects of genetic and epigenetic (environmental) factors during development

---

Individuals are as old as their neurons in the sense that almost all neurons are generated by early postnatal life and are not replaced by new ones during a given lifetime. However, the specific connection patterns within the nervous system appear to be capable of some alteration after infancy under the influence of experience.

The cardiovascular system and the nervous system are the first organ systems to function during embryonic life. In humans, the heart begins to beat late in the third week after fertilization. Before the heart beats, the nervous system begins to differentiate and change in shape. Growth in size occurs after the heart starts to pulsate and blood slowly circulates to bring oxygen and essential nutrients to the developing nervous system. During the second month, when stimuli are applied to the upper lip of the embryo, there is an avoidance reflex withdrawal of the head. A mother may feel life as early as the twelfth prenatal week.

From relatively few primordial cells present several weeks after fertilization of the ovum, the nervous system undergoes a remarkable change to attain its complex and intricate organization. Once a neuroblast leaves the ventricular layer of the generative neural tube, not only is it committed to differentiate into a neuron, but it will never divide again. To generate the estimated 100 billion neurons in the mature brain requires a calculated production of 2,500 neurons per minute during the entire length of prenatal life. The brain of a 1-year-old child has as many neurons as it will ever have. Throughout life, cells are continuously lost at an estimated rate of 200,000 per day in humans. The estimate is based on the observation of the 5 to 10% loss of brain tissue with age. Assuming that there is a 7% loss of neurons over a life span of 100 years and assuming 100 billion neurons are present at 1 year of age, then 200,000 neurons will be lost per day. Because the brain has so many neurons,

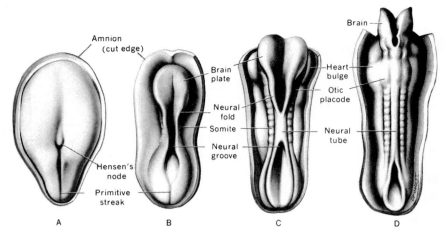

Figure 6.1: Dorsal aspect of human embryo. **A.** Primitive-streak plate stage of a 16-day presomite embryo. **B.** Two-somite keyhole stage of an approximately 20-day embryo. Note the first somites, neural fold, and neural groove. **C.** Seven-somite stage of an approximately 22-day embryo. **D.** Ten-somite neural tube stage of an approximately 23-day embryo. (Adapted from Scammon.)

most individuals get through life without losing enough to become mentally disabled.

The central goal of developmental neurobiology is to gain an understanding of the interactions and resolutions of the forces of "nature" versus "nurture." *Nature* refers to the cell's intrinsic potential, contained in the genetic pool, to mastermind the neuroblast and attain the full repertoire of cellular processes and features of the mature neurons. *Nurture* refers to the extrinsic epigenetic extracellular factors, both tropic and trophic (see below), which shape the development of the neuron and continue to operate, even on the mature neuron.

Differentiation and growth continue postnatally, attaining the organized complexity of the entire nervous system. It continues throughout life as the nervous system is remodeled through plasticity. The totality of events occurring during the development of the brain is not the exclusive property of rigid genetic codes. For example, "The human brain probably contains more than one trillion synapses, and there simply are not enough genes, to account for this complexity."

The normal development of a neuron and its subsequent integration into neuronal circuits result from activities at both (1) the *genetic level* and (2) the *epigenetic level*. The former (genetic) comprises (a) transcription or the transfer of information from DNA molecules into RNA mole-

cules and (b) translation or the transfer of information from the RNA molecules into polypeptides. The latter (epigenetic) includes many environmental and extracellular factors that can modify, regulate, or channel subsequent development. Epigenesis involves the roles of tropic and neurotropic molecules which have critical roles in the structural changes during the ontogeny of the nervous system. Tropic (having affinity for and turning toward) factors are molecules to which, for example, growth cones are attracted (see contract guidance in Neuronal Navigation and Development). Trophic (relating to nutrition for survival) factors are molecules secreted by their targets (target-derived neurotrophic factors) and are essential for the differentiation, growth, and survival of neurons. Even neurons depend upon one another for trophic factors affecting their signaling efficiency and even their survival.

The neurotrophic concept states that during development, neurons are critically dependent for their survival on these target-derived factors. The presence of limited amounts of these factors ensures that only a select proportion of neurons survive and do not succumb to naturally occurring cell death (see apoptosis later) and thus the appropriate innervation density of the target is attained. The scenario during development may be categorized as a competitive yet regulated "battle ground" among many influences.

(1) The genetic impetus is to produce during early development an oversupply of neurons, axons, dendrites (including their terminal branches), and synapses. (2) The growth of the axons to their target is usually attained by a specific route; however, alternate routes are possible. (3) The projections of the axons from several sources to a specific target neuron or structure (e.g., muscle) is generally diffuse and intermingled in the vicinity of their definitive target. (4) Competition occurs among the oversupply of axonal terminals for appropriate targets (neuron or synapses) with the elimination of supernumerary neurons, axons, and synaptic terminals. Experimental evidence indicates that developmental changes continue to occur even in old age. Dendrites and axons of neurons of the cerebral cortex of old rats (equivalent in human terms of roughly 75 years) respond to an enriched environment by forming new axon terminals and synaptic connections. Investigations reveal that the structure and chemistry of the brain can be affected by experiences throughout life, indicating that there is more flexibility and plasticity in neuronal connectivity in old age than previously thought. Thus the debate over nature or nurture as regards the brain and behavior is essentially over. Although many details remain to be resolved, both are involved.

ORIGIN OF THE NERVOUS SYSTEM

When the human embryo is but 1.5 mm long (18 days old), the ectoderm (outer germ layer) differentiates and thickens along the future midline of the back to form the *neural plate* (Fig. 6.1). With the transfer of certain chemical substances from the underlying mesoderm, the induction of this ectoderm occurs so it is now irreversibly committed to form neural tissue. The neural plate is exposed to the surface and to the amniotic fluid; it is continuous laterally with the future skin. Certain portions of the ectoderm differentiate and thicken in the head region to form *placodes*, which are progenitors of the organs of special sense such as the eyes (optic placode), ears (otic placode), and nose (nasal placode). In fact, the neural plate is a giant placode. The neural plate elongates,

and its lateral edges are raised to form the *neural folds* or *keyhole stage* (Fig. 6.1). The anterior end of the neural plate enlarges and will develop into the brain. The lateral edges, or lips, continue to rise and grow medially until they meet and unite in the midline to form the neural tube. This midline union commences in the cervical region and progresses both cephalically and caudally until, in 25 days, the entire plate is converted into the *neural tube* (Fig. 6.1). The tube becomes detached from the skin and sinks beneath the surface (Fig. 6.2). The cavity of the neural tube persists in the adult as the ventricular system of the brain and the central canal of the spinal cord.

The cephalic end of the neural tube differentiates and enlarges into three dilations called the "primary brain vesicles." These three divisions are called the *prosencephalon* or *forebrain*, the *mesencephalon* or *midbrain*, and the *rhombencephalon* or *hindbrain*. A bilateral column of cells differentiates from the neural ectoderm at the original junction of the skin ectoderm and the rolled edges of the neural plate. These two columns of cells become the *neural crests* (Fig. 6.2). The neural tube is the primordial structure for the central nervous system (CNS) (brain and spinal cord), including all neurons in the CNS, oligodendroglia, and astroglia. The neural crest gives rise to a number of neural and nonneural derivatives. The neural derivatives include (1) neurons in all the sensory, autonomic, and enteric ganglia; (2) cells of the pia mater and arachnoid and the sclera and choroid coats of the eye; (3) neurolemma (Schwann) cells and satellite cells of the ganglia; (4) adrenal medullary cells; and (5) receptor cells of the carotid body. Some neurons of sensory ganglia of cranial nerves V, VII, IX, and X are derived from cells of the otic placode.

Several mesodermally derived elements are associated with the nervous system, including the meninges. Those that secondarily invade the CNS include the blood vessels and microglial cells.

DIFFERENTIATION OF NEURONS AND GLIAL CELLS

The embryonic neural tube eventually comprises four concentric zones: ventricular, sub-

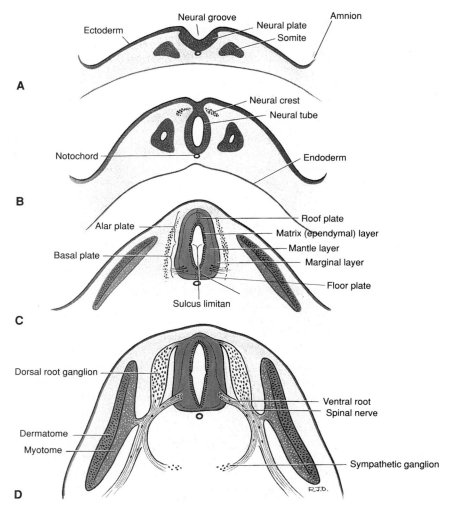

Figure 6.2: Development of the spinal cord, neural crest, somite, and spinal nerve (transverse sections) in a human embryo of the following ages: **A.** Approximately 19 days; **B.** approximately 20 days; **C.** approximately 26 days; **D.** after 1 month of age. The alar plate gives rise to sensory (afferent) neurons, the basal plate to motor (efferent) neurons. The sulcus limitans is the boundary between alar and basal plates.

ventricular, intermediate (mantle), and marginal (Fig. 6.3). The adult nervous system is derived from these basic zones, none of which corresponds precisely to any adult components.

The *ventricular zone* consists of dividing cells. The nucleus of each ventricular cell migrates to the luminal end of the cell (adjacent to the central canal), rounds up, and undergoes a mitotic division; after dividing, the nuclei of the daughter cells migrate to the apical portions of their respective cells, where the replication of its DNA occurs. Thus, the ventricular zone

is known as the lamina of the *to-and-fro nuclear movement*. The mitotic and nuclear migration cycle lasts from 5 to 24 hours. Ventricular cells are the progenitors of neurons and macroglia (astroglia and oligodendroglia) of the CNS.

The precursor cells of glial cells can be distinguished from those of neurons by the presence of glial fibrillary acidic protein (GFAP) in dividing glial precursor cells of the ventricular zone. The first glial cells to be formed appear at about the same time as the first neurons. As previously stated, most, but not all, neurons in

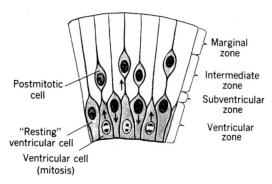

Postmitotic cell

"Resting" ventricular cell

Ventricular cell (mitosis)

Marginal zone

Intermediate zone

Subventricular zone

Ventricular zone

Figure 6.3: The four zones of the embryonic central nervous system. The arrows within the ventricular cells indicate the direction in which their nuclei migrate during a mitotic cycle. Arrow outside the cells indicates the direction in which the postmitotic neuroblasts migrate.

humans are generated during prenatal life. In contrast, the precursors of the glial cells retain some capacity for proliferation throughout life.

The *subventricular zone* in time differentiates from the ventricular zone. It is composed of small cells which proliferate by mitosis but do not exhibit the to-and-fro nuclear movements during the mitotic cycles. This zone persists only a few days in the spinal cord but many months and even years in the cerebrum. The zone generates certain classes of neurons and macroglia of the CNS. It gives rise to (1) the rhombic lips located on the lateral margins of the medulla and (2) the ganglionic eminence located in the floor of each lateral ventricle. The rhombic lips generate certain brainstem and cerebellar neurons including the billions of interneurons of the cerebellar cortex (Chap. 18). The ganglionic eminence generates many of the small neurons of the basal ganglia (Chap. 23) and of some other deep structures of the cerebrum.

After these newly differentiated neurons have apparently lost their capacity to synthesize DNA, the mitotic cycle ceases, and the cells are triggered to migrate from both the ventricular and subventricular zones into the intermediate zone or even farther to form the cortical plates (see later). Never again will these postmitotic cells divide. Those cells that migrate into the rhombic lips and ganglionic eminences, as noted above, retain their capacity to undergo

mitosis. As a rule, the large neurons differentiate before the small neurons. The large neurons are primarily those whose axons extend long distances and small neurons (local circuit neurons) are those whose fibers are confined to the region immediately surrounding the cell body.

The *intermediate (mantle) zone* evolves into the gray matter of the CNS with its complex neural organization. The neurons that migrate and collect to form the cortical plates differentiate into two groups of neurons: those of the cerebral cortex and those of the cerebellar cortex. Most cerebellar cortical neurons are derived from the rhombic lips.

The *marginal zone* is the cell-sparse layer with no primary cells of its own. Eventually it is invaded by axons, both myelinated and unmyelinated, and macroglia to form much of the white matter.

NEURON: EARLY DEVELOPMENT THROUGH MATURITY

Neuronal Navigation and Docking During Early Development

The stages involved in the creation of the neuronal network of the brain and spinal cord and its integration with the peripheral nerves during prenatal development are precise and apparently predetermined to a considerable degree. The first two stages are *pathway selection* and *target selection*. In humans they are instrumental in establishing the basic groundwork of the neuronal networks and pathway systems during prenatal life. The third, or *activity-dependent and experience-dependent stage*, continues throughout life.

Pathway Selection and Target Selection

Evidence is available that identifies some of the factors involved in assembling, integrating, and maintaining the one hundred billion neurons of the human nervous system. Since there are more neurons than genes, each neuron can't possibly have its own gene to regulate the navigational system controlling (1) *pathway selection* or cell migration from the ventricular layer of the neural tube and (2) *target selection* or the guidance of the growth of axons at their tips (growth cones) as their endings "hone in" to make synaptic connections with their target neurons. The development of the nervous system from the neural plate and neural crest stage to the mature nervous system is synchronized by genetic influences and epigenetic factors. In essence, each neuroblast differentiates into a neuron with its axon terminals which must *migrate to and dock in its designated site, and be there at the right time to be integrated into a prescribed circuitry.*

At the time a neuroblast commences to migrate from the ventricular zone of the neural plate it becomes a postmitotic cell that is (1) incapable of dividing and (2) branded to become a neuron. The kinetics of cell migration commences as each neuroblast (and glioblast) leaves the ventricular zone at a definite time to navigate to its port of call in the brain and spinal cord. The differentiation of each immature neuron, and the specific path it takes to reach its destination, is determined (1) by the activation of specific sets of genes combined with (2) a variety of epigenetic external signals from other cells in the environment. Initially the neuroblasts of the brain contact the fibers of the radial glial cells. These are specialized cells, each with a process extending to the ventricular surface and another to the pial surface. The neuroblasts migrate along the scaffolds of these glial fibers by *contact (mechanical) guidance*; however, many neuroblasts migrate without the guidance of the glial fibers. Both of these migratory patterns are apparently accomplished with the aid of *tropic molecular cues* or *markers*, which attract the migrating neuroblast or its growing tip. This establishes the basic structural matrix of the brain and spinal cord (see later, Development of the Cerebellum and Fig. 6.4). In addition, there are *neurotrophic* factors, which are chemical substances released by the targets of neurons. Such factors trigger chemical changes in the neurons that are critical for the survival, differentiation, and growth of neurons. Nerve growth factor (NGF) is the prototypical target-derived neurotrophic factor (family of proteins called neurotrophins)(Chap. 2). Other putative neurotrophins have been proposed. The view that each neuron has a single target-derived neurotrophic factor is being modified;

more than one factor can presumably influence the development and survival of some neurons. In addition, some neurotrophic factors may be derived from sources other than the target.

Once the immature neuron arrives at its destination, the outgrowth of its axon begins. The terminal tip of the elongating axon is the *growth cone*, which is characterized by the presence of finger-like projections (filopodia) or flattened extensions (lamellipodia). The growth cones act as mobile sentinels. Powered by actin microfilaments, the cones actively explore and probe the tissue environment. Filopodia protrude randomly from the leading edge of the growth cone. Those that extend in the "intended" new direction of growth become stabilized, whereas the others are retracted. Stabilization involves the concentration of actin in the filopodia and the local consolidation of the microtubules in the growth cone. This establishes the new direction in which the axis cylinder continues to elongate. Receptor molecules on the cone's plasma membrane, acting as sensors, are responsive to the diffusible molecules in the vicinity. Chemotrophic factors furnish guidance cues leading to the precision of pathfinding as the axon elongates and also sprouts collateral branches. Some guidance cues can be inhibitory and thus modulate and regulate random collateral sprouting of branches and prevent aberrant growth. The glycoproteins *laminin* and *fibronectin* are growth factors present in the extracellular matrix of both the developing peripheral nervous system (PNS) and CNS. The cone responds to molecular cues (chemoaffinity) and *guidepost cells*, which trigger a radical turn (even at a right angle turn) in the trajectory of the axon and also define the location of branching sites for the development of collateral branches. This guided growth is not fully understood; however, it is established that growth cones follow cues and markers that are encoded by the cells with which they are in direct contact, or that diffuse from target cells. Nonetheless, the molecular nature of these cues remains elusive.

One of the primary goals of developmental neurobiology is to identify the chemical signals involved with the accurate guidance of growing axons as they establish the basic circuitry of the nervous system. Directing axons to their mark during development is presently conceived to involve, in part, diffusible chemotropic (neurotropic) factors secreted by cells along the designated pathways and target cells. These factors apparently effect the biochemical and functional properties of the receptor sites on the axonal growth cones. This is an expression of *epigenesis*, in which these chemotropic factors contribute to the patterns associated with axon pathfinding and axon fasciculation (Jessel and Dodd, 1992).

Early differentiation of the nervous system is regulated by a series of chemical inductive signals, some derived from mesoderm. The mesodermal notochord conveys local signals that induce the formation of the floor plate of the neural tube (**Fig. 6.2**). In turn, the cells of the floor plate secrete diffusible proteins (axonguidance factors) called netrin-1 and netrin-2—named for the Sanskrit word for "one who guides" (Kennedy et al, 1994). The axons originating dorsally in the neural tube near the roof plate grow ventrally to the region near the floor plate. These netrins possess commissural outgrowth-promoting activity signals that cause these growing axons to decussate (cross over) as commissural axons to the contralateral side. These factors apparently are released by the floor plate even when the human embryo is as young as 1 month old. Thus, they have a role in the act of designating the sites of the decussation of various fiber systems in the spinal cord and brainstem. Examples include the spinothalamic fibers in the anterior white commissure (**Fig. 9.2**) and the internal arcuate fibers from the dorsal column nuclei that decussate in the medulla to form the medial lemniscus (**Fig. 10.3**).

The glycoproteins, called neural cell adhesion molecules (NCAMs), contribute to the general adhesive properties of neurons that are important as identity sites enabling one neuron to recognize another. An NCAM molecule on one neuron can bind to a counterpart NCAM molecule on another neuron during development of specific populations of neurons; however, NCAM molecules may not have a role in promoting axonal growth. Rather, NCAMs are requisite for anchoring the growth cone to a surface, but not for the directed migration and guidance. The axons and dendrites grow out in a predetermined manner during normal development, with axonal outgrowth preceding dendritic outgrowth. Axons utilizing growth cones as sensors can be conceived as navigating through an epigenetic landscape that guides their growth through reactions to a variety of chemical factors and physical substrates.

In summary, there are presumed to be a variety of (1) outgrowth-promoting protein molecules that stimulate the increase in numbers and lengths of axons, including such chemotropic factors as laminin and nitrins, and (2) outgrowth-suppressing molecules that have the opposite effect. These chemotropic factors combine to influence the directed migration and guidance of the growing axons to their targets. The NCAMs have an anchoring role to bind the axon to a surface.

The goal of each axon is to make functional synaptic connections with such targets as other neurons (dendrites, cell bodies, and axons) and effectors (muscles and glands). Complex interactions between the nerve terminal and the postsynaptic cell are critical for the initially immature synapse to become stabilized and functionally effective. The growth cone matures into the presynaptic nerve terminal by honing its capability to store and release transmitter spontaneously into a mature terminal with a coordinated response to action potentials. Some of this differentiation is required by the postsynaptic cell. In turn, the postsynaptic cell is modified by influences from the presynaptic membrane, that regulates the number and distribution of transmitter receptors and other molecules of the postsynaptic membrane.

The interaction of the axon terminal (growth cone) with the plasma membrane of a myotube (immature striated muscle fiber) at a neuromuscular junction (motor end plate) illustrates the influence of the presynaptic terminal upon the postsynaptic membrane. Prior to the arrival of the motor nerve terminal, the acetylcholine (ACh) receptors are uniformly distributed over the surface of the muscle fiber. Following the arrival of the future synaptic site, the axon terminal induces the accumulation of a new cluster of ACh receptors on the muscle membrane at the point of ACh release. Some receptors are redistributed as they diffuse within the membrane and become immobilized in the cluster. Others are synthesized anew and are inserted within the cluster. Thus, the presynaptic ending controls the synthesis and distribution of receptors on the postsynaptic membrane. A diffusible protein called acetylcholine receptor inducing activity (ARIA) has a role in this transformation. Following the clustering of the receptor sites at the motor end-plate, the receptors outside the vicinity of the end-plate disappear.

In summary, the precision of the molecularly guided navigation during these two stages is coupled by giving rise to the basic neuronal connections specified by recognition molecules. Thus, the basic connectivity of complex circuitry of the nervous system is established in the sensory systems such as the posterior column-medial lemniscal pathways (Chap. 10), the motor systems such as the corticobulbar and corticospinal pathways (Chap. 11), and other integrating circuits such as those associated with the basal ganglia (Chap. 24). These are presumed to have developed independently of activity or experience.

Oligodendrocytes develop relatively late, always after the growth of the axon in the CNS. This timing is essential because these glial cells exert inhibitory influences on axonal growth and regeneration. This results from the action of membrane-bound inhibitors of mature oligodendrocytes and CNS myelin.

Activity-Dependent
and Experience-Dependent Stage

This stage is involved with refining the coarser features of the circuitry by fine tuning the patterns of connectivity of the pathway systems through activity and experience. The impetus to accomplish this is through activity and by the experience gained by responding and adjusting to both external and internal environmental stimuli. Many of these connections continue to be capable of modification throughout life. The activity-dependent and experience-dependent plasticity of the ocular dominance columns of the visual cortex is expressed in the anatomical and physiological changes during the critical period that results in amblyopia (see later). Activity- and experience-induced changes in the nervous system are phenomena responding to and associated with the continuous honing of the skills in proficient athletes and musicians.

Structural plasticity, axonal sprouting, and the changes in number of dendritic spines can be enhanced (or suppressed) in appropriate neurons through an increase (or decrease) in activity. Engaged exposure to sensory stimulation (e.g., touch or visual) during development can lead to significant increases in the number of dendritic spines and synapses in neocortical neurons of the primary sensory areas. Even the cortical map of the primary sensory cortex can be modified by activity and experience (Chap. 25). The ability of axons to regenerate in the adult is an expression of the neuron's retention of an embryonic potential throughout life (Chap. 2). A physiological expression of motor learning and skills by the activity of inhibitory synapses is noted in the "importance of inhibition" (Chap. 3). Changes at the molecular level that are associated with memory presumably involve the second messenger system and modulatory glutamate transmitters acting through NMDA receptors on postsynaptic neurons (Chap. 15).

DEVELOPMENT OF THE CEREBELLUM

The development of the cerebellum presents a dramatic example of the migration of germinal cells (neuroblasts and glioblasts) from two sources navigating along different routes to finally mesh into the intricate circuitry that characterizes the cortex and deep nuclei of the cerebellum (**Figs. 6.4 and 18.2**). Only a few aspects of these precisely timed and integrated sequences will be outlined.

The two sources are: the ventricular zone of the neural (cerebellar) plate and the rhombic lip of the dorsolateral lower pons. The routes are: the direct migration from the ventricular zone to the primordial cerebellum (cerebellar plate) and the migration from the rhombic lip to the outer surface (external granular layer) of the cerebellar plate.

The neuroblasts of the ventricular zone migrate into the cerebellar plate to form two strata: the neuroblasts of the deep stratum differentiate into the neurons of the deep cerebellar nuclei (dentate, emboliform, globose, and fastigial nuclei), while those of the superficial stratum differentiate into the Purkinje cells and Golgi cells (neurons of the cerebellar cortex). Neuroblasts

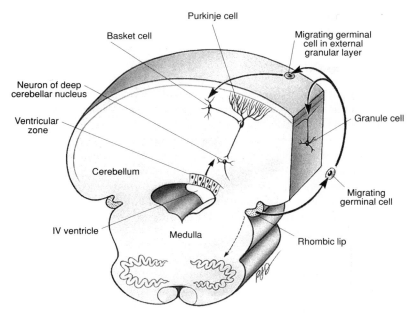

Figure 6.4: The two routes (arrows) of the migration of neuroblasts during the histogenesis of the cerebellum.

from the rhombic lip migrate over the surface of the cerebellar plate to form the external granular layer. This layer gives rise to granule cells, basket cells, and stellate cells (neurons of the cerebellar cortex). Glial cells are derived from the same sites as the neurons.

The events of these migrations from dual sources to the right places and arrivals at the right times, lead to the formation of the complex integrated circuitry involving the neurons of the cerebellum (**Fig. 6.4 and Chap. 18**) (see above, Neuronal Navigation and Development).

The Purkinje cells form their dendritic trees within the molecular layer. At the same time, the granule cells migrate from the external granular layer through the molecular layer to the granular layer (deep to the cell bodies of the Purkinje cells). These cells are guided (contact guidance) along the processes of radial glial cells (Bergmann glial cells). Neurotrophic factors and interactions among the differentiating Purkinje cells and granule cells contribute to the events within the molecular layer. Among these are the formation and orientation of the parallel fibers of the granule cells and the complete differentiation of the dendritic trees of the Purkinje cells, as well as the specific connections of these neurons with each other and with

other neurons. Added to this can be the sequence involving the differentiation, growth, and synaptic connections of the Golgi cells, stellate cells, basket cells, and the climbing and mossy fibers.

NEURAL SPECIFICITY AND PLASTICITY

The structural organization and functional expression exhibited by each neuron at any time results from the continual interactions between intrinsic influences from within the neuron—largely of genetic origin—and extrinsic influences from epigenetic environmental sources. The predictability of the form and connections of a neuron is called *neural specificity*; this is presumably determined genetically. Variations from the predictable patterns are expressions of neural plasticity or the capability of being changed or transformed; this is presumed to be largely determined by epigenetic factors. During differentiation, a substantial complement of genetic information is utilized by the immature neuron with the instructions for expressing neuronal specificity, namely to: migrate to its designated locale in the nervous system, assume the structural identity characteristic for that neuron, and have the potential to develop those biochemical and physiological features normally exhibited by that neuron.

The nervous system exhibits plasticity in that it may modify its morphology and response performance following stimulation by the internal and/or external environments. The fact that humans and other organisms are able to learn and memorize to varying degrees indicates that the nervous system is modifiable. Actually the ever-functioning brain is activity-dependent in order to maintain its integrity; it requires a continuous stream of input. Plasticity is operative as a factor in the ability of the organism to alter its behavior in response to novel epigenetic factors. With respect to learning, the identification of the permanent changes in the nervous system associated with plasticity have been somewhat elusive, for example, the hippocampus has a role in the early stages of memory formation (Chap. 22). Evidence indicates that synaptic transmission can be enhanced for hours and even weeks in the hippocampus following a brief period of high frequency stimulation. This persistent change in synaptic strength is thought to be related, in part, to biochemical (plastic) alterations in the presynaptic transmitter release mechanism, or in the postsynaptic receptors, or in both. The nervous system can adapt to the changing demands of the epigenetic environment by modulating both the properties of the plasma membranes and the "strength" of the synaptic transmission. Furthermore, these adaptations may occur at all levels including sensory inputs, relay nuclei, association areas of the cerebral cortex, and the motor output.

Neuron specificity can be modified by epigenetic influences. Plasticity occurs in the slight alterations in the position of the cell body, in the arborization pattern of the dendritic tree, and in the distribution pattern of terminal synapses of the axon. The general pattern of synaptic connections are presumed to be established at an early stage of development. They become localized on both specific neurons and also on specific locations (cell body dendrites or axon) of other neurons. Each neuron has the capability of generating new dendritic processes and axonal branches to meet functional demands. As the axon matures, many processes and branches remain and many retract and are pruned. Each neuron is integrated into a functional entity as its complement of input synapses and output synapses is resolved. The epigenetic influences exerted on each neuron during development can result in structural and functional alterations; some of these can be severe (see Critical Periods).

Plasticity may be expressed by a drastic change in the type of transmitter released by a neuron. For example, the postganglionic sympathetic neurons innervating the sweat glands have cholinergic endings that release acetylcholine (Table 20.1). During early development, however, prior to innervating the sweat glands, they are adrenergic neurons. Following their innervation of the sweat glands, an interaction occurs between these neurons and a presumed target-derived neurotrophic factor released by the sweat glands, which results in the conversion of these adrenergic neurons into cholinergic neurons. This example illustrates that a neuron's specific role is not irrevocably programmed to produce one transmitter. Rather, the choice of the neurotransmitter synthesized and released by a neuron is acquired at a comparatively late stage developmentally and it can be changed by the epigenetic environment of the neuron. As an illustration, the differentiation of neurons can be dependent upon and biased by multiple diffusible chemical factors. This applies to certain neuroblasts that presumably have an *unrestricted progenitor potential*. Such an embryonic cell may be present in the inner layer of the optic cup. It has been suggested that this cell may be prompted by diffusible factors to differentiate into any of the cells of the adult retina (photoreceptors, bipolar neurons, horizontal, amacrine and retinal ganglion cells, and glial (Muller's) cells (Chap. 19). Cells that differentiate to only one mature neuronal type have a *highly restricted progenitor potential*.

The brain is forever turning over its biochemical constituents, which may be involved with plasticity in order to cope with certain new demands. Isotope studies reveal that the biochemical turnover within the nervous system is rapid. For example, on the basis of their half-life, free amino acids in the brain are incorporated into proteins within half an hour. Depending upon the substance, the rate of turnover ranges from a "fast turnover" of a few hours to a "slow turnover" measured in days. In the case of myelin, the half-life of one of its constituents, lecithin, is about 15 days. Proteins, considered to be stable entities, also turn over to an astonishing degree. Every 30 days a rat has replaced all but about 25% of its brain protein, so that by 6 months only about 1 to 2% of the original protein remains.

Plasticity is active during development as the anatomical and physiological changes of the neurons and their integration mature as functional circuits and pathways. The role of plasticity continues throughout life as one of the mechanisms mediating adjustments required to respond to changing functional demands on circuits. Much evidence demonstrates that the neural connection patterns within the postnatal cerebral cortex are not static, but are dynamically maintained and adjusted by continuous stream of input experience and usage. Drastic changes in the usage are accompanied by alteration in these patterns (Chap. 25). In both the CNS and PNS some alteration may result in the elimination of surplus collaterals. This pruning is one means of enhancing the precision of the neuronal interconnections.

Plasticity is significant because of its role (1) in making the structural physiological and biochemical changes required to make the adjustments to comply with needs of the activity-dependent nervous system and (2) in correcting and ameliorating some features of recovery from injuries to the CNS. Plasticity is expressed by the sprouting of collateral branches from intact neurons toward neurons deprived of much of their afferent input from adjacent neurons that have been injured. This attempt to reinnervate may be due, in part, to a response to trophic factors released by the partially denervated neurons.

The biological expression of each person's individuality is based on a distinctive genetic constitution combined with unique epigenetic modifications involving a degree of plasticity.

INTRANEURONAL TRANSPORT OF SIGNALS

Anterograde and retrograde transport systems convey macromolecules, including trophic fac-

tors, that are involved in such roles as general maintenance of the neuron, axonal growth during development, axonal remodeling as an expression of plasticity, and regeneration of injured neurons (Chap. 2). These transport systems are essential for coordinating the complex functional interrelations between the cell body and the entire axon and dendrites—especially since macromolecules are synthesized in the cell body. Some macromolecules are thought to convey signals (*signal peptides*), that is, they act as messengers with roles in influencing various aspects of the neuronal processes. Macromolecules newly synthesized by each neuron are delivered from the cell body, via the *anterograde transport pathway* in the axon, to sites where these proteins are utilized by the neuron throughout its life, from early development through maturity.

Indications are that neurons utilize the *retrograde transport pathway* to convey signal peptides from the axon to the cell body and then to the nucleus, providing information concerning conditions within the axon. Means of conveying information from the sites of axonal growth, reorganization, and injury are essential because axons have a limited capacity for synthesizing macromolecules. Retrograde communication can influence activity, for example, in the gene transcription essential for supplying macromolecules required for axonal repair, regeneration, plasticity, and even "learning" (Ambron et al, 1995). This rapid retrograde transport is a system by which the needs of each axon are continuously communicated to the biosynthetic centers of the neuron. Another role of signals is to inform the cell body of the neuropeptide transmitter stores in the axon terminals, and to adjust the activity of the biosynthetic centers of the cell body to maintain adequate supplies of transmitters in the terminals (Chap. 3).

RECIPROCAL SCHWANN CELL-AXON INTERACTIONS

From the early stages of development through old age, *reciprocal Schwann cell-axon interactions* occur with profound effects by one upon the other. The vehicles for these activities are signal molecules (information carriers) that are

(1) generated by Schwann cells to act on neu-rons or (2) generated by neurons and their axons to act on Schwann cells. Among these signal molecules are neurotrophic factors involved with growth and survival. Neurons and Schwann cells are critically dependent upon signaling mechanisms of subtle complexity. Although not as well documented, significant glial cell-axon interactions are also presumed to occur.

The Schwann cells are involved with influ-encing the differentiation and growth of axons. Their released soluble factors have roles in guiding the growing axons, promoting their maintenance, and insuring their survival. The ensheathment and myelination of both unmy-elinated and myelinated axons are specially regulated by contact with axons. This relation-ship is essential for the conduction of the nerve impulse. The Schwann cells play a critical role in several aspects of axonal regeneration in the PNS. The ability of these cells to promote the regenerative efforts of the CNS (Chap. 2) has encouraged interest in using Schwann cells as autographs for CNS repair.

The neuron, through its axons, exerts influ-ences by chemical factors that can (a) stimulate differentiation of Schwann cells, (b) induce and repress the proliferation of Schwann cells, and (c) modify the migration and growth of Schwann cells. By this means, the appropriate placement of Schwann cells in functionally relevant num-bers is reached during development, mainte-nance, and regeneration.

The relation of Schwann cells and axons is not stereotypic, as demonstrated in several var-iants from the typical nerve with each fiber en-sheathed with its own Schwann cells. In unmy-elinated fibers, the usual pattern of Schwann cell ensheathment is for the Schwann cell to harbor a number of nerve fibers within individ-ual channels continuous with the Schwann cell surface (**Fig. 2.7**). A variant is shown by the olfactory nerve, where clusters of groups of fine fibers are enclosed in troughs communally within the Schwann cell (**Fig. 2.7**). In the en-teric plexus of the gut (autonomic nervous sys-tem, Chap. 20) there are enteric glial cells (equivalent of Schwann cells). These cells form specialized ensheathing cells that ensheathe both the cell bodies and their processes.

APOPTOSIS OR NATURALLY OCCURRING NEURONAL DEATH

Apoptosis results, in part, from the competition among neurons for neurotrophic factors released by their target. The necessity of an axon to lo-cate the appropriate target cells is critical for the survival of the neuron. If it fails, the neuron may die. The target cells supply certain essen-tial neurotrophic factors that sustain the presy-naptic neurons during their development to be-come mature neurons. Several neurotrophic factors have been identified, each of which sus-tains the survival of specific assemblies of neu-rons. These comprise nerve growth factor (Chap. 2), brain-derived neurotrophic factor, neurotro-phin-3, and ciliary neurotrophic factor. It is pre-sumed that when the number of presynaptic neurons innervating a region exceeds the amount of neurotrophic factor available to sus-tain them, the excess population of presynaptic neurons die. In effect, the quantity of available neurotrophic factors is a means of matching of the appropriate number of presynaptic neurons to the physiological needs of the postsynaptic cells. To achieve functional maturity, neurons normally expire by the billions as the brain re-fines its circuitry during development.

In summary, *apoptosis*, also called *naturally* or *programmed neuronal death*, is expressed as the demise of numerous neurons.

This is conceived to reflect the failure of these neurons to be activated by adequate amounts of neurotrophic factors that are pro-duced by target cells and are essential for the neurons to survive. Apoptosis is distinct from the death resulting from injuries. This role of neurotropic factors, coupled with the emergence of *neurotrophic theory*, emphasizes the signifi-cance of survival signals in vertebrate neuronal development. This is encompassed within an even broader concept that most, if not all, cells, including neurons, require signals from other cells to survive. Thus, cells deprived of this ade-quate stimulation by these signals die.

AGING OF THE BRAIN DURING POSTNATAL LIFE

The number of neurons tends to decrease with age, for as neurons die they are not replaced by new neurons. The consequences of a slight loss are not necessarily noticeable because the remaining neurons may functionally compensate for a small decrease in numbers.

The brain is said to decrease gradually in weight over the years, losing as much as 10% between the ages of 20 and 90 years. This is presumably related to the loss and atrophy of neurons and glia and to the decrease of extracellular spaces. The loss of cells varies from region to region, with the brainstem exhibiting only a slight decline and the cerebral cortex undergoing the greatest loss. Some evidence indicates that the decrease in weight and the degree of cortical atrophy in healthy aged individuals who have no neuropathological condition in the brain are relatively slight. Within the cerebral cortex, the loss of neurons is greatest in neocortex of the frontal pole, precentral gyrus, cingulate gyrus, and primary visual cortex.

Neurons undergo senescence. Aging of the neurons is evidenced by change in size (either decrease or increase), by the accumulation of pigment, or by the decrease in amount of Nissl substance. In humans, for example, the quantity of ribonucleoproteins in the alpha motoneurons of the spinal cord increases significantly from birth to 40 years of age, plateaus from 40 to 60 years, and decreases from 60 years on. In elderly people, decrease in the weight of the brain, increase in the size of the ventricles, and calcification in the meninges are all signs of an aging nervous system.

An indication of the degree of the aging process after the prime of life is obtained by comparing several parameters in the 30-year-old age group with those in the 75-year-old group. In the older group, the reduction in brain weight is about 10%; in the blood flow to the brain, about 20%; in the number of nerve fibers in large nerves, about 33%; in the number of taste buds, about 66%; and in the velocity of nerve conduction, about 10%. The last correlates with the observation that the rate and magnitude of reflex responses to stimulation do decrease with age.

SPINAL CORD AND PERIPHERAL NERVOUS SYSTEM

Up to about the third fetal month, the spinal cord extends throughout the entire length of the developing vertebral column. At this time the dorsal (sensory) roots and the ventral (motor) roots of the spinal nerves extend laterally at right angles from the spinal cord. The roots unite in the intervertebral foramina to form the spinal nerves. The roots and spinal nerves are products of outgrowths from the spinal cord and neural crests (**Fig. 6.2**). Because the growth in length of the bony vertebral column exceeds that of spinal cord during fetal and early postnatal life, the spinal cord after the third fetal month becomes relatively shorter than the vertebral column. This is accompanied by an elongation of the roots of the spinal nerves between the spinal cord and the intervertebral foramina.

At birth the caudal end of the spinal cord is located at the level of the L3 vertebra, and at adolescence, as in the adult, this caudal end is located at the level approximately between the L1 and L2 vertebrae. As a result of this disparity in growth, the lumbar, sacral, and coccygeal roots become directed caudally at an acute angle to the spinal cord. The subarachnoid space below the first lumbar vertebra in the adult is occupied by dorsal and ventral roots of spinal nerves (cauda equina) and the filum terminale, not by spinal cord (**Fig. 7.1**).

Adjacent to the neural tube are 31 pairs of somites. These are the embryonic structures that differentiate into muscles, skeleton (including the vertebral column), and connective tissues (**Figs. 6.1 and 6.2**). The somites are segmental (metameric) structures arranged in sequence from the first cervical through the coccygeal levels. Segments are repeating units of similar composition.

Each pair of nerves develops in association with each pair of somites. The apparent segmentation of the spinal cord is dependent upon the development of the paired segmental spinal nerves. The bilateral neural crest also becomes segmented into paired units, one pair for each future sensory (dorsal root) ganglion of each spinal nerve.

BRAIN

Prenatal Development

Early in the second fetal month, the "three-vesicle brain" differentiates into the "five-vesicle brain" (**Fig. 6.5**). The prosencephalic vesicle is subdivided into the telencephalon, or end-brain, and the diencephalon, or between (twixt) brain. The mesencephalic vesicle remains as the midbrain; the rhombencephalic vesicle is subdivided into the metencephalon, or afterbrain, and the myelencephalon, or spinal brain.

The development of the "contorted" brain from the tubelike structure is the result of the complex integration of several processes: (1) three bends known as flexures, (2) differential enlargements of the different regions, (3) growth of portions of the cerebral hemispheres over the diencephalon, midbrain, and cerebellum, and (4) the formation of sulci and gyri in the cerebral and cerebellar cortices (**Figs. 6.5 to 6.7**). The flexures are the mesencephalic (midbrain) flexure (forming an acute angle on the anterior surface of the brain), the pontine flexure (forming an acute angle on the posterior surface), and the cervical flexure at the lower medulla (forming an acute angle on the anterior surface). The posterolateral margin of the rhombencephalon

is the rhombic lip, which develops into the cerebellum. The differential enlargement is most pronounced in the cerebral and cerebellar hemispheres. The telencephalon during development surrounds most of the diencephalon; there is an intussusception (telescoping) of the diencephalon into the telencephalon (**Figs. 6.5 to 6.7**).

The main outlines of the form of the brain are recognizable and the external surface of the brain is still smooth at the end of the third fetal month. Fissuration commences in the fourth fetal month with the appearance of the lateral sulcus of the cerebrum and posterolateral sulcus of the cerebellum separating the nodulus and attached flocculi from the vermis of the posterior lobe (**Fig. 18.1**). The central sulcus, calcarine sulcus, and parietooccipital sulcus are indicated by the fifth fetal month; all the main gyri and sulci of the cerebral cortex are present by the seventh fetal month. The external structure of the cerebral hemisphere of the 8-month-old fetus is characterized by the prominence of the precentral and postcentral gyri, by a wide-

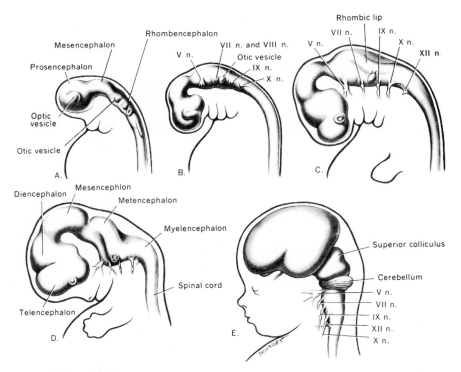

Figure 6.5: Human brain (lateral view): **A.** in a 3-week-old embryo; **B.** in a 4-week-old embryo; **C.** in a 5-week-old embryo; **D.** in a 7-week-old embryo; and **E.** in an 11-week-old fetus. (Adapted from Corliss.)

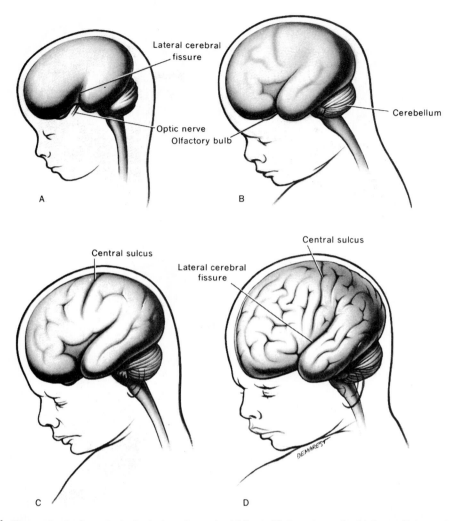

Figure 6.6: Human brain (lateral view): **A.** in a 4-month-old fetus; **B.** in a 6-month-old fetus; **C.** in an 8-month-old fetus; and **D.** in a newborn infant. (Adapted from Corliss.)

open lateral sulcus exposing the insula, and by the presence of all primary and secondary sulci and a few tertiary sulci. The occipital lobe overrides the cerebellum. During the last month of fetal life the frontal and temporal lobes are stubby, the insula is still exposed to the surface, and the occipital poles are blunt. The cortical gyri are broad and plump, and the fissures are shallow. The patterns of the primary and secondary sulci are simple.

The cerebrum of the full-term neonate is more fully developed in the regions posterior to the central sulcus than in the anterior regions. The frontal pole and the temporal pole are rela-

tively short, and the insula is almost completely covered by the adjacent lobes. The number of tertiary sulci is still small. The pia mater is not completely adherent to the brain and does not dip into all the sulci. The superficial blood vessels are straight. The brain has a gelatinous consistency. The cortex is poorly demarcated from the white matter. By the end of infancy, at 2 years of age, the relative size and proportions of the brain and its subdivisions are essentially similar to those of the adult brain. The brain is firmer. The gray cortex is demarcated from the subcortical white matter, which is now myelinated. The superficial cortical blood vessels are

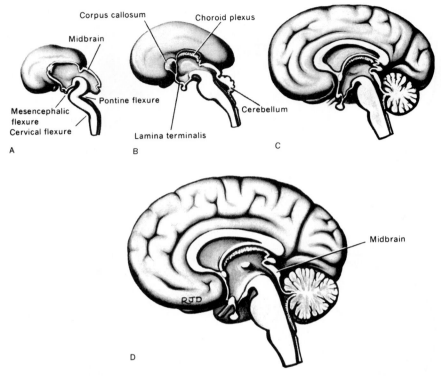

Figure 6.7: Human brain (midsagittal view): **A.** in a 3-month-old fetus; **B.** in a 4-month-old fetus; **C.** in an 8-month-old fetus; and **D.** in a newborn infant. (Adapted from Corliss.)

predominately tucked into the fissures and sulci. After the end of the second year the tertiary sulci dominate the topographic pattern of the cerebral surface. These sulci are variable from brain to brain and thereby put the stamp of individuality on each brain. Tertiary sulcation may continue throughout life.

Postnatal Growth

The large brain in the newborn infant exceeds 10% of the entire body weight; in the adult the brain constitutes only approximately 2% of the total body weight. The postnatal growth of the brain is rapid, especially during the first 2 years after birth. The brain weighs about 350 g in the full-term infant and about 1000 g at the end of the first year. The rate of growth slows down after this, and by puberty the brain weighs about 1250 g in girls and 1375 g in boys. It appears that the brain of a girl grows more rapidly than that of a boy up to the third year, but the brains of boys grow more rapidly after that. This brain

size is reflected in the growth of the cranial skeleton. In contrast to the adult, the young child has a large cranium in relation to the face. Head circumference is a measure of the growth of the brain. The head circumference is approximately 34 cm at birth, 46 cm at the end of the first year, 48 cm at the end of the second year, 52 cm at 10 years, and only slightly larger at puberty and in the adult.

CRITICAL PERIODS: EFFECTS OF GENETIC AND ENVIRONMENTAL FACTORS ON DEVELOPMENT

Of all the malformations and congenital defects in human beings, ranging from minor observable variations from the norm to lethal abnormalities, as many as one-half are estimated to involve the nervous system. Although the entire nervous system develops as an integrated organ system, its various parts and subparts mature at different rates and tempos. During its ontogeny, each structure passes through one or more critical periods, during which it is sensitive to various influences. These periods are generally times of rapid biochemical differentiation. In such a period, the proper influences have a significant role in advancing normal development. When normal influences are wanting or when abnormal influences are exerted at these critical times, subsequent normal development is often impaired. When the impaired development results in anatomic abnormalities which are present at birth, they are called *congenital malformations*. These abnormalities are usually caused by genetic factors (chromosomal abnormalities or mutant genes) and environmental factors.

Genetic Factors

Many cases of congenital mental deficiency and retardation are the result of trisomy of autosomes (three chromosomes instead of the usual pair). *Down's syndrome (mongolism)* is a genetic condition in which there are three of the No. 21 chromosome.

Another genetic disease, *phenylketonuria (PKU)*, is a clinical syndrome of marked mental retardation associated with irritability and abnormal EEG patterns. This condition is due to an inherited inborn error of phenylalanine metabolism (transmitted by an autosomal recessive gene) that results in an excessive accumulation of the amino acid phenylalanine and its metabolites. The basic defect is a deficiency of the enzyme phenylalanine hydroxylase in the liver; it is essential for the conversion of phenylalanine to tyrosine. Treatment consists of placing PKU patients on a low-phenylalanine diet commencing in the first year of life; it must be done at this time because the brain damage caused by this condition is due to the accumulation of excess phenylalanine, which reaches its peak between the second and third years of life.

Nutrition

Malnutrition and undernutrition during fetal life, infancy, and childhood do have an effect on the developing nervous system. Certain nutritional deficiencies, especially those occurring at the critical early rapid period of maturation, can result in permanent damage.

In humans, this critical period extends from the second trimester of pregnancy through most of the first year after birth. During this interval many neurons and macroglia are being replicated and much of the brain growth is taking place. Evidence indicates that under severe protein malnutrition, the rates of proliferation of new neurons and glial cells are reduced. This reduction occurs during fetal life because even the fetus is not protected from maternal malnutrition. The developing brain is vulnerable during the remainder of this critical period of postnatal life; the formation of glial cells is impaired, and myelination is inefficient. Severe malnutrition during this period in human infants is known as *marasmus*. If the child is fed a nutritionally adequate diet after this period, the damage is not completely repaired, even though normal appearance may be achieved in some subjects. Those who appear to be healthy have brains which may have been damaged by the protein deficiency. The functional abnormalities in children reared on nutritionally inadequate diets may consist of transient apathy, lethargy, or hyperirritability, together with a lesser intellectual development as measured by a decrease of some 10 to 20% of mental capacity.

Prolonged protein deficiency in children from 1 to 2 years of age may result in *kwashiorkor*. In this condition, the number of neurons is not reduced, because the deficiency occurs after the full complement of neurons is formed; however, the complete differentiation and connectivity of these cortical cells may be impaired. If, after being subjected to prolonged, severe malnutrition, children with kwashiorkor are fed a normal diet, their IQ test scores are still below those of other children in the same population, even siblings, who were not subjected to severe malnutrition.

The timing of nutritional deprivation is a critical factor in determining whether or not subsequent recovery from the effects of such deficiencies is possible. In contrast to brains of fetuses and young children, the brains of adolescents and adults are most resistant to permanent effects of malnutrition. The young and mature adult victims of starvation during World War II did not show any loss of intelligence after their nutritional rehabilitation.

The effects of malnutrition assume gigantic proportions in the world today. Roughly 60% of the world's preschool population—over 500 million children—is exposed to varying degrees of undernutrition. These children live primarily in underdeveloped lands on diets low in proteins and calories. Malnutrition is contributory to the early death of many of them. Survivors grow up in poverty and become adults with physical and mental handicaps. Therefore, these poverty (nongenetic) conditions are perpetuated through their children—to be passed on from one generation to the next.

Hormones

The mental retardation associated with cretinism in humans is due to a thyroid hormone deficiency at a critical period during the late stages of in utero development (estimated to begin at the seventh fetal month). The cerebral cortex of cretinoid individuals is poorly developed. There is a reduction in number and size of the cell bodies of the neurons, as well as hypoplasia of both their axons and dendrites.

Mental retardation of the cretinoid human child can be prevented or effectively remedied if adequate doses of thyroid hormones are given during the first year of life.

Amblyopia (Lazy Eye)

Amblyopia, or lazy-eye, in humans is a condition of reduced visual acuity caused by inadequate stimulation by formed objects of the macula of one eye between the second and fourth years of age. It results in a defect in the image viewed by the macula of the deviated eye. The slightly cross-eyed child favors one eye over the other to avoid seeing double (diplopia). In response to the altered balance of visual output from the two eyes, long lasting anatomical and physiological changes occur in the ocular dominance columns of visual cortex (Chap. 19). The inadequate input to the visual cortex from the macula of the deviated eye was insufficient during and limited to the critical period to nurture the maturation of the experience-dependent synaptic

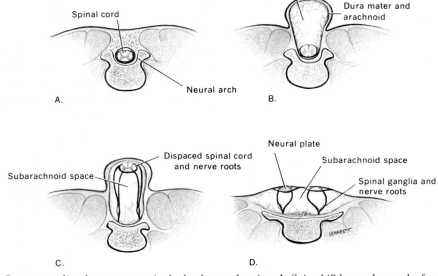

Figure 6.8: Some anomalies that may occur in the lumbosacral region. **A.** Spina bifida occulta results from the failure of the neural arches of the vertebrae to fuse dorsally. **B.** Spina bifida with meningocele is a defect with a subarachnoid fluid-filled meningeal cyst bulging through unfused neural arches. The cyst is covered with skin. **C.** Spina bifida with myelomeningocele is a defect with a meningeal cyst containing spinal cord and nerve roots. **D.** Spina bifida with myeloschisis is a defect in which the neural plate (having failed to close) is exposed to the surface. Devastating neural tube defects commonly are associated with a deficiency in folic acid. (Adapted from Corliss.)

plasticity in the ocular dominance columns. This failure during the critical period results in a permanent amblyopia. Ocular dominance plasticity is one of the best examples of synaptic plasticity in the neocortex.

This concept of the critical period during childhood is the basis for the suggestion that young children should be exposed to rich visual experiences, even more than they can handle intelligently. This should help to ensure the optimal maturation of the child's visual pathways.

Spina Bifida

Spina bifida is one of the more common examples of defects; the term is used to cover a wide range of closure defects, usually located in the lower lumbar region (Fig. 6.8). The most extreme version occurs when the neural plate in the lumbar region remains as a plate exposed to the outside. An infant with this defect has bladder and bowel incontinence, sensory loss, and motor paralysis of the lower extremities. In less severe cases the meninges, or the meninges along with the spinal cord, though displaced backward, are still covered by the skin. In a minor form, only the bony neural arches may be defective and functional impairment is absent.

SUGGESTED READINGS

Ambron R, Dulin M, Zhang X-P, Schmied R, Walters E. Axoplasm enriched in a protein mobilized by nerve injury elicits memory-like alterations in aplysia neurons. *J Neurosci.* 1995;15:14–23.

Bjorklund A, Stenevi U. Intracerebral neural implants: neuronal replacement and reconstruction of damaged circuitries. *Ann Rev Neurosci.* 1984: 7:279–308.

Bowen I. Apoptosis. In: Cuello A, ed. *Neuronal Death and Repair. Restorative Neurology.* Amsterdam: Elsevier; 1993;6:7–23.

Brauth S, Hall W, Dorling R, eds. *Plasticity of Development.* Cambridge, Mass: MIT Press; 1991.

England M. *A Color Atlas of Life Before Birth. Normal Fetal Development.* Chicago, Ill: Mosby Yearbook Pub; 1990.

Gilbert S. *Developmental Biology.* 3rd ed. Sunderland, Mass: Sinauer; 1991.

Goodman C, Bastiani M. How embryonic nerve cells recognize one another. *Sci Am.* 1984;251(6): 58–66.

Harwerth R, Smith E III, Duncan G, Crawford M, von Noorden G. Multiple sensitive periods in the development of the primate visual system. *Science.* 1986;232:235–238.

Jacobson M. *Developmental Neurobiology.* 3rd ed. New York, NY: Plenum; 1991.

Jessell T, Dodd J. Floor plate-derived signals and the control of neural plate patterns in vertebrates. *Harvey Lecture.* 1992;86:87–128.

Kaas J, Merzenich M, Killackey H. The reorganization of somatosensory cortex following peripheral nerve damage in adult and developing mammals. *Annu Rev Neurosci.* 1983;6:325–356.

Kennedy T, Serafini T, de la Torre J, Tessier-Lavigne M. Netrins are diffusible chemotropic factors for commissural axons in the embryonic spinal cord. *Cell.* 1994;78:425–435.

Lam D, Bray G. *Regeneration and Plasticity in the Mammalian Visual System.* Cambridge, Mass: MIT Press; 1992.

LeDouarin N, Smith J. Development of the peripheral nervous system from the neural crest. *Annu Rev Cell Biol.* 1988;4:375–404.

Ludrin S, Norman M. Congenital malformations of the nervous system. In: Davis R, Robertson D, eds. *Textbook of Neuropathology.* Baltimore, Md: Williams & Wilkins; 1985.

Lumsden A, O'Leary D. Development—editorial overview. *Curr Opin Neurobiol.* 1994;4:1–7.

Merzenich M, Nelson R, Stryker M, Cynader M, Schoppmann A, Zook J. Somatosensory cortical map changes following digit amputation in adult monkeys. *J Comp Neurol.* 1984;224:591–605.

Moore K, Persaud T. *The Developing Human. Clinically Oriented Embryology.* 5th ed. Philadelphia, Pa: WB Saunders; 1993.

Nishi R. Neurotrophic factors: two are better than one. *Science.* 1994;265:1052–1053.

Parnavelas J, Stern C, Sternling R, eds. *The Making of the Nervous System.* New York, NY: Oxford University Press, 1988.

Patel A. Undernutrition and brain development. *Trends Neurosci.* 1983;6:151–154.

Patterson P. Neuron-target interactions. In: Hall Z. *An Introduction to Molecular Neurobiology.* Sunderland, Mass: Sinauer; 1992:428–454.

Patterson P. Process outgrowth and specificity of connections. In: Hall Z. *An Introduction to Molecular Neurobiology.* Sunderland, Mass: Sinauer; 1992:388–427.

Purves D. *Body and Brain: A Trophic Theory of Neural Connections.* Cambridge, Mass: Harvard University Press; 1988.

Purves D. *Neural Activity and the Growth of the*

Brain. Cambridge: Cambridge University Press; 1994.

Purves D, Lichtman J. *Principles of Neural Development.* Sunderland, Mass: Sinauer; 1985.

Rakic P, Bourgeois J-P, Eckenhoff M, Zecevic N, Goldman-Rakic P. Concurrent overproduction of synapses in diverse regions of the primate cerebral cortex. *Science.* 1986;232:232–235.

Rowland L, Wood D, Schon E, DiMauro S, eds. *Molecular Genetics in Diseases of Brain, Nerve, and Muscle.* New York, NY: Oxford University Press, 1989.

Russell D. Neurotrophins: mechanisms of action. *The Neuroscientist.* 1995;1:3–6.

Sadler T. *Langman's Medical Embryology.* 6th ed. Baltimore, Md: Williams & Wilkins; 1990.

Sapolsky R. *Stress, the Aging Brain and the Mechanisms of Neuron Death.* Cambridge, Mass: Bradford Books, MIT Press; 1992.

Sladek J, Jr, Shoulson I. Neural transplantation: a call for patience rather than patients. *Science.* 1987;240:1386–1388.

Sperry R. Physiological plasticity and brain circuit theory. In: Harlow H, Woolsey C, eds. *Biological and Biochemical Bases of Behavior.* Madison, Wis: University of Wisconsin Press; 1958: 401–424.

Steller H. Mechanisms and genes of cellular suicide. *Science.* 1995;267:1445–1449.

Steward O. *Principles of Cellular, Molecular and Developmental Neuroscience.* New York, NY: Springer-Verlag; 1989.

Timiris P, Privat A, Giacobini E, Lauder J, Vernadakis A. Plasticity and Regeneration of the Nervous System. *Adv Exp Med Biol.* 1991;296: 1–365.

Volpe J. *Neurology of the Newborn.* 3rd ed. Philadelphia, Pa: WB Saunders; 1994.

Williams R, Herrup K. The control of neuron number. *Annu Rev Neurosci.* 1988;11:423–453.

Spinal Cord 7

The spinal cord is a cylinder of gray and white tissue (matter) that is located in the upper two-thirds of the vertebral canal and is surrounded by the bony vertebral column. It is the central processing and relay station (1) receiving input via the peripheral nerves from the body and descending tracts from the brain and (2) projecting output via peripheral nerves to the body and ascending tracts to the brain.

ANATOMIC ORGANIZATION

The spinal cord extends from the foramen magnum at the base of the skull to a cone-shaped termination, the *conus medullaris*, usually located at the caudal level of the first lumbar centrum. The nonneural *filum terminale* continues caudally as a filament from the conus medullaris to its attachment in the coccyx (Fig. 5.1).

Meningeal Coverings

The spinal cord is surrounded by the three meninges which are continuous with those encapsulating the brain (Chap. 5). All three meninges invest the spinal nerve roots emerging from the spinal cord and are continuous with the connective tissue sheath of the peripheral nerves.

The vascular *pia mater* is intimately attached to the spinal cord, its roots, and the filum terminale. The nonvascular *arachnoid* extends caudally to the sacral-2 vertebral level where it merges with the filum terminale. The *subarachnoid space*, which is filled with CSF and blood

vessels surrounds the spinal cord and is called the *spinal* or *lumbar cistern* between the conus medullaris and the sacral-2 level (Fig. 5.1). The roots of the lumbar and sacral spinal nerves "float" within the CSF of this cistern. To avoid injury to the spinal cord during removal of CSF, spinal taps into the cistern are made in the lower lumbar region. The *dura mater* and the capillary-thin *subdural space* (not containing CSF) surround the arachnoid and merge with the filum terminale. The spinal cord is suspended from the dura mater by a series of 20 to 22 pairs of *denticulate ligaments*, which are flanges extending laterally from the pia mater to the dura mater. The attachment to the dura mater is between two successive spinal nerves. The ligaments are oriented rostrocaudally in a frontal plane between the dorsal and ventral roots.

Between the dura mater (equivalent to inner dura mater surrounding the brain) and the periosteum of the vertebral column (equivalent to outer dura mater surrounding the brain) is the epidural space with its venous plexuses and fat. The *epidural space* caudal to the sacral-2 level is the site for the injection of anesthetics used to modify sensory input (e.g., saddle block for painless childbirth).

Blood Supply

The variably sized spinal arteries are branches of the vertebral, cervical, thoracic, and lumbar arteries. Each artery passes through an intervertebral foramen and divides into an anterior and a posterior spinal root (*radicular arteries*), which form an anastomotic plexus on the surface of the spinal cord. Venous drainage is via a venous plexus, and veins roughly parallel the arterial tree. The large spinovertebral venous plexus is continuous rostrally with that surrounding the brain. Venous pressure within these veins and CSF pressure may become elevated when the outflow of venous blood into the systemic circulation is impeded, as when the pressure in the thoracic and abdominal cavities increases while one is lifting a heavy object or coughing.

SPINAL ROOTS AND PERIPHERAL NERVES

The spinal cord receives its input and projects its output via nerve fibers in the spinal rootlets and roots, spinal nerves, and their branches (Figs. 7.1 and 7.2). Nerve fibers emerge from the spinal cord in an uninterrupted series of dorsal and ventral rootlets which join to form 31 pairs of *dorsal* and *ventral roots*. In the vicinity of each intervertebral foramen, a dorsal root and a ventral root join to form a *spinal nerve*, which supplies the innervation of a segment of the body. In all, there are 8 pairs of cervical (C); 12 of thoracic (T); 5 of lumbar (L); 5 of sacral (S); and 1 of coccygeal (Co) roots and nerves (Fig. 7.1; Table 7.1). (Cervical-1 and coccygeal-1 usually have only ventral roots.)

The thoracic, lumbar, and sacral nerves are numbered after the vertebra just rostral to the foramen through which they pass (e.g., T4 nerve emerges below T4 vertebra); the cervical nerves are numbered for the vertebra just caudal (e.g., C7 nerve is rostral to C7 vertebra). Because the spinal cord is much shorter than the bony vertebral column, the lumbar and sacral nerves develop long roots, which extend as the *cauda equina* (horse's tail) within the spinal cistern

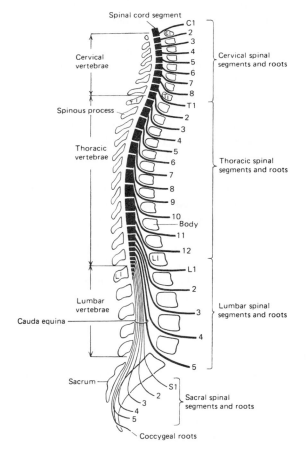

Figure 7.1: Topographic relations of the spinal cord segments, spinous processes, bodies of the vertebrae, intervertebral foramina, and spinal nerves. Refer to Table 7.1. Each spinal cord segment (except upper cervical segments) is located at a higher vertebral level than the site of the emergence of its spinal nerve through the intervertebral foramen.

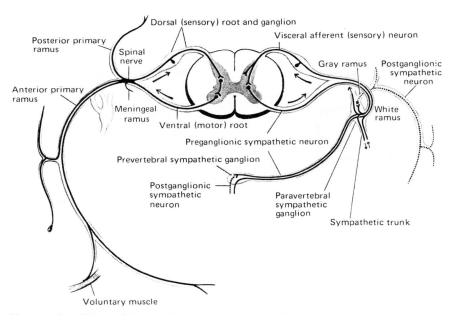

Figure 7.2: Neurons of a reflex arc of the somatic nervous system on the left, and a visceral reflex arc of the sympathetic nervous system on the right. The spinal somatic reflex arcs are described in Chapter 8, and the spinal visceral arcs in Chapter 20.

(Figs. 5.1 and 7.1). The spinal cord is enlarged in those segments that innervate the upper extremities—called the *cervical (brachial) enlargement*, from which emerge the roots of the C5 to T1 spinal nerves—and in those segments that innervate the lower extremities—called the *lumbosacral enlargement*, from which emerge the roots of the L3 to S2 spinal nerves.

Functional Components of Spinal Nerves

Each spinal nerve contains nerve fibers classified into one of four functional components,

namely: (1) *general somatic afferent*, (2) *general visceral afferent*, (3) *general somatic efferent*, and (4) *general visceral efferent*. Those components that are distributed throughout the body are designated *general*, those that innervate the body wall and extremities are somatic, and those that innervate the viscera are *visceral*. Furthermore, sensory fibers are *afferent* and motor fibers are *efferent*.

Dorsal Roots

The *dorsal (sensory) roots* consist of afferent fibers that convey input via spinal nerves from the sensory receptors in the body to the spinal cord (Fig. 7.2). The cell bodies of these neurons are located in the *dorsal root ganglia* within the intervertebral foramina. Despite the term, these ganglia contain no synapses. The fibers of the dorsal root of each spinal nerve supply the sensory innervation to a skin segment known as a dermatome (Fig. 7.3 and Table 7.2). There is usually no C1 or Co1 *dermatome*. Adjacent dermatomes overlap, so that the loss of one dorsal root results in diminished sensation, not a complete loss, in that dermatome (Chap. 9).

The general afferent fibers are classified first

Table 7.1

Spinal Process of Vertebra	Interspace Between Vertebral Bodies*	Spinal Cord Segment
C1		C1–2
C6	C6	T1
T10	T10	L1
T12	T12	S1
	T12–L1	All sacral and coccygeal levels
	S2 or S3	Caudal terminations of subarachnoid space
	Coccyx	Termination of filum terminale

Named from centrum of vertebra above interspace.

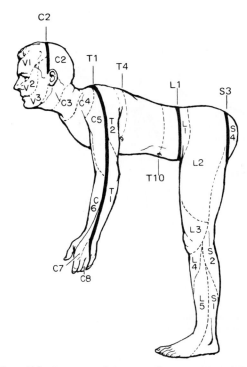

Figure 7.3: Dermatomal (segmental) innervation of the skin. Refer to Table 7.2. The trigeminal nerve is represented by the ophthalmic division (V1), maxillary division (V2), and mandibular division (V3). (Adapted from Haymaker W. *Bing's Local Diagnosis in Neurological Diseases.* St Louis, Mo: Mosby; 1969.)

into (1) *general somatic afferent (GSA)* fibers, conveying influences from sensors in the extremities and body wall and (2) *general visceral afferent (GVA)* fibers, conveying influences from the viscera (e.g., circulatory system).

A classification of sensory receptors and their probable functional roles are presented in

Table 7.2

Dorsal Spinal Root	Body Region Innervated*
C2	Occiput
C4	Neck and upper shoulder
T1	Upper thorax and inner side of arm
T4	Nipple zone
T10	Umbilical girdle zone
L1	Inguinal region
L4	Great toe, lateral thigh, and medial leg
S3	Medial thigh
S5	Perianal region

* Dermatome and region to which radicular parts is referred.

Table 7.3: Classification of Sensory Receptors (Probable Functional Roles)

I. Receptors of general sensibility (exteroceptive)
  A. Endings in epidermis
    1. Free nerve endings (tactile, pain, thermal sense)
    2. Terminal disks of Merkel (tactile)
    3. Nerve (peritrichial) endings in hair follicle (tactile, movement detector)
  B. Endings in connective tissues (skin and connective tissue throughout body)
    1. Free nerve endings (pain, thermal sense)
    2. Encapsulated nerve endings
      a. End bulbs of Ruffini (touch-pressure, position sense, kinesthesia)
      b. Corpuscles of Meissner (tactile, flutter sense)
      c. Corpuscles of Pacini (vibratory sense, touch-pressure)
  C. Endings in muscles, tendons, and joints (proprioceptive)
    1. Neuromuscular spindles (stretch receptors)
    2. Golgi tendon organs, neurotendinous endings (tension receptors)
    3. End bulbs of Ruffini in joint capsule (touch-pressure, position sense, kinesthesia)
    4. Corpuscles of Pacini (touch-pressure, vibratory sense, kinesthesia)
    5. Free nerve endings (pain)
II. Receptors of special senses
  A. Bipolar neurons of olfactory mucosa (olfaction)
  B. Taste buds (gustatory sense)
  C. Rods and cones in retina (vision)
  D. Hair cells in spiral organ of Corti (audition)
  E. Hair cells in semicircular canals, saccule, and utricle (equilibrium, vestibular sense)
III. Special receptors in viscera (interoceptive)
  A. Pressoreceptors in carotid sinus and aortic arch (monitor arterial pressure)
  B. Chemoreceptors in carotid and aortic bodies and in or on surface of medulla (monitor arterial oxygen and carbon dioxide levels)
  C. Chemoreceptors probably located in supraoptic nucleus of hypothalamus (monitor osmolarity of blood)
  D. Free nerve endings in viscera (pain, fullness)
  E. Receptors in lungs (respiratory and cough reflexes)

Table 7.3. Further details concerning sensations, functional significance, reflexes and pathways associated with these receptors are discussed in subsequent chapters. A classification of afferent fibers by conduction velocity recognizes groups I, II, III, and IV fibers (Chap. 8). Furthermore, group I is subdivided into Ia,

Table 7.4: Classification of Nerve Fibers

Fibers	Diameters	Conduction Velocity, m/s	Role/Receptors Innervated
		SENSORY*	
Ia (A-α)	12–20	70–120	Primary afferents of muscle spindle
Ib (A-α)	12–20	70–120	Golgi tendon organ
			Touch and pressure receptors
II (A-β)	5–14	30–70	Secondary afferents of muscle spindle
			Touch, pressure, and vibratory sense receptors
III (A-δ)	2–7	12–30	Touch and pressure receptors
			Pain and temperature receptors
IV (C)	0.5–1	0.5–2	Pain and temperature receptors
			Unmyelinated fibers
		MOTOR†	
Alpha (A-α)	12–20	15–120	Alpha motoneurons innervating extrafusal muscle fibers‡
Gamma (A-γ)	2–10	10–45	Gamma motoneurons innervating intrafusal muscle fibers‡
Preganglionic autonomic fibers (B)	>3	3–15	Lightly myelinated preganglionic autonomic fibers
Postganglionic autonomic fibers (C)	1	2	Unmyelinated postganglionic autonomic fibers

* The fibers of I, II, and III are myelinated and those of IV are unmyelinated. The fibers of I and II are associated with mechanoreceptors and those of III with mechanoreceptors in hair skin.
† Cell bodies of alpha and gamma motoneurons are located in lamina IX.
‡ A lower motoneuron (lower motor neuron, alpha motoneuron, gamma motoneuron) is a motor neuron with its cell body in the CNS and an axon that innervates voluntary (striated, skeletal) muscle fibers.

for nerve impulses from the primary sensory endings of the muscle spindles, and Ib, for impulses from the Golgi tendon organs (**Table 7.4**). Group II fibers transmit impulses from encapsulated skin and joint receptors (e.g., Meissner's and Pacinian corpuscles) monitoring touch, pressure, temperature, and joint movements, and from secondary sensory endings of muscle spindles. Group III and IV fibers transmit impulses arising from unencapsulated endings mediating pain, touch, and pressure. In all cases, those of greater diameter are faster in conduction; thinner fibers and myelinated fibers are faster than unmyelinated ones.

A second classification of fibers by conduction velocity into A, B, and C is also employed for both sensory and motor fibers. The A and B fibers are myelinated and the C fibers are unmyelinated. The A fibers are further divided by conduction velocity (hence fiber size) into alpha, beta, gamma, and delta (**Table 7.4**).

Ventral Roots

The ventral (motor) roots consist of efferent fibers that convey output from the spinal cord.

These fibers contain two functional components: (1) *general somatic efferent* (GSE) fibers, which innervate voluntary striated muscles (**Table 7.5**) and (2) *general visceral efferent* (GVE) fibers, which convey influences to the involuntary smooth muscles, cardiac muscle, and glands.

These fibers are axons of (1) *alpha motoneurons* that convey impulses to the motor end-plates of voluntary muscle fibers, (2) *gamma motoneurons* that convey impulses to the motor endings of intrafusal fibers of the muscle spindles (Chap. 8), and (3) *preganglionic autonomic*

Table 7.5

Ventral Spinal Root	Muscles Innervated
C5–6	Biceps brachii (flexes elbow)
C6–8	Triceps brachii (extends elbow)
T1–8	Thoracic musculature
T6–12	Abdominal musculature
L2–4	Quadriceps femoris (knee jerk, patellar tendon reflex)
L5–S1–2	Gastrocnemius (ankle jerk, Achilles tendon reflex)

neurons that synapse with postganglionic neurons (Chap. 20). Gamma motoneurons are also known as *fusimotor neurons* (innervate the muscles of the fusiform-shaped spindles). In addition, some sensory (afferent) fibers are present in the ventral roots (their cell bodies are in a dorsal root ganglia).

Each alpha motoneuron and the muscle fibers it innervates constitute a *motor unit*. Such units vary widely in the number of muscle fibers they contain, ranging from units innervating 3 to 8 muscle fibers in the small, finely controlled extraocular muscles of the eye to units innervating as many as 2,000 muscle fibers in such postural muscles as the soleus muscle of the leg. The muscle fibers of a motor unit interdigitate with the fibers of other motor units. In general, there are several functional types of muscle fibers, namely, fast (fast-twitch) fibers, slow (slow-twitch) fibers, and intermediate types with some features of each. Each motor unit consists of one type. The fibers of the fast motor units contract forcefully, relax rapidly, and fatigue quickly. They are pale in color, contain few mitochondria, are poorly vascularized, and obtain their energy through glycolysis. World-class sprinters and high jumpers, requiring quick starts and short bursts of speed, may have up to 85% of fast-twitch fibers. The fibers of the slow motor units contract and relax relatively slowly and tend to fatigue less rapidly. They are reddish in color, contain numerous mitochondria, are highly vascularized, and utilize oxidative metabolism for energy. World-class long-distance runners, especially marathoners, may have up to 90% slow-twitch fibers. They have great capacity for running through fatigue.

LAMINAE OF THE SPINAL CORD

The spinal cord is divided into the gray matter (cell bodies, dendrites, axons, and glial cells) and white matter (myelinated and unmyelinated axons and glial cells). The nerve fibers of the gray matter are oriented in the transverse plane, whereas those of the white matter are oriented in the longitudinal plane parallel to the neuraxis. The gray matter has been parceled anatomically, primarily on the basis of the microscopic appearance, into nuclei or laminae

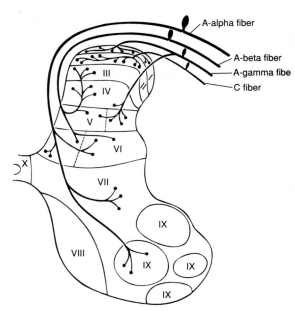

Figure 7.4: The sensory fibers of the dorsal root and the laminae of the spinal cord (Fig. 7.5) in which each terminates. The heavily myelinated A alpha fibers from the neuromuscular spindles and the Golgi tendon organs terminate in laminae VI, VII, and IX (Chap. 8). The myelinated A beta fibers from the cutaneous mechanoreceptors terminate in laminae III through VI (Chap. 10). The thinly myelinated and unmyelinated A delta and C fibers from nociceptors terminate in laminae I, II and V (Chap. 9). (Adapted from Brodal.)

Table 7.6

Lamina	Corresponding Nucleus
I	Posteromarginal nucleus
II	Substantia gelatinosa
III and IV	Proper sensory nucleus (nucleus proprius)
V	Zone anterior to lamina IV
VI	Zone at base of posterior horn
VII	Zona intermedia (includes intermediomedial and intermediolateral nuclei, dorsal nucleus of Clarke, and sacral autonomic nuclei)
VIII	Zone in anterior horn (restricted to medial aspect in cervical and lumbosacral enlargements)
IX	Medial nuclear column and lateral nuclear column

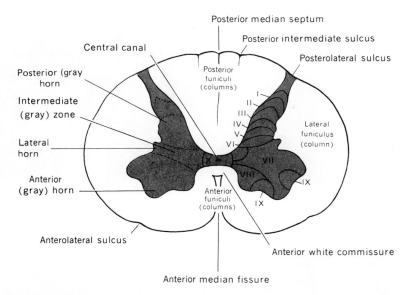

Figure 7.5: Section through a cervical level of the spinal cord to illustrate some subdivisions of the gray matter and white matter. The white matter is composed of three funiculi (columns). The gray matter is divided into two horns and an intermediate zone. Division of the gray matter into Rexed laminae is shown on the right.

(called *Rexed laminae*) (Figs. 7.4, 7.5, and Table 7.6). The gray matter is also divided into a *posterior horn* (laminae I through VI), an intermediate zone (lamina VII), and an *anterior horn* (laminae VIII and IX). The white matter comprises three columns (*funiculi*): posterior, lateral, and anterior (Fig. 7.5).

PATHWAYS AND TRACTS

Sensory signals originating in sensory receptors in the body and limbs are transmitted through the spinal cord to the brain along sensory pathways. Motor commands from the higher centers

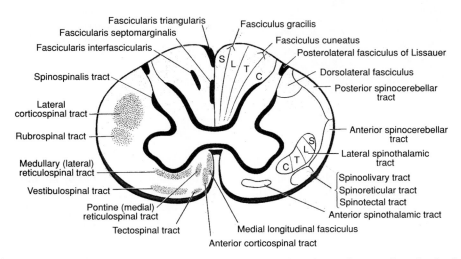

Figure 7.6: The spinal cord tracts. The ascending tracts are represented as plain outlines on the right, the descending tracts as stippled outlines on the left, and the intrinsic spinal tracts (composed of descending and/or ascending fibers) as solid outlines. The representation of the tracts is arbitrarily drawn. The lamination of the posterior columns and lateral spinothalamic tracts is indicated: C, cervical; T, thoracic; L, lumbar; and S, sacral.

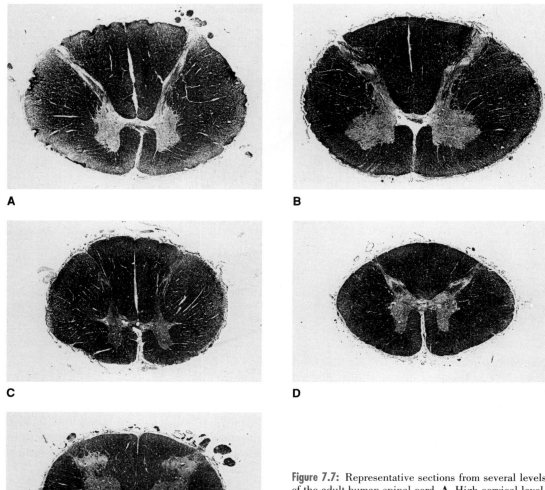

A

B

C

D

E

Figure 7.7: Representative sections from several levels of the adult human spinal cord. **A.** High cervical level. **B.** Cervical enlargement level. **C.** Midthoracic level. **D.** Low thoracic level. **E.** Lumbar level. All photographs of these Weigert-stained sections are at the same enlargement. (Courtesy of Dr Joyce Shriver, Mount Sinai School of Medicine.)

in the brain descend through the spinal cord along motor pathways. Within the white matter of the spinal cord the sensory fibers of the pathways form groups called *ascending tracts* or *fasciculi* and the fibers of the motor pathways form groups called *descending tracts* (Fig. 7.6). The functional significance and location of these pathways form a basis of neurologic diagnosis. Lesions within or impinging upon the nervous

system often are revealed by alterations in sensory perceptions, balance, or reflex activity. Lesions sometimes can be pinpointed by the examiner who has a thorough knowledge of these tracts and the associated roots of the spinal nerves.

Regional differences are present at various levels of the spinal cord (Fig. 7.7). The amount of gray matter at any spinal level is primarily related to the richness of the peripheral innervation. Hence, the gray matter is largest in the spinal segments of the cervical and lumbosacral enlargements innervating the upper and lower extremities; such large structures require a massive innervation. The thoracic and upper lumbar levels have relatively small amounts of gray matter: they innervate the thoracic and abdominal regions.

The absolute number of nerve fibers in the white matter increases at each successively higher spinal level. Stated otherwise, the white matter of a spinal level caudal to another level has fewer fibers. The difference results because (1) additional fibers of the ascending sensory pathways join the white matter at each successively higher level and (2) fibers of the descending motor pathways from the brain leave the white matter before terminating in the gray matter at each successive level.

SUGGESTED READINGS

Abel-Maguid T, Bowsher D. The grey matter of the dorsal horn of the adult human spinal cord, including comparisons with general somatic and visceral afferent cranial nerve nuclei. *J Anat.* 1985;142:33–58.

Bannister L. Sensory terminals of peripheral nerves. In: Landon DN, ed. *The Peripheral Nerve.* London: Chapman & Hall; 1976.

Boyd I, Davey M. *Composition of Peripheral Nerves.* Edinburgh: Livingstone; 1968.

Brown A. The terminations of cutaneous nerve fibres in the spinal cord. *Trends Neurosci.* 1981;4: 64–67.

Coggeshall R. Law of separation of function of the spinal roots. *Physiol Rev.* 1980;60:716–755.

Crock H, Yoshizaua H. *The Blood Supply of the Vertebral Column and Spinal Cord in Man.* New York, NY: Springer-Verlag; 1977.

Gillilan L. Significant superficial anastomoses in the arterial blood supply of the human brain. *J Comp Neurol.* 1958;115:55–74.

Hopkins W, Brown M. *Development of Nerve Cells and Their Connections.* New York, NY: Cambridge University Press; 1984.

Martin J, Jessell T. Modality coding in the somatic sensory system. In: Kandel E, Schwartz J, Jessell T, eds. *Principles of Neural Science.* 3rd ed. New York, NY: Elsevier; 1991:341–352.

Martin J, Jessell T. Anatomy of the somatic sensory system. In: Kandel E, Schwartz J, Jessell T, eds. *Principles of Neural Science.* 3rd ed. New York, NY: Elsevier; 1991:353–366.

Netter F. *Atlas of Human Anatomy.* West Caldwell, NJ: Ciba-Geigy Corp; 1989:plates 148–159.

Ralston D, Ralston H III. The terminations of the corticospinal tract axons in the macaque monkey. *J Comp Neurol.* 1985;242:325–337.

Schiebel A. The organization of the spinal cord. In: Davidoff R, ed. *Handbook of the Spinal Cord,* Vol 2. New York, NY: Dekker; 1984.

Reflexes and Muscle Tone 8

Organization of the somatic motor (efferent) system

Spinal reflex arcs

Muscle spindles

Stretch (myotatic, deep tendon) reflex

Gamma reflex loop

Golgi tendon organ (GTO) and reflex loop

Flexor reflexes

Muscle tone (Tonus)

Coactivation

Integration of spinal reflexes: role of interneurons

Somatic reflexes are the automatic stereotypic motor responses by voluntary muscles to adequate sensory stimuli. From a vast array of external and internal stimuli bombarding the body, selections are made by sensory receptors within the skin, voluntary muscles, tendons, and joints. From them a continuous flow of sensory messages are transmitted via spinal and cranial sensory nerves to the spinal cord and brainstem for processing in order to achieve response goals. These are realized by information conveyed via *alpha motoneurons* to the extrafusal muscle fibers and via *gamma motoneurons* to the intrafusal muscle fibers (see later). The alpha and gamma motoneurons, called *lower motoneurons*, comprise the *final common pathway* that controls striated muscle activities expressed as reflex, postural, rhythmic, and voluntary movements.

The motor apparatus consists of a mechanical arrangement of muscles, bones, and joints organized as levers. Each movement at a joint involves the interplay between agonist muscles and antagonist muscles (including accessory muscles for adjustments). The agonist muscles execute the prime movement and the antagonist muscles counterbalance agonists. The antago-

nist muscles are involved in decelerating and stabilizing the movement. The *spinal reflex responses*, such as the withdrawal of the upper limb when the finger contacts a hot stove, are automatic reactions to stimuli involving a simple, neural sequence of a receptor, sensory neurons, interneurons, lower motor neurons, and voluntary muscles. *Posture* is essential as a foundation for the performance of other movements. This positioning and orientation of the body in space is sustained by the constant compensatory adjustments by the musculature in response to shifts in gravity. *Rhythmic motor patterned movements* such as walking, running, and chewing, once voluntarily initiated, continue to be executed automatically. They combine voluntary and reflex activity. The *voluntary movements* initiated in the highest centers in the brain utilize the above stated movements to express the goals of the skilled volitional actions. These are learned, mastered, honed, and sustained by various amounts of practice. Included are playing a musical instrument, using a word processor, driving a car, riding a bicycle, and participating in such sports as golf, fly casting, and baseball. The proprioceptive receptors are the essential sensors generating a continuous flow of critical information that enables the central nervous system to activate the exquisite coordination of the body musculature required for these reflexes and movements.

Proprioception includes the information sensed by low-threshold mechanoreceptors of the musculoskeletal system comprising muscles, tendons, joint capsules, and ligaments. Their activity results in sensing the position and movements of the limbs, head, jaws, and back. Its two submodalities are sense of stationary position (*position sense*) and sense of movement (*kinesthesia or kinesthetic sense*). The peripheral receptors signaling these senses include (1) neuromuscular spindles (stretch receptors in muscle) and Golgi tendon organs (tension receptors in tendons), (2) mechanoreceptors in joint capsules, and (3) some cutaneous mechanoreceptors (Chapter 10). The information sensed by these somatic receptors is integrated into the spinal reflexes and muscle tone involving the voluntary muscles. This also applies to these activities associated with somatic cranial nerves and the brainstem (jaw reflex, Chapter 10). The *conscious senses* of *position sense* and *kinesthesia* are conveyed via labeled lines of the dorsal column-medial lemniscus system. The *unconscious sense* of *proprioception* is conveyed via the spinocerebellar tracts to the cerebellum (Chapter 10).

ORGANIZATION OF THE SOMATIC MOTOR (EFFERENT) SYSTEM

The somatic nervous system can be conceptualized as a complex integrated assemblage of neural circuits functioning to regulate the activity of the voluntary muscles—those that primarily act through levers of bones and joints. It is only by influencing muscles to contract (or to relax) that the somatic nervous system can express itself. These influences are made manifest through postures and movements. Postures are the body poses from which each movement begins and ends. Each posture is maintained and controlled through a series of reflexes and reactions that utilize continuously acting feedback circuits operating through several segmental levels of control (see later). The flow of voluntary muscle activity from one posture to another

posture is a movement. In this context, posture is the framework for a movement, whether crude, stereotyped, skilled, or volitional.

The motor systems within the CNS are hierarchically organized into (1) the spinal cord, (2) the brainstem, and (3) the cerebral cortical level. The *spinal cord level* is involved in automatic and stereotypic responses to peripheral stimuli—known as *reflex responses*. Reflex activity can be modulated from higher levels—that is, either enhanced by excitatory influences or suppressed by inhibitory influences. The *brainstem level* includes the nuclei of origin and their descending motor pathways that project to influence the motor activity of the spinal cord reflex circuits (Chap. 11). The brainstem centers process neural influences from the cerebral cortex, spinal cord, and cranial nerves (particularly the vestibular nerve). They are integrated into the motor systems projecting to the spinal cord, that include the corticoreticulospinal pathways, corticorubrospinal pathway, vestibulospinal pathways, corticotectospinal pathway, and raphe-spinal and ceruleus-spinal projections. The *cerebral cortical level* comprises the motor areas from which, in addition to those mentioned above, originate the corticobulbar and the corticospinal tracts (Chaps. 11 and 25). From this level, motor commands stimulate nuclei in the brainstem and spinal cord that activate skilled movements such as speech and writing.

The basal ganglia and cerebellum are major neural structures that participate in modulating the activity of the motor systems. The basal ganglia are specifically involved with movements formulated at the cortical level, including planning of synergies among the muscles during movements (Chap. 24). These ganglia receive influences from all neocortical areas and, following processing, direct their activity to influence the motor and premotor cortical areas. The cerebellum has a critical role in acting as a modulator during the on-going motor activity in coordinating the sequence and strength of muscular contractions (Chap. 18).

SPINAL REFLEX ARCS

Reflex responses are mediated by neuronal linkages called *reflex arcs* or *loops*. The struc-

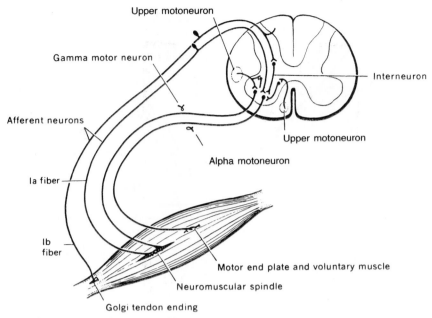

Figure 8.1: Three types of reflex loops are illustrated: (1) The myotatic reflex loop consists of a muscle spindle, Ia afferent neuron, alpha motoneuron, and voluntary muscle fiber. (2) The gamma reflex loop consists of the sequence gamma motoneuron, muscle spindle, Ia afferent neuron, alpha motoneuron, and voluntary muscle fiber. (3) The Golgi tendon organ (GTO) loop consists of the sequence GTO, Ib afferent neuron, spinal interneuron, alpha motoneuron, and voluntary muscle fiber.

ture of a spinal somatic reflex arc can be summarized in the following manner: (1) A sensory receptor responds to an environmental stimulus. (2) An afferent root neuron conveys influences via the peripheral nerves to the gray matter of the spinal cord. (3a) In the simplest reflex arc the afferent root neuron enters the spinal cord in order to synapse directly with the lower motoneurons (*monosynaptic reflex*; Fig. 8.1). (3b) In the more complex and more common reflex arcs, the afferent root neuron synapses with interneurons which, in turn, synapse with lower motoneurons (polysynaptic reflex; Figs. 8.1 and 8.3). (4) A lower motoneuron transmits influences to effectors—the striated voluntary (skeletal) muscles (Fig. 8.2, Table 7.4).

Spinal reflexes are also classified as (1) intrasegmental, (2) intersegmental, and (3) suprasegmental reflexes. A *segmental reflex* comprises neurons associated with one or even a few spinal segments. An *intersegmental reflex* consists of neurons associated with several to many spinal segments. A *suprasegmental reflex*

involves neurons in the brain that influence the reflex activity in the spinal cord.

Reflexes in which the sensory receptor is in the muscle spindle of any muscle group are known as the *myotatic, stretch,* or *deep tendon reflexes* (DTR). These are intrasegmental reflexes. Examples are: (1) the biceps reflex—tapping the biceps brachii tendon results in flexion of the forearm at the elbow, (2) the triceps reflex—tapping the triceps tendon results in extension of the forearm at the elbow, (3) the quadriceps reflex (knee jerk)—tapping of the quadriceps tendon results in extension of the leg at the knee, and (4) the triceps sural reflex (ankle jerk)—tapping of the Achilles tendon results in plantar flexion of the foot.

Reflexes in which the sensory receptor is the Golgi tendon organ (GTO), located in a tendon at its junction with a muscle, are known as *Golgi tendon reflexes* (Fig. 8.1 and later discussion).

A third kind of reflex, with sensory receptors variously located, is a *flexor reflex* (Fig. 8.3). In this reflex, for example, the upper extremity

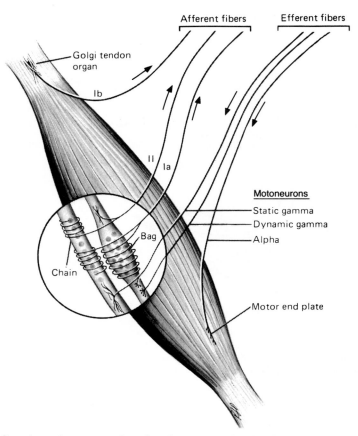

Afferent fibers   Efferent fibers

Golgi tendon
organ

Ib

II   Ia

Motoneurons
Static gamma
Dynamic gamma
Alpha

Bag

Chain

Motor end plate

Figure 8.2: Nerve endings in a voluntary muscle and tendon associated with reflexes. The Golgi tendon organ (GTO) consists of afferent terminals intertwined among braided collagenous fibers. The intrafusal muscle fibers in the muscle spindle (enlarged section) are innervated by Ia and Group II afferent fibers and by static and dynamic gamma motoneurons. The Ia fiber forms a spiral ending in the bag region of a nuclear bag fiber and in the midregion of a nuclear chain fiber. The Group II fiber commences on either side of the primary endings of chain and static bag fibers. Gamma motoneurons terminate in the contractile polar regions of the intrafusal fibers. The static gamma motoneuron terminates as trail endings mainly on the chain fiber and occasionally on a bag fiber. The dynamic gamma motoneuron terminates as plate endings on a bag fiber. The alpha motoneuron terminates as a motor end-plate on an extrafusal muscle fiber.

The muscle spindle is a stretch-gated receptor (responds to muscle stretch) and the GTO is a tension-gated receptor (responds to muscle tension).

withdraws from a noxious stimulus such as a hot stove. The reflex comprises (1) sensory receptors, (2) afferent neurons, (3) spinal interneurons, (4) alpha motoneurons, and (5) voluntary muscles. The flexor reflex is a protective reflex initiated by a diverse group of receptors in the skin, muscles, joints, and viscera and is conveyed by A-delta and C pain fibers, as well as Group III and IV fibers (called flexor reflex afferents [FRAs]). Intense stimulation can elevate the level of excitability within the spinal cord to a point at which a *crossed reflex* is

evoked, with such responses as leaning or jumping away from a stimulus (Fig. 8.4).

MUSCLE SPINDLES

A *muscle spindle (neuromuscular spindle)* is a 3- to 4-millimeter long spindle-shaped (fusiform) receptor consisting of a capsule encasing 2 to 12 modified striated muscle fibers known as *intrafusal fibers* (Fig. 8.2). The spindles are oriented parallel (said to be *in parallel*) to the skel-

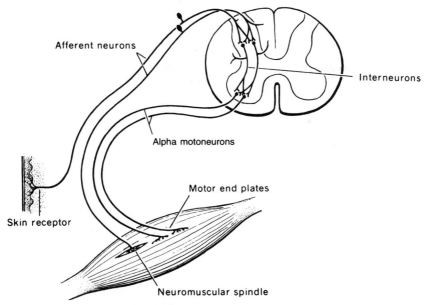

Figure 8.3: The flexor (withdrawal) reflex. This loop consists of the sequence skin receptor, afferent neuron, spinal interneuron, alpha motoneuron, and voluntary muscle fiber.

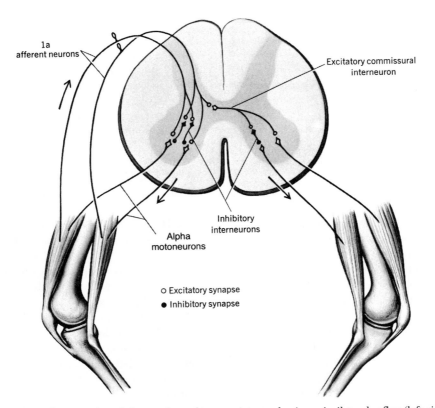

Figure 8.4: Reciprocal innervation of the agonist and antagonist muscles in an ipsilateral reflex (left side) and in a contralateral crossed reflex (right side).

etal *extrafusal fibers*, called this because of their location outside the spindles. Extrafusal fibers are the voluntary muscles that perform the work of contraction. The capsule of the spindle is continuous with the connective tissue between the extrafusal fibers and, in turn, with the tendon of the muscle.

Muscle spindles are sensory receptors that monitor the length and rate of change in length of the extrafusal fibers, and, thus, are called *stretch receptors*. They have both a motor and a sensory innervation. The motor innervation of the intrafusal fibers is by *gamma motoneurons (fusimotor neurons)* and the extrafusal fibers by the *alpha motoneurons*. The sensory innervation of the intrafusal fibers is by Group Ia fibers and Group II fibers. Alpha motoneurons and gamma motoneurons are also called lower motoneurons.

Three types of intrafusal fibers are located within a muscle spindle: (1) dynamic nuclear bag fibers, (2) static nuclear bag fibers, and (3) nuclear chain fibers (**Fig. 8.2**). Each fiber is a specialized muscle fiber with a central region that is not contractile. The bag fibers are relatively long and large with each containing numerous nuclei in a central enlargement or bag—hence, bag fibers. The chain fibers are thinner and shorter with each containing a row of nuclei in the central region resembling a chain—hence, chain fibers. The nuclear bag fibers are apparently accountable for the dynamic sensitivity of the primary sensory endings, while the nuclear chain fibers are accountable for the static sensitivity of both the primary and secondary sensory endings.

The sensory endings are associated with the central regions of the intrafusal fibers and are responsive to the stretch of these muscle fibers. The gamma motor neurons innervate the contractile polar regions of the intrafusal fibers. Contractions of these intrafusal fibers tug at the central non-contractile region from both ends and increase the sensitivity of the sensory endings to stretch.

The spindles are innervated by two types of sensory endings—(1) *primary* or *annulospiral endings* derived from Group Ia fibers and (2) *secondary* or *flower-spray endings* derived from Group II fibers (**Fig. 8.2**). The primary endings terminate as spiral endings on the bag region of the bag fibers and the equatorial region of the chain fibers. The secondary endings terminate as a spray (flower spray endings) on either side of the primary endings on both types of fibers (**Fig. 8.2**). The gamma motoneurons terminate on the bag and chain fibers as *plate endings* (motor end-plates) and *trail endings*. Plate endings terminate primarily on the bag fibers and infrequently on the chain fibers. Trail endings also terminate on both fiber types, but primarily in the chain fibers.

The Group Ia afferent (large myelinated) nerve fibers innervates all 3 types of intrafusal muscle fibers to form primary endings (**Fig. 8.2**). The Group II afferent (small myelinated) nerve fibers innervate both chain and bag fibers to form secondary endings. The gamma motoneurons and their axons enable the CNS to control the sensitivity of the muscle spindles to length and changes in length. Two types of gamma motor neurons innervate the three types of intrafusal fibers. (1) Dynamic gamma motoneurons only innervate dynamic bag fibers. This type increases the dynamic sensitivity of the muscle spindle (gamma dynamic). This is important in reacting to external forces that upset body balance and on-going movements. (2) Static gamma motoneurons innervate combinations of static bag fibers and chain fibers. These static motoneurons act to increase the static sensitivity of the muscle spindle (gamma static). This acts to increase the firing rate of the afferent fibers to the muscle spindle during constant and maintained muscle length.

The muscle spindle is specialized to sense muscle length and the velocity of muscle length change. Thus the spindle is a stretch-gated receptor responding to muscle stretch. In contrast, the GTO of a muscle tendon is a tension-gated receptor responding to muscle tension (see later).

Each Ia sensory neuron has direct monosynaptic connections with alpha motoneurons within the spinal cord (**Fig. 8.1**). Group Ia fibers from the primary endings of spindles can synapse monosynaptically with alpha spindles that innervate the same muscle containing the spindle—called a *homonymous muscle*—or can synapse monosynaptically with alpha motoneurons that innervate a synergistically acting muscle—called a *heteronymous muscle*. The Group II afferent fibers have direct monosynaptic connections with alpha motoneurons innervating homonymous muscles. Some gamma motoneurons, called *dynamic gamma motoneurons*, are thought to terminate only on bag fibers as plate endings. They are named for their involvement in phasic (motion) reflexes. The other gamma motoneurons, called *static gamma motoneurons*, terminate on bag and chain fibers as trail endings. These neurons are important in tonic (i.e., static or postural) reflexes.

Much of the information from the spindles is conveyed via ascending tracts for processing in the CNS especially in the cerebellum and the cerebral cortex (somatosensory cortex; Chap. 25).

STRETCH (MYOTATIC, DEEP TENDON) REFLEX

Stretch reflexes have an essential role in the maintenance of muscle tonus and posture (**Fig. 8.1**). The simple knee jerk is a *stretch (extensor) reflex* initiated by tapping the tendon of the relaxed quadriceps femoris muscle. Stretch reflexes are *two-neuron* (involving the sequence of an afferent neuron and an efferent alpha motoneuron), *monosynaptic* (only one set of synapses between the two neurons), *ipsilateral* (reflex restricted to one side of the body), and *intrasegmental* reflexes. The tap on the tendon stretches the quadriceps muscle and many of the neuromuscular spindles. When stretched, the spindles stimulate the Group Ia afferent fibers to convey volleys of impulses, that (1) monosynaptically excite the alpha motoneurons, that in turn stimulate the quadriceps muscle to contract and (2) through interneurons, inhibit the alpha motoneurons innervating the antagonistic hamstring muscles. Thus the leg extends at the knee joint as the quadriceps suddenly contracts and the hamstrings relax. The brisk knee jerk is initiated by the sudden *synchronous* stretch of many quadriceps muscle spindles. In contrast, the slow continuous contractions maintaining postural muscle tonus are sustained by the *asynchronous* stretch and discharge of many spindles over a period of time.

GAMMA REFLEX LOOP

The myotatic reflex acts in the coarse adjustments of muscle tension; the fine adjustments in muscle activity are dependent upon the integrity of the gamma reflex loop. Influences from the brain (supraspinal influences) and some peripheral receptors regulate the "set" of the muscle spindles through the gamma motoneurons.

The *gamma loop* (**Fig. 8.1**) comprises the (1) efferent gamma motoneuron, (2) muscle spindle within the voluntary muscle, (3) Group Ia afferent neuron for feedback, (4) alpha motoneuron, and (5) voluntary muscle fibers. The influences conveyed by the gamma motoneuron alter the sensitivity of the muscle spindle by altering the length of the intrafusal fibers and the tension they exert. As gamma motoneuron activity increases, the set of the muscle spindles can be raised to a higher level. This can increase the firing rate of the Ia fibers, stimulating the alpha motoneurons. Many of the descending supraspinal influences from the brain do not act directly on alpha motoneurons, but, rather, through this gamma reflex loop.

The *static gamma neurons* are involved preferentially with tonic reflexes (muscle tone). The rigidity associated with increased tonic stretch reflexes (as in Parkinson's disease) may be due to heightened activity of the static gamma neurons. The *dynamic gamma neurons* are involved with the phasic stretch reflexes, i.e., contraction of muscles for movement. The spastic signs expressed in upper motoneuron paralysis (Chap. 12) may be due primarily to increased activity of the dynamic gamma neurons. In effect, this gamma system is critical for continuous fine muscle control. This permits the spindle to maintain its delicate sensibility over a wide range of muscle lengths that are constantly occurring during reflex and voluntary contractions.

GOLGI TENDON ORGAN (GTO) AND REFLEX LOOP

The GTOs (neurotendinous spindles) are encapsulated mechanoreceptors located at the junctions of muscles with tendons (**Fig. 8.1**).

Within the capsule of the GTO are endings of Ib afferent fibers intertwined among collagenous fibers of the tendon (Fig. 8.2). The shortening of the muscle during contraction tightens the braided collagenous fibers which, by squeezing the nerve endings, generate action potentials. In general, the GTOs in a tendon respond to various degrees of muscle tension. Specifically, the GTOs within each tendon respond differentially because each GTO is linked through collagenous fibers to a different number of muscle fibers and to different types of motor units. Thus, different degrees of "squeezing" exerted within a GTO on the Ib ending contribute to the subtlety of the neural influences conveyed from a variety of GTOs to the spinal cord.

This loop comprises (1) the GTO in muscle tendons, (2) Group Ib afferent fibers, (3) interneurons within the spinal cord, (4) alpha motoneurons, and (5) striated muscle fibers. As the tension within the tendon of a contracting muscle increases, the GTOs increase the number of action potentials conveyed via the Ib afferent neurons to an interneuron pool of the spinal cord. These influences tend to inhibit the activity of the alpha motoneurons. The exquisite balance between the excitatory gamma loop and the inhibitory GTO reflex loop is basic to the precise integration of reflex activity. The GTO reflex loop acts to prevent the over-contraction of the agonist muscle and facilitate the contraction of the antagonist muscles through reciprocal inhibition.

FLEXOR REFLEXES

Flexor reflexes are associated with (1) such behavioral responses as protection against a potentially harmful noxious stimuli and (2) such locomotor activities as walking and running. These reflexes are initiated by pain receptors (nociceptors) in the skin (cutaneous), fasciae, and joints, as well as touch, pressure, and other receptors.

Withdrawal, Protective, and Escape Responses

The flexor reflex is fundamentally a withdrawal response from a noxious stimulus. Depending on the seriousness of this potentially threaten-

ing act, an individual reacts with protective and even escape responses. Cutaneous receptors in skin and deep receptors in muscles and joints react to intense touch/pressure, heat, cold, and tissue trauma, along with the associated pain. These stimuli are conveyed via Group II, III, and IV (called FRAs) fibers to interneurons in the CNS. The effect of these inputs results in flexion through (1) excitation of the alpha motoneurons to the flexor muscles and (2) inhibition of the alpha motoneurons to the antagonistic extensor muscles. The high intensity of the stimuli results in the spread of the activity via commissural neurons and intersegmental circuits to the contralateral side to evoke the crossed extensor reflexes (Fig. 8.4) with the synchronous excitation of the extensor lower motoneurons and the inhibition of the flexor lower motoneurons. This occurs, for example, in the act of withdrawing an upper limb following touching a hot object accompanied by shifting the weight to the contralateral lower limb to support the body.

Locomotion

In this activity, the brain contributes by influencing the integrated rhythms of the reflexes of flexion and extension of the upper and lower limbs as in locomotion. The FRAs contribute through multineuronal reflex circuits to inhibit the extensor motoneurons and to excite the flexor motoneurons of a lower limb and to excite the extensor motoneurons and to inhibit the motoneurons of the contralateral limb (Fig. 8.4). Through spinal intersegmental circuits, the rhythmic activity of the lower limbs is integrated with the rhythmic activities of the upper limbs as is characteristic in walking and running.

MUSCLE TONE (TONUS)

Muscle tone is the minimal degree of contraction exhibited by a muscle without conscious effort; it exists even when the muscle is "at rest." When an examiner manipulates an extremity (e.g., flexion and extension) of a relaxed, normal individual, the muscle tone is the amount of resistance that is not related to any conscious effort by the patient. Abnormalities of muscle tone are expressed as *hypotonia* (decreased resistance to passive movement) and *hypertonia* (increased resistance to passive movement; Chap. 11).

Hypotonus is not an expression of the isolated muscle so much as an expression of reflex nervous activity upon the muscle. Hypotonia can be produced (1) by severing the ventral roots containing the motor fibers to a muscle or (2) by severing the dorsal roots containing the sensory fibers from a muscle. Lesions of the cerebellum can also result in hypotonia.

Hypertonia is expressed in two forms: spasticity and rigidity. Spasticity combines an increase in resistance to passive manipulation with the "clasp knife" phenomenon along with an increase in DTRs (hyperreflexia). The "clasp knife" phenomenon is so-called because there is a marked increase in resistance during the initial phases of action, but suddenly the resistance disappears (as when opening the blade of a jack knife). *Rigidity* is expressed as increased tone (hypertonia) in all muscles although the strength and reflexes are not affected. The rigidity may be uniform throughout the range of movement imposed by the examiner (called *plastic* or *lead pipe rigidity*) or it may be interrupted by a series of jerks (called *cog-wheel rigidity* as in Parkinson's disease, see Chap. 24).

COACTIVATION

Neural influences from the brain via the descending motor pathways to the brainstem and spinal cord circuits stimulate the *simultaneous* discharge of both alpha and gamma motoneurons of a particular muscle (Chap. 3). This is known as the *coactivation* of these lower motoneurons. Coactivation is essential in the performance of a smooth coordinated muscular activity and in sustaining a voluntary contraction. The voluntary activities, ranging from the exquisite movements of a figure skater on ice to the lifting and holding of a heavy object, are largely dependent upon the coordinated contractions of muscle fibers.

The following is the sequence of events in coactivation: The stimulation of the alpha motoneurons results in the contraction of a muscle with the accompanying shortening of its muscle

spindles. This brings about a reduction in the firing rate of the Ia afferents and of the excitatory influences to the alpha motoneurons. This reduction is offset by the stimulation (*coactivation*) of the gamma motoneurons innervating the intrafusal fibers of the muscle spindles. By stimulating the intrafusal fibers, these neurons maintain the appropriate firing rate of the Ia afferent fibers, which excite the alpha motoneurons innervating the extrafusal muscle fibers.

The alpha and gamma motoneurons innervating a specific muscle or muscle group are simultaneously stimulated by neurons receiving their influences from segmental and intersegmental circuits and from upper motoneurons originating in the brain.

As compared to the alpha motoneurons, the gamma motoneurons (1) only innervate intrafusal muscle fibers, (2) have smaller cell bodies and thin myelinated fibers, (3) are not excited monosynaptically by afferent fibers from peripheral receptors, (4) are not integrated into the inhibitory Renshaw cell feedback circuit, and (5) tend to discharge spontaneously. The gamma motoneurons are influenced through the descending tracts by the activity of the cerebellum (Chap. 18), reticular system (Chap. 22), and basal ganglia (Chap. 24).

INTEGRATION OF THE SPINAL REFLEXES: ROLE OF INTERNEURONS

Somatic movements are the motor expressions of the integrated activity of the supraspinal pathways from the brain (Chap. 11) and many reflex loops; all are realized through the lower motoneurons. The placement of the interneurons within most of these reflex loops adds to the complexity and versatility of the motor control.

The descending motor supraspinal pathways from the brain influence either (1) indirectly, by synapsing with interneurons integrated into spinal neural circuits or (2) directly, by synapsing with the lower motoneurons. The alpha motoneurons are stimulated primarily through indirect supraspinal connections. Some fibers of the corticospinal tract, lateral vestibulospinal tract, reticulospinal tracts, and raphe spinal tract make monosynaptic connections with the alpha motor neurons. These alpha motoneurons contribute to the intrinsic spinal circuitry through collateral branches that excite interneurons called *Renshaw cells* (Fig. 3.10). In turn, the excited glycinergic Renshaw cells are intercalated in a negative feedback circuit that directly inhibits the alpha motoneuron. This tends to turn off the firing activity of the alpha motoneuron so that it will be ready to respond to firing again in response to excitatory stimulation. *Intersegmental interneurons* convey influences from one spinal segment via axons to one or more other spinal segments on the same side of the spinal cord. These neurons are connected with commissural interneurons (see later) and together they act in integrated rhythmic movements of the upper and lower extremities such as walking and running. However, interneuronal circuits are crucial in all movements. For example, in a smooth flexion movement, the flexor (agonist) muscle group contracts while the extensor (antagonist) muscle group relaxes for this type of action; this is a consequence of reciprocal innervation, which is a form of neural processing. The neurons involved with reciprocal innervation have axons (1) that make excitatory synaptic connections with the lower motoneurons innervating agonist muscles, and collateral branches (2) that synapse with inhibitory interneurons. In turn, these interneurons inhibit lower motoneurons innervating the antagonistic muscles. In effect, this coordinates the action of the opposing muscles—the one contracts while the other relaxes. Other forms of neural processing are noted in Fig. 3.11.

Commissural interneurons relay influences from one side across the midline to the gray matter of the contralateral side. These are important in *crossed reflexes*, also known as *crossed extensor reflexes* (Fig. 8.4). The extremity opposite to that in which the FRA fibers are stimulated responds in the reverse fashion. That is, the extensor muscles contract and the flexor muscles relax. This crossed (extensor) reflex utilizes the commissural neurons to relay neural information to the opposite side. A painful stimulus to the foot (stepping on a tack) evokes a reflex flexor withdrawal of the ipsilateral extremity and especially an enhancement of ex-

tensor musculature contractions of the contralateral extremity enabling the contralateral extended limb to support the body, while the flexed ipsilateral extremity is off the ground. The interplay of these crossed reflexes is utilized in the alternate rhythms of both upper and lower extremities during running and walking.

The afferent neurons innervating the sensory receptors are integrated into the spinal reflexes for feedback purposes. In addition to their role as monitors of new and naive information, the receptors sense the effects of motor activity and feed this information back to the CNS. Through this input, the circuitry within the CNS is continuously informed of its effects on muscular activity. In this role, these neurons are known as feedback (reafferent or reentry) neurons. The receptors at work in this feedback schema are known as direct receptors and indirect receptors. Direct receptors—the muscle spindles—are directly innervated by gamma motoneurons from the CNS and, thus, are integrated into direct feedback circuits. *Indirect receptors*, such as the GTO, joint, and cutaneous receptors, do not have a direct efferent innervation from the CNS and, thus, are integrated into so-called indirect feedback circuits.

SUGGESTING READINGS

Brooks V. *The Neural Basis of Motor Control.* New York, NY: Oxford University Press; 1986.

Desmedt J, ed. *Motor Control Mechanisms in Health and Disease.* New York, NY: Raven Press; 1983.

Freund H. Motor unit and muscle activity in voluntary motor control. *Physiol Rev.* 1983;63: 387–436.

Hasan Z, Stuart D. Animal solutions to problems of movement control: the role of proprioceptors. *Ann Rev Neurosci.* 1988;11:199–223.

Henneman E. Organization of the spinal cord and its reflexes. In: Mountcastle V, ed. *Medical Physiology.* 14th ed. St Louis, Mo: CV Mosby; 1980; 1:762–786.

Jewett D, Rayner M. *Basic Concepts in Neuronal Function.* Boston, Mass: Little Brown & Co; 1984:329–388.

Matthews P. *Mammalian Muscle Receptors and Their Central Actions.* London: Edward Arnold; 1972.

Phillips C. Motor apparatus of the baboon's hand. *Proc R Soc Lond B Biol Sci.* 1969;173:141–174.

Pain and Temperature

Environmental energies from both inside and outside the body stimulate sensory receptors which are located throughout the organism. Following the conversion (transduction) of these energies to nerve impulses by the receptors and their nerve terminals, this information is transmitted by fibers in the spinal and cranial nerves to nuclei within the spinal cord and brainstem for neural processing. Some processed inputs are transmitted along the ascending pathways (nerve fiber tracts), linking processing centers (nuclei) until information eventually reaches the higher centers in the brain, e.g., the cerebral cortex and cerebellar cortex.

FEATURES OF SENSORY SYSTEMS

The term *sensory* is used to include all afferent input from the peripheral nerves, whether consciously perceived or not. *Sensations* are conscious perceptions and experiences associated with stimuli arising directly from the stimulation of receptors of the sense organs. The *sensory systems* are involved in (1) the awareness of sensations, (2) the unconscious inputs that underlie the control of movements and many bodily functions, and (3) neural activities associated with arousal. The sensory systems have evolved to provide information from both the internal and external environment of the organism. *Receptors* are the monitors sensing the environment. They are involved with *transduction*, which is conversion of stimulus energy into neural activity. The quality of each stimulus results in a form of sensation called a *modality* such as pain, thermal sense, touch, or vision. Each modality has submodalities (e.g., vision has several, such as color and perception of form and depth). The three receptor types and some associated modalities are (1) *mechanoreceptors* such as temperature (thermal), noxious (pain or nociceptors), auditory (sound), and touch receptors, (2) *chemoreceptors* (taste and smell), and (3) *photoreceptors* (light). The transduction in a mechanoreceptor is brought about by the direct mechanical interaction of the stimulus with the channels on the receptor membrane. Only a few channels are open in the unstimulated membrane. When the receptor membrane is deformed by the stimulus, the channels open and Na^+ and K^+ shift to produce a depolarization called the receptor potential. The transduction in a chemoreceptor results from the interaction of a chemical with a receptor linked to a second messenger system to mediate channel openings. This is the means utilized by olfactory receptors and certain gustatory receptors. The transduction in a photoreceptor is associated with the absorption of light by the membranous disks of the rods and cones of the retina. The resulting change in receptor membrane permeability involves a second messenger system.

Four distinct elementary general somatic modalities are recognized: (1) *pain* elicited by noxious stimuli in damaged tissue, (2) *thermal sensations* elicited by warm and cool stimuli, (3) *touch* elicited by mechanical stimuli applied to the body (Chap. 10), and (4) *proprioceptive sensations* elicited by the mechanical displacement of muscles and joints (Chap. 10).

Two major *general sensory systems* are associated with sensory input from the spinal nerves from the body. Equivalent systems are associated with similar input from the head (e.g. from the trigeminal nerve). They are (1) the anterolateral system of pathways for pain and temperature, and somewhat for touch; and (2) the dorsal column-medial lemniscal system of pathways for touch and proprioception (Chap. 10). Each of the systems is organized (a) with most of the sensory submodalities conveyed by functionally separate pathways, (b) hierarchically with successive serial processing centers (called relay nuclei) terminating with the cerebral cortex, and (c) for parallel processing at each level of centers (Chap. 3). These two systems and their pathways converge on distinct and separate populations of neurons within the ventral posterior nucleus (ventrobasal nucleus) of the thala-

mus. From the thalamus, neural information is projected to the sensory areas of the cerebral cortex where the various submodalities are integrated into the experience of perception. It is at these higher centers that the several aspects of sensations are finely honed, including (1) quality (e.g., pain), (2) intensity, (3) location on body, (4) duration, and (5) affect (e.g., range from pleasant to unpleasant). It is these attributes that make a perception more than a sensation.

The pathways of the general sensory systems consist, with exceptions, of first order, second order, and third order neurons. The *first order neurons* are those peripheral sensory neurons with cell bodies in the spinal dorsal root or cranial nerve ganglia and axons that terminate in the spinal cord or brainstem. The *second order neurons* are those with cell bodies in the nuclei of the spinal cord and brainstem and with axons that ascend to terminate in the thalamus. The *third order neurons* are those with cell bodies in the thalamus and axons that terminate in the somatosensory cortex (areas 3, 1, and 2) of the parietal lobe.

The centers and nerve fibers involved with the processing and conveying of information resulting in the conscious appreciation of pain and temperature are in such close proximity that their pathways are collectively called the *pain and temperature pathways*.

RECEPTORS

Receptors have been variously classified. The *exteroceptors*, located near the body surface, are generally stimulated by external environmental energies. They are sensed as touch, light touch, pressure-touch, pain, temperature, odor, sound, taste, or light. The *proprioceptors* are located within deep structures of the head, body wall, and extremities. Proprioception includes such modalities as position sense, vibratory sense, balance, and sense of movement. The *interoceptors* monitor the viscera and then project information sensed as cramps, pain, and fullness and are utilized in visceral reflexes (e.g., carotid sinus reflex). *Mechanoreceptors* respond to mechanical stimuli (touch, hearing). *Chemoreceptors* respond to chemical stimuli (taste, smell).

Thermoreceptors (temperature receptors) respond to various degrees of warmth and cold.

Pain

Receptors of "painful" stimuli are collectively referred to as *nociceptors*. They are free (naked) nerve endings that respond to direct stimulation and to chemical products associated with local injury (noxious stimuli) (**Figs. 10.1 and 10.2**). Three types of free nerve ending receptors are associated with two types of afferent nerve fibers. On the basis of functional criteria, they are: (1) mechanosensitive nociceptors with A-delta fibers, (2) mechanothermal nociceptors with A-delta fibers, and (3) polymodal nociceptors (respond to thermal, mechanical, and both thermal and chemical stimuli) with C fibers (**Fig. 9.1**). Each of these receptors contributes uniquely to the quality and intensity of pain. Thus, pain is a product of concurrent inputs from a combination of receptors. Pain has been defined as an unpleasant sensation that is per-

ceived as arising from a specific region of the body and is commonly produced by processes that damage or are capable of damaging bodily tissue.

Following trauma or inflammation, chemical mediators are released locally from the damaged tissues that can sensitize and, at times, activate the A-delta and C nociceptors. Two such agents are the peptide bradykinin and such eicosanoids as prostaglandins. The responsive nociceptors release the peptide substance P. This can activate local mast cells to release histamine, which, in turn, excites the nociceptors. In addition, substance P stimulates the dilation of blood vessels, which is followed by edema and the further release of bradykinin. The effectiveness of aspirin and anti-inflammatory analgesics in the control of pain is because these agents inhibit an enzyme involved in the synthesis of prostaglandins. The well-known subjective perception is that of a brief, strong stimulus that evokes a brief, intense sharp pain (first pain) followed by a dull, prolonged pain (second pain). First pain is associated with A-delta activity and the second pain with C fiber activity.

To distinguish between nociception and pain is basic to an understanding of sensory systems. *Nociception* implies the reception by nociceptors of stimuli that form signals to provide information to the central nervous system (CNS) of tissue damage eliciting a noxious stimulus. Pain is the perception of an unpleasant sensation. *Perceptions*, such as pain, are abstractions of the sensory input by the CNS. Pain is said to be a subjective perception with a psychological dimension. A noxious stimulus that triggers a nociceptor to respond is not necessarily perceived as pain.

Neurologists usually test for cutaneous pain simply by pricking the skin with a safety pin. Thermal sensibility is evaluated by applying a tube containing ice (40°F) and another containing warm water (110°F) to a body part. Temperature differences of 5° to 10° are normally detected subjectively.

The thermal receptors sensing heat and cold are located in free nerve endings. Small shifts in the skin temperature, of about 0.2° F, are sufficient to alter the firing rate of the endings. In essence, the thermoreceptors are not objec-

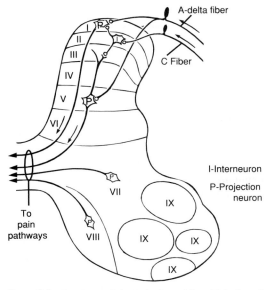

Figure 9.1: Laminae of the spinal cord in which dorsal root fibers terminate. The A-delta fibers (pain and touch) terminate in laminae I and V, where they synapse with projection neurons (P) with axons that ascend in the pain pathways (Fig. 9.2). The C fibers (pain and temperature) terminate in lamina II. Interneurons (I) in lamina II have axons that synapse with projection neurons in laminae I and V (Refer to Table 7.6). Laminae VII and VIII have neurons that project via pain pathways.

tive sensors of actual skin temperature; rather, their role is to signal information resulting in adjustments to the environment. For example, the perception is especially vigorous when the change is rapid. For example, the perception of hot occurs when the "cold" hand is placed in lukewarm water. The momentary distorted perception of coolness is perceived when a foot is placed in a bathtub with hot water.

FIRST-ORDER NEURONS

The pain and temperature inputs are conveyed via two types of first-order afferent neurons with their cell bodies in the dorsal root ganglia, or the cranial nerve equivalent: (1) fast-conducting, lightly myelinated A-delta fibers and (2) slow-conducting, unmyelinated C fibers (Fig. 9.1). The A-delta afferents from low-threshold receptors conduct influences, perceived as sharp localized pain. The C fiber afferents, stimulated by high threshold receptors, are involved in diffuse pain that persists and may have aching, burning, or itching qualities. Often this diffuse pain, presumably due to released chemicals, is preceded by a sharp stabbing pain.

The modalities of pain and temperature are conveyed to the spinal cord via two types of fibers of *first order neurons*. These are (1) fast-conducting, lightly myelinated A-delta fibers and (2) slow-conducting, unmyelinated C fibers (Fig. 9.1). The same modalities are conveyed to the brainstem primarily via the first order neurons of the trigeminal ganglion. Those neurons of fibers excited exclusively by nociceptors are called *nociceptive-specific neurons*. Other first order neurons involved with the pain pathway conveying input from low-threshold mechanoreceptors are called *wide dynamic range neurons*. Both the A-delta and C fibers release the excitatory transmitters glutamate and various neuropeptides, especially substance P.

The A-delta afferents, with low-threshold receptors, conduct influences perceived as sharp, pricking sensations that are accurately localized, known as *fast or initial pain*.

The C afferents, with high threshold receptors, sense pain as a burning sensation with a slower onset and as a more persistent and less distinctly localized modality known as *slow or delayed pain*. Both the fast pain and the slow pain are essentially somatic sensations from superficial receptors in the body. In addition, a *deep or visceral pain*, at times subjectively characterized as aches with a burning quality, results from the stimulation of deep somatic and visceral receptors. This form of pain is associated with inputs conveyed by A-delta and C fibers in both somatic and visceral nerves.

Stimulation of *mechanoreceptor nociceptors* (e.g., from the cut of a knife or the prick from a pin) and *thermal nociceptors* in free nerve endings evokes a neural code that is conveyed via A-delta fibers and perceived as sharp and pricking pain (or temperature). Stimulation of thermal and *polymodal nociceptors* (mechanical, heat, and chemical noxious stimuli) in free nerve endings evokes codes that are conveyed by C fibers and perceived as slow, burning pain (or temperature). Thermal nociceptors respond selectively to heat and cold. In humans, heat receptors respond selectively when the temperature exceeds the heat pain threshold of 113°F. Cold receptors respond to noxious cold stimuli.

PATHWAYS FROM THE BODY, LIMBS, AND BACK OF HEAD

Pain and temperature pathways from the body, limbs, and back of the head (posterior to the coronal plane through the ears, Fig. 9.2) are components of the *anterolateral pathway* (located in the white matter of the anterolateral quadrant of the spinal cord). They are the (1) *(lateral) spinothalamic tract* terminating in the thalamus, (2) *spinomesencephalic tract* terminating in the periaqueductal gray (PAG) of the midbrain, and (3) *spinoreticular tract* terminating in the brainstem reticular formation (Fig. 9.2). The *anterior spinothalamic tract* conveying light touch is included in the anterolateral pathway (Fig. 10.3). Additional fibers of nociceptive neurons are incorporated in the spinocervicothalamic pathway located in the dorsal columns of the lemniscal system (Chap. 10).

The A-delta and C fibers enter the spinal cord as the lateral bundle of the dorsal root. These fibers bifurcate into branches that ascend

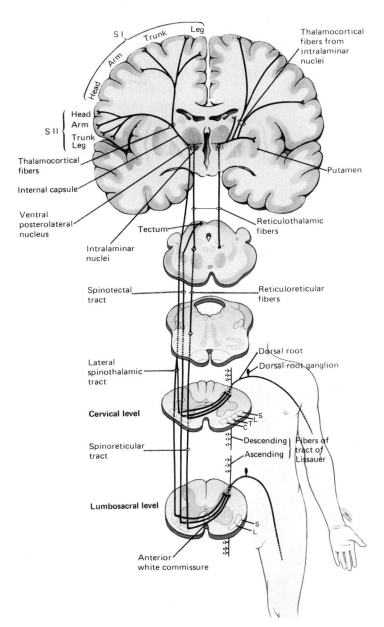

Figure 9.2: The pain and temperature pathways originating in the spinal cord. They are the lateral spinothalamic tract, spinomesencephalic (spinotectal), and spinoreticulothalamic fibers. Note that the VPL thalamic nucleus projects to the body regions of both SI and SII of the somatosensory cortex and that the intralaminar thalamic nuclei project diffusely and widely to the cerebral cortex. On the right side of the cross-sections of the spinal cord, note the lamination of the lateral spinothalamic tract (C = cervical, T = thoracic, L = lumbar, and S = sacral levels).

and descend one or two spinal levels in the *posterolateral fasciculus (tract of Lissauer)* from where they enter and terminate in the dorsal horn (Fig. 9.1). The A-delta fibers have excitatory synapses with projection neurons. The C fibers synapse with interneurons interacting with (1) projection neurons whose axons ascend to higher centers in the brain and (2) inhibitory interneurons that modulate the flow of nociceptive information to higher centers. The A-delta fibers synapse with neurons in laminae I, II, and V, and C fibers synapse with neurons in lamina II. The branches of each main fiber terminate in several spinal levels. According to the gate control theory (Fig. 9.3), processing of these inputs occurs within the dorsal horn by interactions involving nociceptive-specific neurons, wide dynamic range neurons, interneurons, and projection neurons. Descending control mechanisms also are important in pain modulation (Fig. 9.4).

The pain and temperature pathways terminate in several thalamic nuclei. These include the ventral posterior lateral nucleus (VPL), posterior nucleus (PTh), and intralaminar nuclei (Chap. 23). The VPL and ventral posterior medial nucleus (VPM) (receives information from the head) are called the ventrobasal nucleus (VB). In terms of the nature of their nociceptive inputs, there are two major subdivisions of these nuclei. (1) The intralaminar nuclei receive input from neurons of spinal laminae VI, VII, and VIII stimulated via the spinoreticulothalamic pathway, conveying information from large complex nociceptive fields. (2) The lateral nuclear thalamic group consists of the VB and PTh nuclei. It receives input from laminae I and V via the spinothalamic pathway conveying

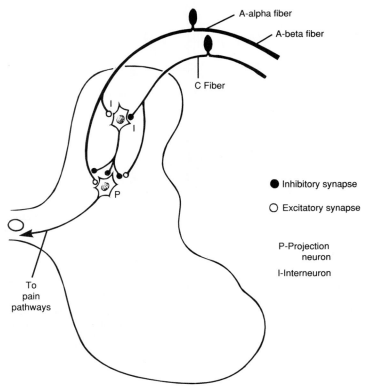

A-alpha fiber

A-beta fiber

C Fiber

● Inhibitory synapse

○ Excitatory synapse

P-Projection neuron

I-Interneuron

To pain pathways

Figure 9.3: Gate Control Model for pain modulation. The model postulates the interaction of (1) the C pain fibers that have inhibitory synapses with an interneuron and excitatory synapses with a projection pain neuron, (2) the myelinated A-alpha and A-beta non-nociceptive fibers that have excitatory synapses with both the interneuron and the projection pain neuron, and (3) the interneurons that have inhibitory synapses with the projection pain neuron. See page 133 for further explanation.

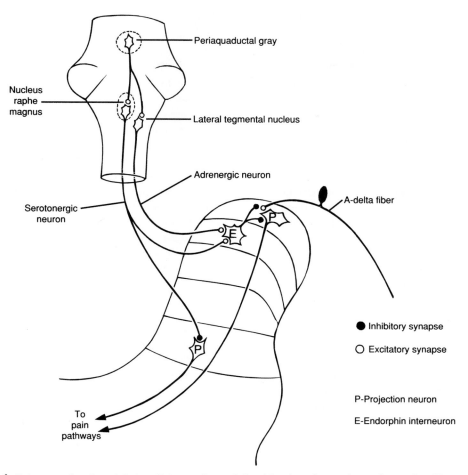

Periaquaductal gray

Nucleus raphe magnus

Lateral tegmental nucleus

Adrenergic neuron

Serotonergic neuron

A-delta fiber

P

E

P

To pain pathways

● Inhibitory synapse

○ Excitatory synapse

P-Projection neuron

E-Endorphin interneuron

Figure 9.4: Pain control and modulation. Pain can be modulated by the release of opioid peptides. Neurons of the periaqueductal gray (PAG) matter of the midbrain have excitatory synaptic connections with serotonergic neurons in nucleus raphe magnus and with noradrenergic neurons in the lower brainstem reticular formation. The serotonergic neurons (1) have inhibitory synapses with the nociceptive projection neurons and (2) excitatory synapses with the endorphin-containing interneurons (E) which have inhibitory synapses with the nociceptive projection neurons (P). The noradrenergic (norepinephrine) neurons also have excitatory synapses with these endorphin-containing interneurons. These activities modulate the excitatory synaptic influences of the glutamate and substance P transmitters of the A-delta fibers with the nociceptive projection neurons. See page 133 for further explanation.

information primarily from nociceptive-specific and wide dynamic range neurons.

The *(lateral) spinothalamic tract* originates from projection neurons of laminae I, V, VI, and VII. After the axons of its *second order neurons* decussate (cross over) in the *anterior white commissure* (anterior to central canal), they ascend in the anterolateral pathway and terminate primarily in VPL and PTh thalamic nuclei (lateral nuclear thalamic group) (Fig. 9.2). Some collateral branches terminate in the brainstem reticular formation. This tract conveys informa-

tion perceived with an overlay of the discriminative aspects associated with various subtleties identified with the sensation of sharp pain and, in addition, thermal sense (temperature).

At successively higher levels of the spinal cord, new fibers join the tract on its medial aspect; this produces a laminated *somatotopically organized* tract, i.e., each body segment (or dermatome) is represented in a portion of the tract (Fig. 7.6). As a consequence, in the upper cervical spinal cord, pain and temperature fibers from the sacral region are located posterolaterally and those from the cervical region anteromedially. The VPL thalamic nucleus is also somatotopically organized with the sacral and lumbar (lower body) levels located laterally and the thoracic and cervical levels located medially. This tract is also called the *lateral pain system* or *neospinothalamic tract* (meaning new phylogenetically).

The axons of the pain and temperature neurons located in the thalamus ascend through the posterior limb of the internal capsule and corona radiata and terminate in the parietal lobe of the cerebral cortex (Chap. 25). Fibers from VPL terminate in lamina IV of the *primary somatosensory cortex* (SI; areas 3, 1, and 2 of the postcentral gyrus). Those fibers from PTh nucleus terminate in lamina IV of the secondary somatosensory cortex (SII; areas 3, 1, and 2 near the lateral fissure; Chap. 25). The thalamus may be associated with the vague perception of the awareness of pain, while the parietal lobe and other cortical areas are involved in the appreciation and the localization of pain, and of the integration of stimuli from the pain pathways with that from the other sensory modalities. The *spinomesencephalic (spinotectal) tract* is composed of the fibers of projection neurons in laminae I and V, decussating in the anterior white commissure and ascending in the anterolateral pathway. Its fibers terminate in the PAG of the midbrain (Fig. 9.4). It has roles in the modulation of pain and in the functioning of the reticular system (Chap. 22).

The *spinoreticular tract* is integrated into the *spinoreticulothalamic* pathway terminating in the medial thalamic nuclear group noted above. The spinoreticular fibers originate from neurons in laminae VII and VIII, which receive input from large complex receptive fields in the periphery. The spinoreticular tract consists of crossed and a few uncrossed fibers that, along with collateral fibers from the spinothalamic tract, terminate in the multineuronal, multisynaptic complex known as the brainstem reticular formation (Chaps. 13 and 22). From here reticulothalamic fibers terminate in the intralaminar nuclei of the thalamus and, additionally, in the hypothalamus and limbic structures. This slowly conducting multisynaptic pathway conveys diffuse poorly localized pain from both somatic and visceral sources. The intralaminar

nuclei project to widespread areas of the cerebral cortex, including that of the frontal lobes. The influences exerted by this pathway are integrated into autonomic and reflex responses to pain and to affective-motivational responses. As a consequence, this pathway is also called the *paramedian pain pathway* or the *paleospinothalamic pathway* (old phylogenetic pathway) of the *medial pain system*.

The neospinothalamic pathway, via the VPL nucleus, projects to the primary and secondary somatic sensory areas of the cerebral cortex. These are essential for spatial and temporal discrimination of painful sensations. In contrast, the paleospinothalamic pathway mediates the autonomic and reflexive responses associated with pain and, in addition, the emotional and affective responses.

The roles of the cerebral cortex and the thalamus in the perception of pain are intriguing to decipher. Several clinical observations following certain surgical procedures are relevant to an understanding of the perception of pain. Surgical intervention in various locations, both of the peripheral nervous system and CNS, has not proven to be effective in permanently relieving pain. Surgery can abolish pain temporarily, but the perception of pain subsequently returns with new manifestations. These are unpleasant and frequently different than any pain the patient has ever perceived previously. These include shooting pain, numbness, cold, burning, and aching sensations. Some procedures in the brain can elicit more distress to the patient than the original pain. Such spontaneous lesions can result in marked distortions of pain and pain related symptoms (Thalamic Syndrome, Chap. 23). The bizarre sensations perceived by an amputee in the phantom limb are expressions of processing within neural centers deprived of normal stimulation (see later). Destructive surgical lesions of the intralaminar and posterior thalamic nuclei can alleviate intractable pain; in time, the pain may return.

Several surgical interventions suggest some functional roles for various regions of the brain. (1) Nociceptive information from one half of the body is conveyed to the same side of the spinal cord and then crosses over to the contralateral side to ascend as the neospinothalamic pathway to where aspects of perception occur in the thalamus and the somatosensory areas of the cortex. Painful stimuli can be perceived on the contralateral side of the body following ablation of the somatosensory cortex of a hemisphere. This is accomplished when the entire thalamus and other subcortical structures are intact. (2) The cortex of the frontal lobe and cingulate gyrus are involved in some way with the psychological responses to pain (Chap. 25), as are the dorsomedial and anterior thalamic nuclei with connections to the cortex of the frontal lobe (Chap. 23). Lesions of these nuclei, or of the nerve fibers linking them to the frontal lobe (called prefrontal leukotomy), lower the agony associated with the persistent pain by altering the psychological response to the painful stimuli. The downsides to this approach are the negative changes in the personality and intellectual status of the patient (Chap. 25). Bilateral severing of the fibers linking the cingulate gyrus to the frontal lobe (cingulotomy) can relieve the response to pain without the concomitant personality changes.

PATHWAYS FROM THE ANTERIOR HEAD

Pain and temperature pathways from receptors in the head and scalp, anterior to a coronal plane through the ears are the (1) trigeminothalamic and (2) trigeminoreticulothalamic tracts, both of which terminate in nuclei of the thalamus. These tracts convey impulses from the three divisions of the trigeminal nerve (ophthalmic, maxillary, and mandibular) and cranial nerves VII, IX, and X (Fig. 9.5).

The cell bodies of the first-order fibers (A-delta and C fibers) are located in the trigeminal ganglion (V), the geniculate ganglion (VII), and the superior ganglia (IX and X). The fibers enter the brainstem and descend as the *spinal tract of n. V* (spinal trigeminal tract) on the lateral aspect of the lower pons, medulla, and upper two cervical spinal cord segments. The spinal trigeminal tract is somatotopically organized: the sequence from anterior to posterior includes the fibers from the ophthalmic nerve together with nerves VII, IX, and X (most anterior), maxillary nerve, and mandibular nerve; fibers from each of these nerves extend to the C2 level.

They terminate in the *spinal nucleus of n. V* (spinal trigeminal nucleus), which is located medial to the tract. The spinal tract and nucleus of n. V are the brainstem's counterpart of the posterolateral tract of Lissauer and substantia gelatinosa (lamina II) of the spinal cord, respectively.

The spinal nucleus of n. V is a continuous structure that is subdivided into (1) the rostrally located *pars oralis* (nucleus oralis) which receives touch input from the mouth, lip, and nose; (2) the intermediately located *pars interpolaris* (nucleus interpolaris), which receives pain input from the tooth pulp (dental pain); and (3) the caudally located *pars caudalis* (nucleus caudalis), which receives pain, temperature, and light touch input from the face, mouth, and tooth pulp. The pars caudalis extends caudally to the C2 level (Fig. 9.5).

From cell bodies in the spinal nucleus of n. V, axons of second-order neurons decussate through the lower brainstem reticular formation, and ascend near the medial lemniscus as the *anterior trigeminothalamic tract* (anterior trigeminal tract) to terminate in the VPM nucleus of the thalamus and in the posterior thalamic region.

Third-order neurons pass from the thalamus through the posterior limb of the internal capsule and corona radiata before terminating in the head region in the primary and secondary somatosensory cortices (SI and SII). The trigeminothalamic tract is included in the lateral pain system.

Diffuse, poorly localized pain from the head is probably conveyed by means of the *trigeminoreticulothalamic pathway*, in which second-order fibers end in the reticular formation, from where third-order fibers reach the thalamic intralaminar nuclei (except the centrum medianum). The trigeminoreticulothalamic pathway is part of the medial pain system.

In summary, two pain and temperature pathways are recognized. They are called (1) the anterolateral and trigeminothalamic pathways and (2) the spinoreticulothalamic and trigeminoreticulothalamic pathways.

TEMPERATURE (THERMAL) SENSE

Free nerve endings are the peripheral receptors for the sensations of warmth and cold. Sensory

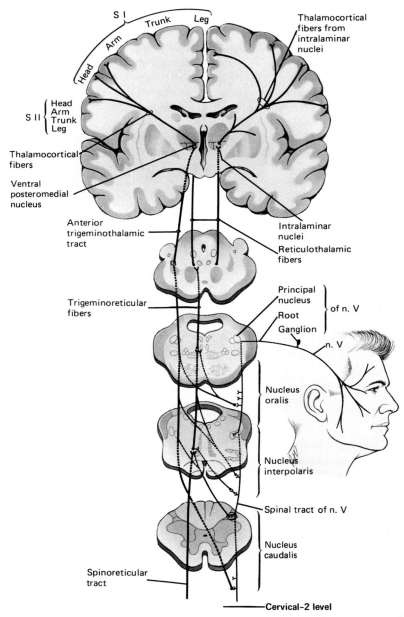

Figure 9.5: The pain and temperature pathways originating in the brainstem. They are the anterior trigeminothalamic tract and the trigeminoreticulothalamic pathway. Note that the ventral posterior medial thalamic nucleus projects to the head regions of both SI and SII of the somatosensory cortex and that the intralaminar thalamic nuclei project diffusely and widely to the cerebral cortex. For details of structures in the brainstem sections, refer to figures 13.6, 13.8, 13.10, and 13.15.

inputs associated with these modalities are conveyed via lightly myelinated A-delta and unmyelinated C fibers. Cold is associated with both types of fibers and warmth with C fibers. An intense heat stimulus can evoke the perception of cold, as can occur when one places a hand in hot water; this is called the *paradoxical cold sensation*. It results because heat does, at times, stimulate cold receptors.

Although thermal pathways are virtually indistinguishable from those for pain, some researchers contend that the thermal senses are conveyed only by fibers of the anterolateral pathway and trigeminothalamic tract.

PERCEPTION OF PAIN

Pain is primarily a warning signal to the organism; it is often accompanied by withdrawal from a noxious stimulus via the flexor reflex. In a phylogenetic sense pain must be one of the oldest protective responses of living organisms. The awareness of pain may be centered in the thalamus, as are certain associated aspects. For instance, a lesion of the dorsomedial nucleus can reduce the intensity or anguish of the pain experience. A lesion of the ventral posterior and intralaminar nuclei may relieve intractable pain, but in many patients this is temporary, suggesting the existence of alternative pathways. Portions of the cortex seem to be important as well. The various nuances of pain (sharpness, dullness) seem to require activity of the secondary somatosensory area (SII). Portions of the parietal lobe seem to be necessary for the subject to locate the source of pain. On the other hand, large cortical ablation, including all of SI and SII, leaves chronic pain undiminished. The interplay of cortex and thalamus is uncertain, and some authorities conclude that the responses to a pain stimulus are indivisible. A dissociation between the perception and tolerance of pain has been noted following psychosurgical treatment of patients suffering from chronic pain. The surgery consists of a lobotomy of the prefrontal cortex (Chap. 25) or lesions of the dorsomedial and anterior thalamic nuclei (nuclei having connections with the prefrontal cortex). These patients report the perception of the pain, but are no longer bothered by it.

Itching is related, in some unknown way, to pain. It originates from the stimulation of free nerve endings within or just deep to the epidermis of the skin. It is transmitted by C fibers and relayed to the brain via the anterolateral pathway.

THE GATE CONTROL THEORY OF PAIN MODULATION

A clinical method used to relieve pain (produce analgesia) is by stimulation of the appropriate peripheral nerve with surface electrodes. The procedure is called *transcutaneous nerve stimulation* (TNS). An explanation for the success of this therapy is based on the Gate Control Theory. In this concept, pain can be modulated by the balance of the interactions among the (1) *nociceptive C fibers* and (2) *non-nociceptive A-alpha* (proprioception) and *A-beta afferent* (touch) *fibers* of the peripheral nerves, and the (3) *interneurons* and (4) *projection neurons* of the dorsal horn. The latter are the neurons of the pain pathways (Figs. 9.2 and 9.3).

The following describes the presumed actions of the neurons comprising the circuitry of this Gate Control Model (refer to Fig. 9.3). The unmyelinated nociceptive C (pain) fiber inhibits the inhibitory interneuron and the projection neuron. The interneuron, which normally inhibits the projection neuron, is spontaneously active and thus, reduces (inhibits) the intensity of the noxious input from the C fibers. The influences exerted by the spontaneous activity of the interneuron on the projection neuron are modulated by excitation from the non-nociceptive A fibers and inhibition from the nociceptive C fibers. In essence nociceptive C fibers tend to keep the gate open (enhancing perception of pain) by inhibiting the inhibitory interneuron and exciting the projection neuron. The non-nociceptive A fibers tend to keep the gate closed (suppression of pain) by exciting the inhibitory interneuron. In addition, the reflected feedback descending influences from the brain can modulate the excitability of these neurons (Figs. 9.4 and 3.11; Chap. 3).

DESCENDING CONTROL MECHANISMS—PAIN MODULATION

Pain and other sensory systems can be modulated and biased by influences conveyed from higher centers via descending tracts, known as *reflected feedback pathways*, to lower levels of the ascending pathways. Through these connections, the sensitivity of receptors and processing centers can be enhanced or suppressed. For example, the gamma motor neurons do modify the responsiveness of the muscle spindles (Chap. 8).

The descending influences from higher centers modulating pain are presumed to be organized in the following way (**Fig. 9.4**). Output from the frontal cortex and hypothalamus activates centers in the PAG and adjacent areas of the midbrain, which have connections with tegmental nuclei of the rostromedial medulla. Another area involved with pain modulation is located in the tegmentum of the dorsal and dorsolateral pons. Fibers from these pontine and medullary tegmental nuclei project (1) to the spinal trigeminal nucleus, and (2) via the pain-modulating dorsolateral tract (located in the lateral funiculus adjacent to the dorsal horn) to laminae I and II of the spinal cord. Many of these neurons in the pons are adrenergic neurons (contain norepinephrine), and those of the medulla are serotonergic neurons (contain serotonin) (Chap. 15). Both of these biogenic amines have been implicated in pain modulation. The effect of the release of these biogenic amines and opioid peptides is that they bind to receptor sites and thereby suppress the activity of the "pain" neurons.

Opioid peptides and opiate drugs (e.g., morphine) are powerful analgesic agents. They produce analgesia by direct action upon specific receptor sites (opiate-binding receptors) on the cell membrane of neurons. It is likely that the opioid-mediated analgesic system is activated by stress, pain itself, and suggestion (see later, stress-produced and stimulus-induced analgesia). Certain neurons in the brain can release neurotransmitters, called endogenous opioid peptides, that result in analgesia. Three families of these peptides are recognized: (1) enkephalins, derived from proenkephalin A; (2) beta-endorphin, from pro-opiomelanocortin (POMC); and (3) dynorphins, from prodynorphin. These opiates are presumed to be the natural pain relievers, because they do so when microinjected into the PAG and the superficial layers of the dorsal horn of the spinal cord. Endogenous opiate peptides are located in various structures of the CNS associated with transmission or modulation of pain. Enkephalins are located in the amygdala, hypothalamus, PAG, rostroventral tegmentum of the medulla, and the dorsal horn of the spinal cord. Less widely distributed are beta-endorphins, located in the hypothalamus (arcuate nucleus), PAG, and in small amounts in the medulla and spinal cord. Dynorphin peptides are roughly similar to the enkephalins in their distribution.

ENDOGENOUS PAIN CONTROL

The natural variability of pain thresholds can be further affected by the emotional state of the individual and by pharmacological agents such as aspirin and morphine. The control and modulation of nociception involves descending influences involving several descending neurotransmitter systems (**Fig. 9.4**). Aspirin apparently acts peripherally, presumably by inhibiting transduction, and thereby minimizes the nociceptive signal. Aspirin is a true analgesic because it affects the entire sensation of pain. In contrast, morphine acts at synaptic sites in the CNS that reduce and modulate nociceptive signals. Morphine and other narcotics seem to mimic the effects of the endogenous opioids (Chap. 15).

The following pathway contributes to the control of nociceptive neurons in the spinal cord (**Fig. 9.4**). Stimulation of the PAG of the midbrain (e.g., from the limbic system following a stressful episode such as a fire-fight in a battle) activates some of its neurons that descend and have excitatory synapses with serotonergic neurons in the nucleus raphe magnus and with groups of noradrenergic neurons in the reticular formation of the lower brainstem. The descending fibers from these neurons (a) directly inhibit the nociceptive projection neurons in the dorsal horn and (b) excite the endorphin-containing interneurons in laminae I and II of the dorsal horn. These interneurons can then, through both presynaptic and postsynaptic connections, also inhibit the nociceptive projection neurons (**Fig. 9.4**). Evidence indicates that endorphin-containing interneurons in both the PAG and dorsal horn are active in pain modulation.

SUMMARY OF THE PAIN SIGNALING SYSTEMS

Two pathway systems are involved with pain: (1) *lateral pain system* and (2) *medial pain system*. The *lateral pain system* is composed of the sequence of (1) A-delta neurons of the peripheral nerves, (2) dorsal horn and spinal nucleus of nerve V, (3) lateral spinothalamic tract and trigeminothalamic tract, (4) ventral posterior thalamic nucleus, and (5) somatosensory cortex (**Figs. 9.2 and 9.5**). This system conducts signals (impulses) rapidly. Functionally, it is associated with sharp, suddenly felt, and discriminating aspects of pain (called phasic pain). Sharp pain is the pain that is readily identified as occurring at a precisely defined site on the body. Because the signal is conveyed to the cerebral cortex, this system probably accounts for most of the sensory qualities associated with pain (such as throbbing or burning).

The observation that phasic pain often subsides rather promptly indicates that the lateral system is dampened quickly. Two means have been proposed to account for this phenomenon. (1) Following an injury, the body's intrinsic opioids, such as endorphins and enkephalins, are apparently activated. (2) Inhibition of the transmission of pain signals from the peripheral nerves to the ascending lateral tracts may occur in the dorsal horn or spinal trigeminal nuclei. These inhibitory influences are derived from the descending (reflected) pathway from neurons in the PAG matter whose axons terminate in these nuclei.

The *medial pain system* is composed of the sequence of (1) C fiber neurons of the peripheral nerves, (2) dorsal horn and spinal nucleus of nerve V, (3) spinoreticulothalamic pathway and trigeminoreticulothalamic pathway, (4) intralaminar thalamic nuclei, and (5) widespread areas of the cerebral cortex (**Figs. 9.2 and 9.5**). In addition, this system has connections with structures of the limbic system (Chap. 22). The system conducts signals relatively slowly through a multineuronal pathway. Functionally, this system is involved with persistent (tonic) pain and diffuse unpleasant feelings for some time after the injury has ceased. Through its connections with the limbic system (the system involved with affect and motivation), it is probably associated with the actions and reactions one takes in response to such feelings.

REFERRED (TRANSFERRED) PAIN

Pain of visceral origin is usually vaguely localized. The site of the visceral irritation and the locale where the pain is felt are not necessarily the same. The pain can be *referred* (transferred) from the visceral source to a corresponding dermatomal segment on the body, extremity, or head. *Referred pain* may also apply to pain of a somatic source.

The brain and the parenchyma of visceral organs do not have pain receptors. Such receptors are primarily in the walls of arteries, meninges, and all the pleural and peritoneal membranes. They are often the sources of severe pain when they are inflamed, irritated, or subjected to mechanical friction. Excessive contraction (cramps) or dilation (distention) of the body's hollow viscera (e.g., intestines) can also produce pain.

The following are examples of referred pain from visceral sources. The pain of coronary heart disease can be referred to the chest wall, left axilla, and the inside of the left arm. The spinal cord segments of T1 and T2 innervate the heart and the skin (dermatomes) areas of the chest, axilla, and left arm. An inflammation of the peritoneum on the diaphragm (often related to the gallbladder) can be referred to the shoulder region. The spinal segments C3 to C5 supply sensory, as well as motor, innervation to the diaphragm (via the phrenic nerve) and to the shoulder region. The source of headaches is not the brain per se. Headaches are thought to be referred from irritated nerve endings in the intracranial (meningeal) and other blood vessels.

Referred pain with a somatic source is some form of back pain. The sources of the pain can be the receptors associated with the ligaments and muscles attached to the bony vertebral column. The pain is often referred to another spinal level.

One concept to explain the phenomenon of referred pain is based on the demonstration that the nociceptive fibers conveying information from a cutaneous site may converge to synapse with the same pool of projection neurons in the dorsal horn. In turn, these projection neurons of the pain pathways receiving these dual inputs project to higher centers, which cannot discriminate the precise source. The pain can be incorrectly attributed to the skin, which is normally the source of greater nociceptive input.

Pain in Dermatomes

A dermatome is the sensory segment of the skin innervated by the fibers of one dorsal root. Dermatomes of successive spinal segments overlap. Hence, the interruption of one complete dorsal root may result in only the diminution (not loss) of sensation in part of a dermatome; however, the irritation of a dorsal root can produce pain over an entire dermatome (Fig. 7.3). In herpes zoster (shingles) there is an intense and persistent pain in one or more dermatomes. This pain is a consequence of the activation of pain fibers by varicella zoster virus, which primarily affects one or more dorsal root ganglia. Mechanical compression, e.g., following a slipped disk, of a dorsal root can irritate a dorsal root and produce pain over a dermatome.

STIMULUS-INDUCED AND STRESS-INDUCED ANALGESIA

Severely wounded soldiers, athletes injured in sports, and professional boxers state that they do not feel pain during and even just after the stressful events of combat. During the race, marathon runners undergo the feeling state of "running through pain." Electric stimulation of the PAG in humans does produce a drastic reduction in clinical pain, called stimulus-induced analgesia. Patients describe a pain that fades away over a few minutes, and even a feeling of warmth and relaxation. The stimulation presumably activates the pain-modulating networks including the biogenic amine analgesic system and the opioid-mediated modulating system.

The ability to respond during emergency situations and to stressful demands by suppressing or reducing the sensitivity to pain is known as behavioral stress-produced analgesia. It is likely that pain stimuli evoke some of this response by influences from the frontal cortex, limbic system, and hypothalamus activating the nonopiate biogenic amine analgesic system and the opiate-mediated analgesic system to action.

Conceptually, the withdrawal reflex is a response of drawing back from a noxious stimulus and that pain is a sensation correlated with the reflex. In this respect, pain reflex withdrawal is a normal reaction to protect the organism, and the analgesic systems are the organism's means of controlling the pain system.

TRACTOTOMY

To abolish intractable pain, neurosurgeons may transect the pain tracts in a procedure known as tractotomy. After the transection of an anterior quadrant of the spinal cord at some level, the lateral spinothalamic tract and other tracts are interrupted. Pain and temperature sensation should be lost on the opposite side of the body beginning one or two levels below the transection. Bilateral tractotomy of the pain tracts (cordotomy) should abolish visceral and somatic intractable pain below the level of the incision. Tractotomy of the descending uncrossed fibers of the spinal trigeminal tract above the level of the obex (medulla) should result in loss of pain and temperature on the same side of the face and nasal and oral cavities (Chap. 17, "Region of the Cerebellopontine Angle," page 247).

PHANTOM LIMB SENSATION

The phantom limb is an expression of activity in nuclei deprived of normal stimulation. An amputee may feel a diffuse pain in his amputated extremity. The phantom limb "moves" easily, even through objects and the remaining limb. The wristwatch, formerly worn, may still be felt on the nonexistent wrist. An explanation is that the nuclear complexes that previously received input from the phantom limb are still present in the nervous system; when these complexes are stimulated in some way, they set in motion neural activities which produce sensations felt as though coming from the absent limb.

SOMATOTOPIC ORGANIZATION OF THE LATERAL SPINOTHALAMIC TRACT

The laminated, somatotopic organization of the lateral spinothalamic tract, with fibers from successively higher levels being located anteromedial to those from lower levels, has significance in analyzing distributions of pain sensation (Fig. 7.6). Pressure on the lateral aspect of the cervical spinal cord (e.g., from an extramedullary tumor in the cervical region) would interrupt pain and temperature fibers from the contralateral sacral region first and then, as the tumor enlarges, those from lumbar, thoracic, and cervical regions. Pressure from the middle of the spinal cord (central canal region) in the cervical region (e.g., from an intramedullary tumor) would interrupt pain and temperature fibers from the contralateral cervical region first and then those from the thoracic, lumbar, and sacral regions as the tumor enlarges and extends further laterally.

SUGGESTED READINGS

Basbaum A, Fields H. Endogenous pain control systems: brainstem spinal pathways and endorphin circuitry. *Ann Rev Neurosci.* 1984;7:309–338.

Beecher H. Pain in men wounded in battle. *Ann Surg.* 1946;123:96–105.

Besson J, Chaouch A. Peripheral and spinal mechanisms of nociception. *Physiol Rev.* 1987;67:67–186.

Bonica J, ed. *The Management of Pain.* 2nd ed. Philadelphia, Pa: Lea & Febiger; 1990.

Dubner R, Bennett G. Spinal and trigeminal mechanisms of nociception. *Ann Rev Neurosci.* 1983;6:381–418.

Fields H. *Pain: Mechanisms and Management.* New York, NY: McGraw-Hill; 1987.

Fields H, Heinricher M, Mason P. Neurotransmitters in nociceptive modulatory circuits. *Ann Rev Neurosci.* 1991;14:219–245.

Höllt V. Multiple endogenous opioid peptides. *Trends Neurosci.* 1983;6:24–26.

Iggo A. Sensory receptors in the skin of mammals and their sensory functions. *Rev Neurol.* 1985;141:599–613.

Jessell T, Kelly D. Pain and analgesia. In: Kandel E, Schwartz J, Jessell T, eds. *Principles of Neural Science.* 3rd ed. New York, NY: Elsevier; 1991:385–399.

Light A. *The Initial Processing of Pain and Its Descending Control: Spinal and Trigeminal Systems.* New York, NY: Karger; 1992.

Mantyh P. The spinothalamic tract in the primate: reexamination using wheat-germ agglutinin conjugated to horseradish peroxidase. *Neuroscience.* 1983;9:847–862.

Melzack R. Phantom limbs and the concept of a neuromatrix. *Trends Neurosci.* 1990;13:88–92.

Nu J, Sessle B. Comparison of responses of cutaneous nociceptive and nonnociceptive brain stem neurons in trigeminal subnucleus caudalis (medullary dorsal horn) and subnucleus oralis to natural and electrical stimulation of tooth pulp. *J Neurophysiol.* 1984;52:39–53.

Shigenaga Y, Chen I, Suemune S, et al. Oral and facial representation within the medullary and upper cervical dorsal horns in the cat. *J Comp Neurol.* 1986;243:388–408.

Turk D, Melzack R. *Handbook of Pain Assessment.* New York, NY: Guilford Press; 1992.

Wall P, Melzack R. *Textbook of Pain.* 2nd ed. Edinburgh: Churchill Livingstone; 1989.

Willis W. *The Pain System. The Neural Basis of Nociceptive Transmission in the Mammalian Nervous System.* Basel: Karger; 1985.

Willis W Jr, Coggeshall R. *Sensory Mechanisms of the Spinal Cord.* New York, NY: Plenum; 1991.

Discriminative General Senses, Light Touch, and Unconscious Proprioception 10

Lemniscal system
Pathways serving discriminative general senses
Pathways serving light (crude) touch
Proprioceptive pathways of the head
Proprioceptive pathways to the cerebellum
Functional correlations

Touch and the discriminative general senses (DGS) cover a number of sensory modalities. Touch by itself refers to *light* (sometimes called *crude*) *touch*, which yields little information apart from the fact of contact with an object. The DGS include as well, "pressure touch," which enables an awareness of shape, size, and texture. Also under DGS is *stereognosis*, that is, appreciation of an object's three dimensionality; perception of an object's weight; vibratory sense (as stimulated by a tuning fork); position sense (a subject's awareness of body parts, especially joints); and body and limb movement awareness. The last two are often grouped as *kinesthetic sense*.

These modalities are monitored by exteroceptors, located in the surface layers of the skin and oral mucosa, and by proprioceptors, located in the deeper skin layers, joint capsules, ligaments, tendons, muscles, and periosteum. With the proviso that the correlation of a specific modality of sensation with a morphologically identifiable nerve ending is, as yet, inconclusive, it is possible to assign the following receptors to modalities.

Somatosensory Receptors (Mechanoreceptors)

Four types of somatosensory receptors are located in the skin and subcutaneous tissues. These mechanoreceptors are the encapsulated nerve endings called the Meissner, Ruffini, and pacinian corpuscles and Merkel disks (**Figs. 10.1 and 10.2, Table 7.3**). The mechanical transduction (mechanotransduction) from the application of stimuli to these receptors through to the generation of action potentials in the sensory neurons is conventionally viewed as a three-stage process. (1) The stimulus (touch or movement) is mechanically applied to the cells encapsulating the receptor nerve ending. (2) The deformation is transduced into an electrical signal—the receptor (generator) potential. (3) The receptor potential is encoded into an action potential (at first node of Ranvier) for transmission by the sensory neuron to the central nervous system (CNS). Each receptor may be characterized by quality of the modality perceived, size of its receptive field, its stimulus threshold, its speed of adaptation, and its first order fiber type projecting to the CNS.

The *receptive field* is the region of the skin

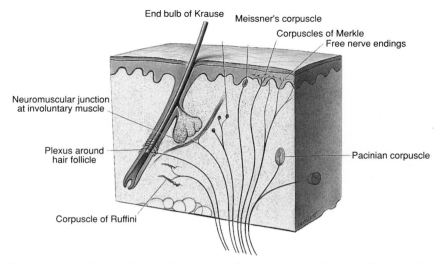

End bulb of Krause   Meissner's corpuscle

Corpuscles of Merkle
Free nerve endings

Neuromuscular junction
at involuntary muscle

Plexus around
hair follicle

Pacinian corpuscle

Corpuscle of Ruffini

Figure 10.1: Sensory nerve endings with roles in sensations. Receptors located in the epidermis include free nerve endings associated with pain and thermal sense and Merkel's corpuscles (also called Merkel's cells) responding to steady skin indentation, a form of touch. Receptors located in dermal papillae, at the junction of the dermis and epidermis, are Meissner's corpuscles monitoring touch, especially sensing fine spatial differences. The hair receptors (plexus around each hair follicle) subserve tactile sense and flutter. Receptors located in the dermis comprise the pacinian corpuscles and corpuscles of Ruffini. Pacinian corpuscles are involved with sensing flutter and vibratory sense. The corpuscles of Ruffini, and a variant called the end bulbs of Krause, subserve touch-pressure and vibratory sense.

capable of activating the receptor. The *stimulus threshold* is the intensity level required to activate the receptor. *Adaptation* is the response and adjustment a receptor makes to a stimulus. Some receptors generate action potentials when the stimulus starts and then soon ceases to respond. This type of receptor, called a *rapidly adapting receptor* provides information primarily when the stimulus changes. When an object (e.g., clothes) touches our skin, we soon are not aware of the object because the reacting sensors are rapidly adapting receptors. Other receptors that continue to respond as long as the stimulus is applied are called *slowly adapting receptors*. Such receptors are nociceptors that are responsible for the warning that is the perception of pain.

Merkel disks respond to a steady skin indentation tactile stimulus. Each has a small receptive field and is a slowly adapting receptor. *Meissner corpuscles* are associated with the tactile sense called fluttering (felt as a gentle trembling of the skin). Each has a small receptive field and is a rapidly adapting receptor. *Merkel*

disks and *Meissner corpuscles* are of significance to the blind in "reading" Braille, because these receptors, with their small receptive fields, can resolve fine spatial differences. The *pacinian corpuscle* is involved with the vibratory sense (felt as a diffuse humming sensation). Vibratory sense is poorly localized because pacinian corpuscles have large receptive fields. In addition, they are rapid adapting receptors. (Pacinian corpuscles are also located in the connective tissues of mesenteries, muscles, and interosseous membranes.) *Ruffini corpuscles* are associated with the sense of touch-pressure and the vibratory sense. Each has a large receptive field and is a slow adapting receptor. Each of these four receptor types has a low stimulus threshold and conveys information to the CNS via A-beta nerve fibers of first order neurons. Of the rapidly adapting receptors, the polymodal nociceptors of free nerve endings may act as somatosensory receptors (Chap. 9).

Receptors, especially the muscle spindles and Golgi tendon organs, are continuously monitoring the degree of stretch within the muscles

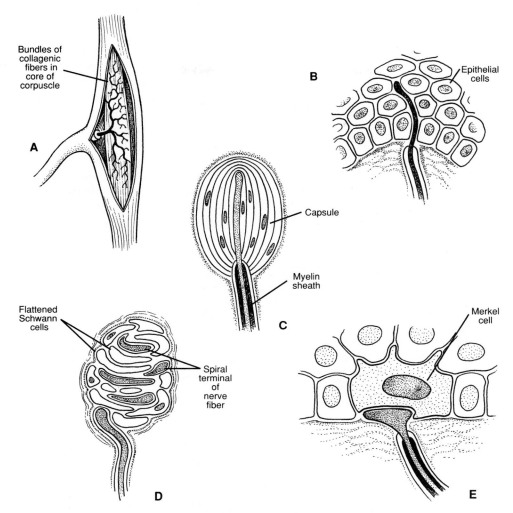

Figure 10.2: Sensory receptors of the skin. A. Corpuscle of Ruffini, an encapsulated receptor, is supplied by a single myelinated axon that branches repeatedly to form diffuse unmyelinated terminals among bundles of collagenic fibers in the core of the capsule. These terminals are presumably stimulated by the displacement of these collagenous fibers among which they are intertwined. Modified Schwann cells are absent. B. Free nerve endings in the epidermis where they lie between contiguous epithelial cells. C. Pacinian corpuscle, an encapsulated receptor, is innervated by a single myelinated axon that extends as an unmyelinated ending through the center of the bulb. The flattened cells surrounding the axon in the core of the capsule are presumably modified Schwann cells. D. Meissner's corpuscle, an encapsulated receptor, is innervated by a myelinated axon that forms an unmyelinated spiral ending amid flattened, transversely oriented Schwann cells. E. Merkel's corpuscle is a modified epidermal cell located in the basal layer of the epidermis. It is innervated by a myelinated nerve fiber "synapsing" as a free nerve ending with a Merkel's cell. (Adapted from Ham and Cormack).

and tension within the tendons (Chaps. 8, 11). The resulting "unconscious proprioception" is utilized in reflex arcs and by many processing centers, especially the cerebellum. It is now recognized that influences from the spindles and GTOs are also integrated into the lemniscal system and contribute to the conscious appreciation of position and movement sense.

The major somatic modalities elicited by mechanoreceptors are (1) *tactile sensations* evoked by the application of mechanical stimuli on the body surface, and (2) *proprioceptive sen-*

sations evoked by the mechanical displacements of muscles, ligaments, and joints. *Proprioception* is the sense of balance, position, and movement.

The two types of tactile sensations are *light (crude) touch* and *tactile discrimination*. *Light touch* is that felt by lightly stroking the skin with a wisp of hair or cotton. It can be tested by having an individual, with eyes closed, identify the location of being touched. *Tactile discrimination* or *pressure-touch* is often called *two-point discrimination*, which is the ability to distinguish between two points at which point-pressures are applied. It is also expressed as the ability to localize and to perceive the shape, size, and texture of an object by palpation, otherwise known as *stereognosis*. Proprioception takes on various forms including vibratory sense, static proprioception, and dynamic proprioception. The *vibratory sense* can be tested by perceiving the vibrations when the stem of a vibrating tuning fork is placed on a joint or other body part. *Static proprioception* is expressed as the ability to sense the position of a body part from information received from that part (called *position sense*). *Dynamic proprioception* or *kinesthetic sense* is the ability to sense movement and balance.

LEMNISCAL SYSTEM

The *lemniscal system* is the major pathway for stimuli contributing to kinesthetic sense and stereognosis. The latter is a complex sense that is based on such qualities as location, spatial form, and the sequence of inputs over time: integrating these qualities results in the perception of form and shape of objects that are touched, felt, and held. The lemniscal system serves DGS stimuli from the body, limbs, and posterior scalp. Stimuli from the rest of the head take the trigeminothalamic pathway. In addition, the *lateral cervical system* (also called the spinocervical tract) is utilized for certain touch and DGS stimuli. Light touch is also mediated by fibers of the *anterior spinothalamic tract*, part of the anterolateral pathway.

The lemniscal pathway, like other sensory systems, is serially organized in sequences of central neurons conveying information to the higher centers. Within these centers are interneurons that contribute to neural processing within the pathway. Each central neuron, including those in the somatosensory cortex, responds to a specific receptor field composed of a group of sensory receptors. The sizes of the receptive fields vary in relation to the sensitivity of the body area. The greater the sensitivity of an area, the greater is the density of small receptive fields in the area. For example, central neurons in the primary somesthetic cortex responding to stimuli from touch receptors in the sensitive tips of the fingers and tongue have large numbers of small receptive fields per unit area of skin or tongue. In contrast, the central neurons responding to the touch receptors in the small of the back have large receptive fields with a small number of fields per unit area of skin. Each central neuron responding is surrounded by a ring of inhibition; the ring is an expression of lateral inhibition (contrast inhibition) to increase the signal to noise ratio (Chap. 3). This lemniscal system terminates in five somatotopic modality-specific representations upon the primary (SI) and secondary (SII) somatosensory cortex. Those of SI are located in Brodmann areas 3a, 3b, 2, and 1 of the postcentral gyrus (Chap. 25), with the neurons in each area responding to a different aspect of the somatic sensation. Thus, a lemniscal pathway comprises a number of sensory channels projecting from the thalamus to terminate in lamina IV of the somatosensory cortex (Chap. 25).

Several cortical areas process somatic sensory information. These include (1) the primary somatosensory (SS) cortex and (2) the secondary SS cortex, (3) the posterior insular cortex of the central lobe (insula), and (4) the posterior parietal cortex (areas 5 and 7). The primary SS cortex has a somatotopic representation of the head and body surface of the contralateral side. The secondary SS cortex has a bilateral somatotopic representation of the head and body surface. The posterior insular cortex receives projections from the secondary SS cortex; it may be involved with object recognition by touch. Areas 5 and 7 receive SS input from the SS cortical areas. Area 5 may be a tertiary SS area; it has a somatotopic representation of the body surface (Chap. 25)

PATHWAYS SERVING DISCRIMINATIVE GENERAL SENSES (DGS)

Lemniscal Pathway from the Body, Limbs, and Back of Head

Information from the body, limbs, and back of head (scalp posterior to a coronal plane through the ears) is conveyed from the peripheral receptors over first-order neurons of the spinal nerves with cell bodies in the dorsal root ganglia. Their heavily myelinated fibers enter the spinal cord as the *medial bundle of the dorsal roots* (Fig. 10.3) and branch into (1) collaterals which terminate mainly in laminae III and IV of the posterior horn, and (2) fibers which ascend in the *fasciculi gracilis* and *cuneatus* of the posterior column before terminating in the *nuclei gracilis* and *cuneatus* of the lower medulla. Some of the collaterals ending in the posterior horn synapse with interneurons involved with spinal reflex arcs; other collateral branches are involved in the light touch component of the anterolateral pathway (see later, "Anterior Spinothalamic Tract").

The lemniscal pathway or system is also called the *posterior column-medial lemniscal pathway* because it begins in the posterior column of the spinal cord and continues as the medial lemniscus of the brainstem. As the fasciculi gracilis and cuneatus it consists of uncrossed fibers.

The first-order neurons form the label lines of the dorsal column-medial lemniscus pathway in a somatotopically organized lamination (Fig. 7.6). Fibers are added to the lateral aspect of the dorsal column (fasciculi gracilis and cuneatus) at each succeeding higher spinal level. The lamination from dorsomedial to lateral in the cervical levels consists, in order, of fibers from the sacral, lumbar, thoracic, and cervical segments of the body. The fibers from the sacral, lumbar and lower six thoracic levels compose the *fasciculus gracilis* of the posterior column and those of the upper six thoracic and all cervical levels (includes innervation of the back of head) compose the *fasciculus cuneatus*. The fibers terminating in the nucleus gracilis originate from below T6 (including the lower extremity) and those in the nucleus cuneatus originate

from above T6, including the upper extremities. The proprioceptive fibers of the lower extremity ascend in the *dorsolateral fasciculus* (a group of fibers located dorsally in the lateral column between the posterior gray horn and the posterior spinocerebellar tract, Fig. 7.6) with the fibers of the lateral cervical system to the lateral cervical nucleus (see later). The neural processing within the nucleus gracilis and nucleus cuneatus preserves and modifies the label lines that project to the thalamus. The processing consists of both feedback inhibition and feedforward inhibition and modulation by distal (reflected) inhibition from the somatosensory cerebral cortex (Chap. 3; Fig. 3.11). The new labeled lines project via the axons of second order neurons that emerge from the nuclei gracilis and cuneatus. They arc anteriorly as the *internal arcuate fibers*, decussate in the lower medulla, ascend as the somatotopically organized *medial lemniscus*, and terminate in the *ventral posterior lateral nucleus and posterior nucleus of the thalamus*. As it ascends, the medial lemniscus gradually shifts from a medial location in the medulla to a posterolateral location in the upper midbrain.

Axons of neurons of the third order emerging from the ventral posterolateral thalamic nucleus, pass through the posterior limb of the internal capsule and corona radiata before terminating in the postcentral gyrus and the adjacent paracentral lobule. The projections into these cortical areas (Brodmann areas 3, 1, and 2; Fig. 25.5) result in two sensory homunculi (Fig. 25.4). These figures are expressions of the relative density of sensory receptors in the various body parts. For these somatic senses, the greatest representation is in such structures as the tongue, lips, face, thumb, and index finger. The large homunculus is the primary somatosensory cortex (SI; areas 3, 1, and 2) and the small one is the secondary somatosensory cortex (SII). The body representation is also found in the nuclei gracilis and cuneatus and in the ventral posterior thalamic nucleus. SI receives inputs originating from the opposite side and SII from both sides of the head, body, and limbs. From SI and SII, fibers project to the somatosensory association cortex of the parietal lobe (Brodmann areas 5, 7, and 40) (Chap. 25).

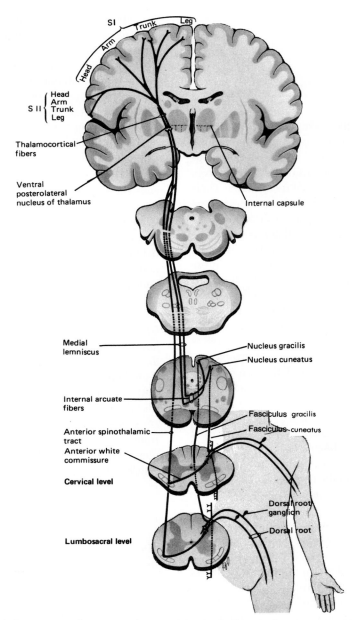

SI

Trunk
Arm
Head
Leg

S II { Head
Arm
Trunk
Leg

Thalamocortical fibers

Ventral posterolateral nucleus of thalamus

Internal capsule

Medial lemniscus

Nucleus gracilis

Nucleus cuneatus

Internal arcuate fibers

Fasciculus gracilis

Fasciculus cuneatus

Anterior spinothalamic tract

Anterior white commissure

Cervical level

Dorsal root ganglion

Dorsal root

Lumbosacral level

Figure 10.3: The discriminatory general sensory pathways originating in the spinal cord comprise the posterior column-medial lemniscus pathway and the anterior spinothalamic tract. Note that the ventral posterior lateral thalamic nucleus (VPL) projects to body regions of both SI and SII. For details of structures in the brainstem, refer to figures in Chapter 13.

Thalamus and Somatic Sensory (Somatosensory) Cortex

The *ventral posterior lateral thalamic nucleus (VPL)* receives sensory input from the body via the labeled lines in the medial lemniscus and spinothalamic tract. These inputs terminate in these nuclei to influence the third order neurons in a somatotopic pattern. These nuclei are parcelled functionally as follows: the *central core* of the nucleus is responsive to stimuli from cutaneous receptors; and the surrounding *shell* of the nucleus is responsive to stimuli from deep receptors (e.g., muscle spindles) (Fig. 10.4). In addition, these nuclei receive reflected (distal) inhibitory influences from the somatosensory cortex.

Axons of third order neurons emerge from the VPL, pass through the posterior limb of the internal capsule and corona radiata, and terminate in lamina IV of the somatosensory cortex located in postcentral gyrus and adjacent paracentral lobule and parietal lobe (see laminar organization of cortex in Chap. 25). The somatic sensory cortex consists of the *primary somatosensory cortex* (SI; areas 1, 2, 3a and 3b), *secondary somatosensory cortex* (SII) (both located in the postcentral gyrus), and the posterior parietal cortex (areas 5 and 7) (see homunculi in Chap. 25).

Five precise somatotopic representations of the body surface are present in the cortex in an orderly but distorted homunculus of the cortex; one each for areas 1, 2, 3a, and 3b of SI and one for SII. Distorted because the receptive field sizes are inversely related to the density of the receptors on the body. The back with its low density of receptors has a small cortical representation of a finger tip with its high density of sensory receptors.

There are somatotopic projections (a) from the medial lemniscus and spinothalamic tracts to the VPL and (b) from the core and shell of VPL to the somatosensory (areas 1, 2, 3a, and 3b) cortex (Fig. 10.4). (1) The *core neurons* receive cutaneous receptor input from slow and rapidly adapting receptors involved with the discrimination of texture. The third order thalamic neurons of the core receiving inputs from these receptors have substantial projections that terminate in area 3b. Those thalamic neurons of the core receiving inputs from rapidly adapting receptors involved with sensing texture have sparse projections that terminate in areas 1, 3b, and SII (Fig. 10.4). (2) The *shell neurons* receive inputs from the deep tissue receptors monitoring muscle stretch, deep pressure, and joint sense. Those thalamic neurons of the shell receiving inputs from muscle spindle stretch receptors have substantial projections that terminate in area 3a. Those thalamic neurons of the shell receiving stimuli from deep pressure and joint receptors involved with sensing size and shape of objects held in the hand have sparse projections that terminate in areas 3a, 2, and SII (Fig. 10.4). In turn, neurons from areas 3a and 3b project to areas 1 and 2. All of these four areas project to SII, which is involved in the discrimination of shape, size, and texture. All five areas of SI and SII have connections with parietal lobe association areas 5 and 7 (Chap. 25).

A similar structural and functional organization is presumably expressed in the ventral posterior medial thalamic nucleus (VPM), which is the nucleus receiving somatosensory input from the head primarily from the trigeminal nerve (see later). The VPM receives its input from the trigeminothalamic pathway and projects its output to the head region of the somatosensory cortex.

The Paths From Receptors to Columns of the Cortex

The sensory pathways involved with sensation are composed of sequences of neurons forming paths transmitting labeled line codes and pattern codes. The lemniscal and trigeminal pathways consist primarily of label lines extending from the somatic receptors in the body to the functional columns (slabs) in the postcentral gyrus of the parietal lobe (Chap. 25). Each receptor exhibits specificity, in that, it responds to a specific stimulus energy. Each line conveys a specific stimulus quality (e.g., position sense) and processes the message in each nucleus of the pathway before arriving for more processing in a cortical column. The stimulus feature encoded by the receptor in the body is faithfully reproduced by the signal received by that line in the cortex. For example, slowly adapting re-

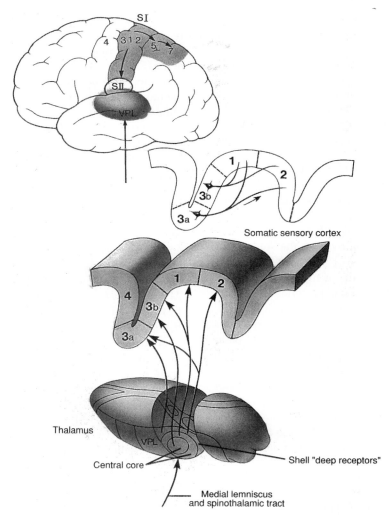

Figure 10.4: Schema illustrating the projections from the ventral posterior lateral and the ventral posterior medial thalamic nuclei (VPL and VPM, repectively) to the somatosensory cortex. The VPL receives input from the medial lemniscus and spinothalamic tracts, and the VPM from the trigeminothalamic tracts. These nuclei are organized into a central core consisting of two zones each responsive to cutaneous stimuli and an outer shell responsive to deep stimuli. Neurons of the central core project to cortical areas 3b and 1 (cutaneous). Neurons of the outer shell project to cortical area 3a (muscle spindles) and to area 2 (deep receptors). These projections are somatotopic.

The somatosensory cortex of the parietal lobe consists of three major subdivisions: primary somatosensory cortex (SI of areas 3, 1 and 2), secondary somatosensory cortex (SII of areas 3, 1, and 2) and posterior parietal cortex (5 and 7). Neurons in areas 3a and 3b project to areas 1 and 2. Neurons of SI (areas 3a, 3b, 1, and 2) project to the secondary sensory cortex (SII). Neurons from SI and SII and some thalamic neurons project to area 5 and the latter to area 7. (Adapted from Jones and Friedman, 1982.)

ceptors are coupled to slowly adapting neurons of the thalamus that are, in turn, coupled with slowly adapting neurons in a column of areas 3a and 3b of the somatosensory cortex. It is of significance that all six layers in each cortical column represent the same modality. Thus,

many lines transmitting different features of each sensation are paths where parallel processing of the stimulus features occurs. It is in the highest centers in the cortex that the features are integrated into a sensation. The paths are not redundant because they accent different features. Parallel processing of the stimulus features in several lines has a significant role in the generation of the variety and subtleties associated with our perceptions.

Trigeminothalamic Pathway from the Facial Region

The DGS from the facial region (head anterior to a coronal plane through the ears) are served via neurons of the trigeminal nerve, which enter the brainstem through the lateral midpons. Most fibers terminate in the principal (sensory) trigeminal nucleus. Other fibers bifurcate into collaterals which branch and terminate in the principal trigeminal nucleus and/or descend for a short distance in the spinal tract of n. V (spinal trigeminal tract) and terminate in the pars oralis of the spinal nucleus of n. V (spinal trigeminal nucleus). The principal trigeminal nucleus is the cranial equivalent of the nuclei gracilis and cuneatus. In all these nuclei are located the cell bodies of the second order neurons of the DGS (**Fig. 10.5**).

From cell bodies of neurons of the second order, located in the principal trigeminal nucleus and rostral portion of the spinal trigeminal nucleus, axons decussate in the pontine tegmentum and ascend as the trigeminothalamic tract (anterior trigeminal tract) before terminating in the VPM (**Fig. 10.5**). Some axons of second-order neurons of the principal trigeminal nucleus ascend *uncrossed* as the posterior trigeminothalamic tract (posterior trigeminal tract) to the same thalamic nucleus.

Axons of the neurons of the third order of the VPM pass through the posterior limb of the internal capsule and corona radiata before terminating in the head area of the postcentral gyrus. Following processing within this gyrus, connections via association fibers are made with areas 5 and 7 of the parietal lobe (**Fig. 10.4**; Chap. 25).

This trigeminal pathway is structurally and functionally the same as the dorsal column-medial lemniscal pathway: (1) The labeled lines from sensory receptors to columns in the postcentral gyrus are similar. (2) These lines are maintained and sharpened by the same processing circuits. (3) The projections from the VPM are similar to those of the VPL. The projection fibers terminate in areas 1, 2, 3a and 3b of the

postcentral gyrus. Subsequent connections with SII and areas 5 and 7 of the parietal lobe are equivalent (**Fig. 10.4**).

PATHWAYS SERVING LIGHT (CRUDE) TOUCH

Pathway from the Body, Limbs, and Back of Head

Light touch from the body and the back of the head (C2 dermatome) is conveyed from peripheral receptors via first-order neurons with cell bodies in the dorsal root ganglia of the peripheral nerves to the posterolateral tract of Lissauer, where the fibers bifurcate and ascend and descend several spinal levels before terminating on interneurons of the posterior horn (**Fig. 10.3**). Some first-order neurons may pass through the medial bundle and terminate in the posterior horn (bypassing the posterolateral tract of Lissauer). Processing occurs within the interneuronal circuits of the posterior horn.

The axons of neurons of the second order, with cell bodies presumably in laminae VI and VII, decussate through the anterior white commissure and then ascend as the anterior spinothalamic tract and terminate in the VPL. This pathway is somatotopically organized, with fibers from the sacral levels located laterally, and those from cervical levels medially within the tract (**Fig. 7.6**). In the lower brainstem this tract is located close to the lateral spinothalamic tract (**Fig. 10.6**). The anterior and lateral spinothalamic tracts together are referred to as the anterolateral tract or system (Chap. 9) and in the brainstem as the spinothalamic tract (**Fig. 13.9**).

The axons of the neurons of the third order pass through the posterior limb of the internal capsule and the corona radiata before terminating in the postcentral gyrus. After neural processing in the gyrus, pyramidal neurons of the cortex project information to the parietal association cortex. Light touch is also conveyed via the posterior column-medial lemniscus pathway and the spinocervical thalamic pathway (**Fig. 10.6**).

Pathways from the Facial Region

From receptors in the facial region (anterior to coronal plane through the ears), light (crude)

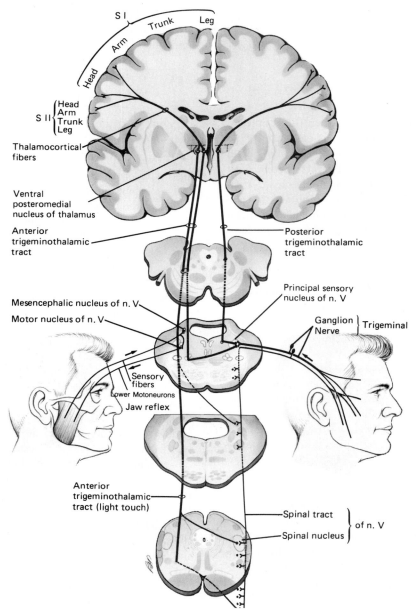

Figure 10.5: The discriminatory general sensory pathways originating in the brainstem are the anterior and posterior trigeminothalamic tracts. Note that the ventral posterior medial thalamic nucleus (VPM) projects to head regions of both SI and SII. The jaw reflex, illustrated on the left side of figure, comprises (1) the afferent fibers with cell bodies in the mesencephalic nucleus of n. V, and (2) efferent (lower motoneurons) fibers with cell bodies in the motor nucleus of n. V. For details of structures in the brainstem, refer to Figs. 13.9, 13.11–13.13, and 13.16.

touch fibers convey impulses via the three divisions of the trigeminal nerves (ophthalmic, maxillary, and mandibular) and cranial nerves VII, IX, and X. The cell bodies of these first-order fibers are located in the trigeminal ganglion,

geniculate ganglion and superior ganglia of nerves IX and X. Upon entering the brainstem, some of these fibers terminate in the principal trigeminal nucleus and others descend in the spinal tract of n. V and terminate in the spinal

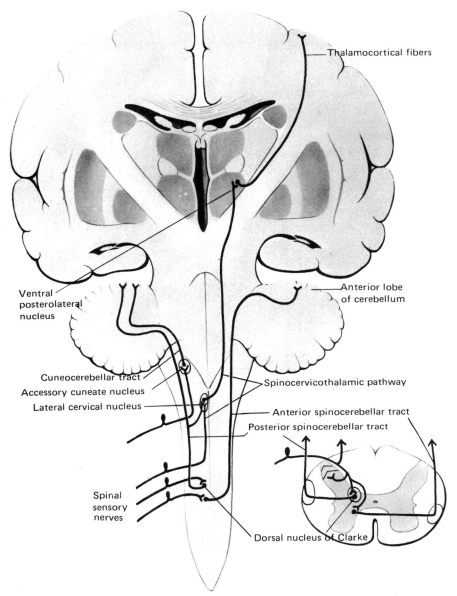

Figure 10.6: Ascending tracts from the spinal cord including the anterior and posterior spinocerebellar tracts, cuneocerebellar tract, and spinocervicothalamic pathway.

nucleus. Second-order neurons from these nuclei have axons which decussate and join the ascending anterior trigeminothalamic tract and terminate in the VPM. From this thalamic nucleus, axons pass through the internal capsule before terminating somatotopically as a homunculus in both the primary and secondary somatosensory cortex. In turn, SI and SII project

to the parietal association cortex, where more processing occurs **(Fig. 10.5)**.

Lateral Cervical System (Spinocervicothalamic Pathway)

The lateral cervical system mediates touch, proprioception, vibratory sense, and to a small degree noxious stimuli. This system is a fast-conduction four neuron pathway (Fig. 10.6).

The first-order neurons, with their cell bodies in the dorsal root ganglia, have axons that terminate in laminae III, IV, and V of the dorsal horn. From these laminae originate the second order neurons whose axons ascend without decussating in the dorsolateral fasciculus of the lateral column to the lateral cervical nucleus (Fig. 7.6). From this nucleus, located in the upper two cervical levels and the lower medulla, originate third order neurons. Their axons decussate in the lower medulla, ascend in the contralateral medial lemniscus and terminate in the VPL. The fourth order neurons project from this thalamic nucleus to the somatosensory cortex (SI and SII).

PROPRIOCEPTIVE PATHWAYS OF THE HEAD

Mesencephalic Nucleus of the Trigeminal Nerve; Jaw Jerk Reflex

Information from proprioceptive endings (e.g., muscle spindles) in the extraocular muscles and muscles of mastication and facial expression are conveyed to the CNS by Ia nerve fibers of cranial nerves III to VII. These Ia fibers have their cell bodies in the *mesencephalic nucleus of the trigeminal nerve*. This nucleus is unique, in that, it is the *only nucleus of primary sensory neurons located in the CNS* and is actually composed of *unipolar dorsal root (trigeminal) ganglion cell bodies* (Fig. 14.2).

The jaw jerk is a two-neuron reflex, similar to the knee jerk reflex (Fig. 10.5), which involves the temporalis, masseter, and internal pterygoid muscles. This reflex can be evoked by tapping the chin of the slightly opened mouth with a reflex hammer. The afferent limb of this reflex arc is composed of neurons with cell bodies of the mesencephalic nucleus. These neurons convey influences from the muscle spindles directly via collateral fibers to the lower motoneurons in the motor nucleus of the trigeminal nerve. These lower motoneurons comprise the efferent limb innervating the muscles of mastication.

PROPRIOCEPTIVE PATHWAYS TO THE CEREBELLUM

The cerebellum plays an essential role in body movement and maintenance of equilibrium. Voluntary muscles are coordinated in their contraction and relaxation so as to permit smooth movement. For this, the cerebellum requires a continuous supply of unconscious information from muscles, tendons, and joints to which receptors throughout the body and limbs contribute. The pathways for this input are outlined here; the main discussion of the cerebellum is in Chap. 17. The information that arrives from muscle spindles (Ia fibers) and Golgi tendon organs (Ib fibers) is primarily unconscious and proprioceptive in nature, but there are, in addition, inputs from exteroceptors for crude touch, pressure, and pain.

There are direct and indirect pathways for impulses from these receptors. The direct pathways convey input directly from the spinal neurons to the cerebellum. They are (1) the posterior spinocerebellar tracts for information from the lower limbs and lower half of the body and (2) the cuneocerebellar tracts for information from the upper limbs and upper half of the body (Figs. 7.6 and 10.6). The indirect pathways are (1) the spinocervicocerebellar pathway, with a synaptic relay in the lateral reticular nucleus of the medulla (Fig. 13.7), and (2) the spinoolivocerebellar pathway, with a synaptic relay in the inferior olivary nucleus of the medulla (Fig. 13.8).

Two complete somatotopic representations can be traced on the cerebellar cortex, one homunculus on the anterior lobe and the other (in halves) on the posterior lobe (Fig. 10.7).

Posterior Spinocerebellar Tract

First-order neurons that convey impulses from peripheral receptors into the spinal cord terminate in the dorsal nucleus (Clarke's nucleus), found in lamina VII (Fig. 10.6). Second-order neurons arise from this nucleus located at levels T1 through L2 and ascend uncrossed as the posterior spinocerebellar tract. The fibers enter the cerebellum by way of the inferior cerebellar peduncle, one of the three fiber bundles on each side giving access to the cerebellum (Fig.

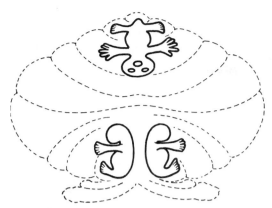

Figure 10.7: Somatotopic map of the anterior and posterior lobes of the cerebellum illustrating the somatic general sensory homunculi.

13.2). The posterior spinocerebellar tract is primarily concerned with conveying information from muscles and joints of the lower limbs.

Cuneocerebellar Tract

First-order neurons ascend in the ipsilateral fasciculus cuneatus of the spinal cord and terminate in the accessory cuneate nucleus (equivalent to the dorsal nucleus of Clarke), which is located lateral to the cuneate nucleus (**Fig. 13.9**). Second-order neurons, identified now as the cuneocerebellar tract, enter the cerebellum through the inferior cerebellar peduncle and terminate in portions of the anterior and posterior lobes dedicated to the upper extremities (**Fig. 10.3**). This pathway is the rostral equivalent of the posterior spinocerebellar tract.

Anterior Spinocerebellar Tract

This tract (**Fig. 10.6**) originates from cells, called *spinal border cells*, located on the periphery of the anterior horn and other cells in the intermediate gray zone. These cells are located in thoracolumbar levels. Axons of these cells decussate in the spinal cord and ascend as the anterior spinocerebellar tract through the medulla and brainstem, entering the superior cerebellar peduncle and recrossing within the cerebellum before terminating in the area of the homunculus in the anterior lobe of the cerebellum (**Fig. 10.7**).

Rostrospinocerebellar Tract

This tract is presumed to arise from cells in the intermediate gray zone of the cervical enlargement. It ascends as an uncrossed tract that passes through both the inferior and superior cerebellar peduncles before terminating in the area of the homunculus in the anterior lobe of the cerebellum (**Fig. 10.7**).

The pattern of termination of the posterior spinocerebellar and cuneocerebellar input to the cerebellum is somatotopic to form separate homunculi rostrally in the anterior lobe and caudally in the posterior lobe (**Fig. 10.7**). The anterior spinocerebellar and rostrospinocerebellar tracts were previously thought to convey somatic sensory information from the lower and upper limbs, respectively. They are now conceived as acting to relay *internal feedback signals* to the cerebellum. The latter reflects the amount and quality of neural activity in the descending motor pathways rather than conveying information from the periphery (Chap. 18).

Indirect Pathways

The spinoreticular fibers of the anterolateral pathway include a population of fibers originating at all spinal levels and terminating in the lateral cervical nucleus and other small nuclei in the medulla. This *spinocervicocerebellar pathway* is completed by neurons arising from such nuclei and terminating in the cerebellum. In this way, the exteroceptors send their input to the cerebellum.

Spinoolivary fibers originate from cell bodies located at all spinal levels, and ascend in the spinoolivary tract (**Fig. 7.6**), that terminates in the inferior olivary nuclei of the medulla (**Fig. 13.10**). They are activated by cutaneous and proprioceptive afferent fibers of the spinal nerves. *Olivocerebellar* fibers cross on their way to the cerebellum, which they enter through the inferior cerebellar peduncle.

Tickling

Tickling is related in some way to light touch and, possibly, pressure sense. It is produced by a light, external moving stimulus. It is transmitted within the CNS through the anterolateral pathway.

FUNCTIONAL CORRELATIONS

The general sensory pathways conveying pain and temperature, tactile sensibility, and discriminative senses have, with a few exceptions, similar features. The neurons of the first order extend from receptors in the periphery and terminate within nuclei (or laminae) in the ipsilateral half of the spinal cord or brainstem. The cell bodies of these neurons are located in ganglia (with no synapses within them) just outside the CNS: dorsal root ganglia, trigeminal ganglion, geniculate ganglion, and superior ganglia of cranial nerves IX and X. The neurons of the second order have cell bodies in a nucleus on the ipsilateral side and axons that decussate to the contralateral side and ascend as tracts which terminate in the thalamus (ventral posterior nucleus and posterior thalamic region). The neurons of the third order project from the thalamus to the postcentral gyrus (primary somatic area) and adjacent secondary somatic area (Fig. 25.3). Note that the spinothalamic fibers (neurons of the second order) decussate at all levels of the spinal cord, with each fiber crossing at a spinal level near the location of its cell body, whereas all second-order neurons of the posterior column-medial lemniscal pathway have axons that decussate at a common level in the lower medulla, where they become known as internal arcuate fibers.

Light touch may be conveyed via two pathways: (1) the anterior spinothalamic tract (and its cranial equivalent, the anterior trigeminothalamic tract), and (2) the posterior column-medial lemniscal pathway (and its cranial equivalent, the anterior and posterior trigeminothalamic tracts).

The loss of tactile sensibility is known as *tactile anesthesia*. Diminution is *tactile hypesthesia* and an exaggeration, which is often unpleasant, is *tactile hyperesthesia*. The last-mentioned may be accompanied by *paresthesias*—the sensations of numbness, tingling, prickling and feeling of discomfiture.

Impairment of the Posterior Column-Medial Lemniscal Pathway

The interruption of this discriminative general pathway results in disturbance in the appreciation of certain sensations and in the regulation and control of movements.

The alterations in the appreciation of the DGS include:

1. Diminution, not loss, of *light touch*. This modality is partially retained because the anterior spinothalamic tract is intact and functional.
2. Loss of *vibratory sense*. The perception of the "buzz" of vibrations is tested by placing the base of a vibrating tuning fork on a joint or bone (e.g., knee, elbow, finger, or spinous process of vertebra).
3. *Astereognosis*—literally meaning not knowing solids—refers to loss of the ability to recognize a common object by feel and palpation. For example, a patient with astereognosis is unable to identify a key, coin, or pencil by handling or touch. The ability to recognize objects by sight is unimpaired.
4. Loss of *two-point discrimination*—the ability to recognize two blunt points as two points when applied simultaneously.
5. Loss of *position sense*—the ability to know where a part of the body is located or to appreciate movement of a joint.

Ataxia (without order) refers to unsteady, awkward, and poorly coordinated movements. It can be caused by lesions in the pathways for proprioceptive stimuli, that is, the posterior column-medial lemniscal pathway including the dorsal roots, posterior column (posterior column ataxia), nuclei gracilis and cuneatus, and medial lemniscus. Patients show an unsteady gait while walking or turning; to reduce the unsteadiness, they walk with a broad base. In severe cases the patient may stagger and fall while the eyes are closed. The signs of the ataxia are more pronounced in patients in the dark or with eyes closed. The severity of the symptoms is reduced when the subject can use visual cues; this is consistent with the concept that two of three of the following sources of sensory input are essential for adequate regulation of posture and movement: proprioceptive general senses, vision, and vestibular sense. *Romberg's sign* is often used to detect posterior column ataxia. In the erect position with feet close together, the ataxic patient will sway when the eyes are closed; swaying is reduced or abolished when the eyes are opened. *Cerebellar ataxia* is another form of this disorder (Chap. 18).

Spinal Cord Lesions and the Light (Crude) Touch Pathways

Following a lesion in the spinal cord, the appreciation of light touch is less apt to be impaired than any of the other sensory modalities. This is because light touch is conveyed by the posterior column, anterolateral pathway, and the lateral cervical pathway. A unilateral lesion of the posterior column results in the loss of two-point discrimination on the same side of the body as the lesion while light touch persists, though it may be marginally lowered, because the anterolateral pathway is intact. A unilateral lesion of the anterolateral pathway results in loss of pain perception on the opposite side of body, but again, light touch persists or may be marginally lowered because the posterior columns are intact.

SUGGESTED READINGS

Brown A. The spinocervical tract. *Prog Neurobiol.* 1982;17:59–96. Burgess P, Wei J-Y, Clark F,

Simon J. Signaling of kinesthetic information by peripheral sensory receptors. *Annu Rev Neurosci.* 1982;5:171–187.

Chouchkov C. Cutaneous receptors. *Adv Anat Embryol Cell Biol.* 1978;54:1–62.

Darian-Smith I. Touch in primates. *Annu Rev Psychol.* 1982;33:155–194.

Fields H, Besson J, eds. Pain Modulation: Progress in Brain Research, Vol 77. Amsterdam: Elsevier; 1988.

Norrsell U. Behavioral studies of the somatosensory system. *Physiol Rev.* 1980;60:327–354.

Proske U, Schaible H, Schmidt R. Joint receptors and kinaesthesia. *Exp Brain Res.* 1988;72:219–224.

Roland P, Mortensen E. Somatosensory detection of microgeometry, macrogeometry and kinesthesia in man. *Brain Research Reviews.* 1987;12:1–42.

Schmidt R, ed. *Fundamentals of Sensory Physiology.* 3rd ed. New York, NY: Springer-Verlag; 1985.

Sinclair D. *Mechanisms of Cutaneous Sensation.* 2nd ed. New York, NY: Oxford University Press; 1981.

Vallbo A, Hagbarth K-E, Torebjörk H, Wallin B. Somatosensory, proprioceptive, and sympathetic activity in human peripheral nerves. *Physiol Rev.* 1979;59:919–957.

Motoneurons and Motor Pathways 11

Lower motoneurons (lower motor neurons)
Upper motoneurons (upper motor neurons)
Motor areas of the cerebral cortex
Motor pathways
Voluntary movements

The brain exerts both powerful and subtle influences upon the activity of the voluntary musculature through descending motor pathways. Originating from neurons with cell bodies located in the cerebral cortex and brainstem, these pathways act by regulating, modulating, and biasing the activity of the lower motoneurons of the cranial and spinal nerves. The neurons of these pathways are controlled directly or indirectly by the cerebral cortex, basal ganglia, and cerebellum.

LOWER MOTONEURONS (LOWER MOTOR NEURONS)

The voluntary (striated, skeletal) muscles are innervated by alpha motoneurons, which have heavily myelinated, fast-conducting axons terminating in the motor-end plates of extrafusal striated muscle fibers. Because these neurons are the only pathway through which the sensory systems and the descending upper motoneuron pathways of the central nervous system (CNS) exert their influences upon striated muscles, they function as the *final common pathway*, the final link between the CNS and the voluntary muscles. The intrafusal striated muscles of the muscle spindles are innervated by gamma motoneurons, which have lightly myelinated, slow-conducting axons.

The term *lower motoneuron*, as used in clinical neurology, refers to motor neurons that innervate the voluntary muscles. Destruction of the lower motoneurons supplying a muscle results in abolishing the voluntary and reflex responses of that muscle, rapid atrophy of the muscles innervated and a flaccid paralysis; these are signs of a lower motoneuron paralysis (Chap. 12). The lower motoneurons have their cell bodies within the anterior horn of the spinal cord (innervates voluntary muscles of the body) and in the motor nuclei of the brainstem (innervates voluntary muscles supplied by the cranial nerves) (Figs. 8.1 and 8.3).

The term *upper motoneuron* refers to the descending motor pathways within the CNS that either directly or indirectly exert influences on the lower motoneurons.

The activities of the alpha and gamma motoneurons are affected by inputs from the peripheral receptors through the spinal and cranial nerves and from the upper motoneurons of the brain. Most influences, both excitatory and inhibitory, are exerted through local interneurons of intrasegmental and intersegmental circuits within the gray matter. On the basis of inputs and other features, several differences exist between alpha and gamma motoneurons:

1. The alpha motoneurons can be stimulated monosynaptically (directly, not through in-

terneurons) by Groups Ia and II afferent fibers from the muscle spindles and by a few fibers of the corticospinal, rubrospinal, vestibulospinal, reticulospinal, and tectospinal tracts. Gamma motoneurons are not stimulated monosynaptically.

2. From the alpha motoneurons, collateral fibers make synaptic contact with Renshaw cells which, in turn, have inhibitory synapses with the same alpha motoneurons thus forming a negative feedback circuit that serves to turn off the active alpha motoneuron so that it can be excited again (**Fig. 3.10**). Gamma motoneurons are not linked to Renshaw cells.

The *lower motoneurons* are the general somatic efferent (GSE) components of the spinal nerves and of cranial nerves III, IV, VI, and XII, which innervate the extraocular and tongue musculature. They are also the special visceral efferent (SVE) components of cranial (branchiomeric) nerves V, VII, IX, X, and XI, which innervate the muscles of mastication and facial expression as well as the pharyngeal and laryngeal musculature (Chap. 14).

The lower motoneurons of the spinal cord are often called *anterior horn motoneurons* (cell bodies located in the anterior horn of the spinal cord). It is important to recognize that lower motoneurons are located in both cranial and spinal nerves.

Location of Cell Bodies of Lower Motoneurons

The cell bodies of the alpha and gamma motoneurons are organized into functionally defined groups in lamina IX of the ventral horn and into general somatic cranial motor nuclei in the brainstem (Chap. 14). The dendrites of these neurons extend beyond the designated borders of lamina IX.

1. The motoneurons are arranged according to the medial-lateral rule (pattern) in the anterior horn (**Fig. 11.1**). The medial group comprises the motoneurons that innervate the axial muscles (neck and back). It is flanked laterally by the intermediate group that innervates the proximal muscles of the limbs (shoulder and arm, hip and thigh). The most lateral group comprises those neurons that innervate the distal muscles of limbs (forearm and hand, leg and foot).

2. The motoneurons are arranged according to the flexor-extensor rule (pattern) (**Fig. 11.1**). The flexor muscle group is located dorsally and the extensor muscle group is located ventrally in the anterior horn.

3. The motoneurons innervating a specific muscle or related muscles are clustered in a narrow longitudinally oriented three-dimensional column. This column extends through more than one spinal segment. As a consequence, each muscle is innervated by axons originating from more than one spinal segment. Thus, a lesion limited to one spinal root or nerve will result in only a partial lower motor neuron paralysis.

4. The alpha motoneurons are presumed to be organized into groups on the basis of their functional attributes as (a) phasic motoneurons and (b) tonic motoneurons. The phasic motoneurons are large and fire with brief bursts at high frequencies. They are active during rapid movements of short duration that exert great force. The tonic motoneurons are relatively small and fire with brief bursts at low frequencies. They are active during delicate movements requiring little force and that sustain moderate tension for an extended period of time.

5. The *intersegmental interneurons* (*propriospinal interneurons*, Chap. 6) coordinating these alpha and gamma motoneurons at different spinal segments have axons located in the white matter (**Fig. 11.1**). The medial motoneurons (axial muscles) are interconnected by intersegmental neurons with long axons. The latter extend through many spinal levels in the anterior funiculus. The lateral motoneurons (limb muscles) are interconnected by intersegmental neurons with shorter axons. The latter extend through a lesser number of spinal segments in the lateral funiculus.

UPPER MOTONEURONS (UPPER MOTOR NEURONS)

The facilitatory (excitatory) and inhibitory influences stimulating the lower motoneurons are

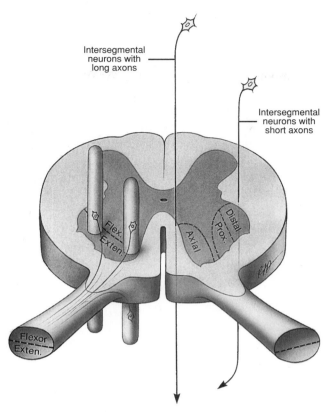

Figure 11.1: The alpha and gamma motoneurons are arranged in functionally defined groups in lamina IX of the ventral horn. The motoneurons located medially innervate axial (neck and back) musculature and those located laterally innervate the proximal and distal limb musculature respectively. The motoneurons located dorsally innervate the flexor muscles and those located ventrally innervate the extensor muscles. The medial motoneurons are interconnected by intersegmental neurons with long axons, and the lateral motoneurons by intersegmental neurons with shorter axons. The cylinder extending through more than one spinal segment in lamina IX represents the distribution of lower motoneurons innervating a specific muscle or related muscles.

conveyed via fibers from two general sources: (1) the head and body via the cranial and spinal nerves—information from these sources is integrated in reflex activity and (2) the brain via descending supraspinal pathways—these are generally called "voluntary" pathways. These are motor control pathways that mediate voluntary motor control of movement and regulate reflexes.

The *descending supraspinal pathways* project influences that modify the activity of the lower motoneurons; they are called *upper motoneurons* (UMNs). These include the neurons and their fibers of (1) the *corticospinal (pyramidal)* and *corticobulbar tracts* originating in the cerebral

cortex **(Figs. 11.2 and 11.3)**; (2) the *rubrospinal* and *tectospinal*, originating in the midbrain; and (3) the *reticulospinal* and *vestibulospinal tracts*, originating in the lower brainstem (pons and medulla) **(Figs. 11.4 and 16–7)**.

Clinicians usually equate the term *upper motoneurons* with the lateral *corticospinal tract* and sometimes include the *corticobulbar tract* (cortical fibers that end in the brainstem). In another usage, the term *pyramidal tract (system)* refers to the corticospinal tract and the term *extrapyramidal tracts (system)* is a collective term referring to all other descending motor tracts and their processing centers.

In contrast to a lower motoneuron, which is

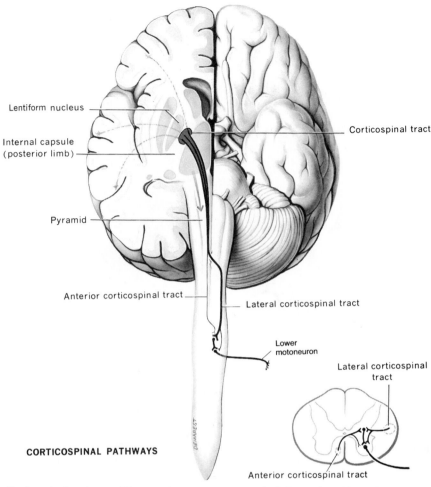

Lentiform nucleus

Internal capsule
(posterior limb)

Pyramid

Corticospinal tract

Anterior corticospinal tract

Lateral corticospinal tract

Lower
motoneuron

Lateral corticospinal
tract

Anterior corticospinal tract

CORTICOSPINAL PATHWAYS

Figure 11.2: Corticospinal pathways. These pathways are composed of descending fibers that originate from wide areas of the cerebral cortex and pass through the posterior limb of the internal capsule, crus cerebri, pons, pyramid, and spinal cord. Many of these fibers terminate upon spinal interneurons that, in turn, synapse with the lower motoneurons. Some fibers terminate directly upon lower motoneurons. The lateral corticospinal tract crosses over at the lower medulla as the pyramidal decussation, and the anterior corticospinal tract crosses over in upper spinal cord levels.

partially present in both the CNS and peripheral nervous systems, an upper motoneuron is located wholly within the CNS. The upper motoneurons have significant roles in voluntary motor activity and the maintenance of posture and equilibrium, control of muscle tone and reflex activity. In general, the influences conveyed via the descending supraspinal pathways exert their effects (1) on groups of muscles and movements (e.g., flexion, extension, adduction) and not primarily on one specific muscle and (2) reciprocally upon agonist and antagonist muscle groups (e.g., they facilitate flexion and inhibit extension or inhibit flexion and facilitate extension). The upper motoneurons exert their influences via both direct monosynaptic connections and indirect multisynaptic connections through interneurons with lower motoneurons.

Other Supraspinal Neurons

Two other types of descending supraspinal pathways are functionally significant. (1) Some fibers of reflected feedback pathways descend

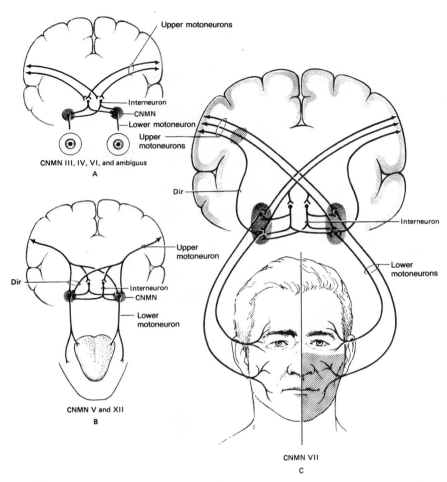

Figure 11.3: The three groups of cranial nerve motor nuclei (CNMN) according to their upper motoneuron innervation. **A.** CNMN III, IV, VI, and ambiguus. The upper motoneurons exert influences through direct bilateral projections to interneurons which, in turn, innervate the lower motoneurons of these motor nuclei. **B.** CNMN V and XII. The upper motoneurons exert influences both through (1) indirect bilateral projections to interneurons and (2) direct (Dir) bilateral projections to the lower motoneurons of these motor nuclei. **C.** CNMN VII. The upper motoneurons exert influences through indirect bilateral projections to lower motoneurons. Of importance, (1) the lower motoneurons innervating muscles of upper face and forehead receive direct bilateral upper motoneuron projections and (2) the lower motoneurons innervating muscles of lower face receive predominantly direct crossed upper motoneuron projections. The upper motoneuron lesion (shaded) results in a paralysis limited to muscles of facial expression of the contralateral lower face (shaded). (See Weber's syndrome, Chap. 17.)

and terminate in the sensory relay nuclei of the ascending pathways (e.g., posterior horn, nuclei gracilis and cuneatus, and spinal trigeminal nucleus). These reflected feedback pathways modulate sensory input and modify the processing within these nuclei (see section regarding descending control mechanisms, Chap. 9). (2) The descending fibers of the autonomic nervous system influence and regulate visceral activity through connections with the preganglionic

neurons of the sympathetic and parasympathetic systems (Chap. 20).

MOTOR AREAS OF THE CEREBRAL CORTEX

Several areas of the cerebral cortex have been designated as motor areas. These include the (1) *primary motor cortex* (area 4, motor strip,

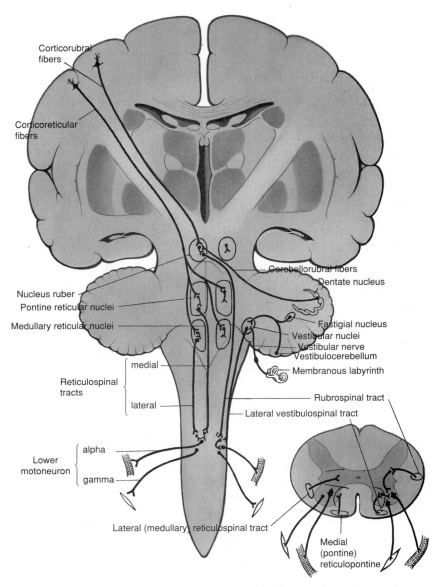

Figure 11.4: Descending motor pathways to the spinal cord including the reticulospinal tracts (corticoreticulospinal pathways), rubrospinal tracts (corticorubrospinal pathways), and vestibulospinal tracts. The corticoreticular fibers terminate bilaterally but (not illustrated) with a slight contralateral preponderance.

MI), (2) *premotor cortex* (areas 6 and 8), (3) *supplementary motor cortex* (portion of area 6), and (4) *second motor cortex* (MII) **(Figs. 25.3 and 25.4)**.

The *primary motor cortex* (area 4) is located in the precentral gyrus and the rostral half of the paracentral lobule. Direct electrical stimulation of this area evokes movements associated with the voluntary muscles. A map of this electrically excitable cortex produces a somatotopi-

cally organized *motor homunculus* (little man, **Fig. 25.4**). The homunculus hangs upside down with the larynx and tongue in the lowest part adjacent to the lateral fissure followed upward by the head, upper limb, thorax, abdomen, and lower extremity; the latter is located in the rostral paracentral gyrus. The amount of motor cortex devoted to specific regions is roughly proportional to the skill, precision, and control of the movements in that region (e.g., large area for larynx, tongue, thumb, and lips). The role of area 4 is to participate in the execution of skilled and agile voluntary movements. Although this motor cortex does contribute to the regulation of axial and proximal limb musculature, it has a more critical role in the control of the distal muscles of the extremities on the contralateral side of the body.

The *premotor cortex*, located rostral to area 4, consists of areas 6 and 8. Area 8, known as the *frontal eye field*, influences eye movements. Stimulation of this area results in conjugate movements of the eyes directed to the opposite side. The *premotor cortex* on the lateral surface of the lobe has (1) a primary role in the control of the proximal limb and axial musculature and (2) an essential role in the initial phases of orientation movements of the body and upper limbs directed toward a target. The *supplementary motor cortex*, located on the medial aspect of area 6, has a somatotopic organization. It plays a significant role in the programming of patterns and sequences of movements. For example, the response to electric stimulation on one side of this area activates complex patterns of movement not only of the contralateral limbs, but also includes bilateral movements of limbs of both sides. Both the premotor cortex and the supplementary motor cortex project to the primary motor cortex. The role of the *second motor cortex* is unknown.

General Statements

The primary motor cortex (area 4), premotor cortex, and supplementary motor cortex are somatotopically organized. Area 4 and the supplementary motor cortex have direct projections via the corticospinal tracts to the spinal cord. The premotor cortex projects primarily to the reticular formation of the pons and medulla. The premotor cortex and the supplementary motor cortex are higher ordered motor cortical regions that have connections with the primary motor cortex.

MOTOR PATHWAYS

General Statement

The descending motor pathways may be subdivided into systems called (1) the corticospinal tract and corticobulbar fibers, (2) corticoreticulospinal pathways, (3) corticorubrospinal pathway, (4) corticotectospinal pathway, (5) vestibulospinal tracts, and (6) raphe-spinal and ceruleus-spinal pathways (aminergic pathways). In addition to being involved with motor circuits associated with the spinal cord and the spinal nerves, these systems also have equivalent roles influencing the local motor circuits of the brainstem and the cranial nerves. Many of the fibers of the systems have significant roles in feedback circuits that modulate the activities of the ascending sensory pathways (Chaps. 9 and 10).

Corticospinal Tract

The upper motoneuron tracts and pathways originate from pyramidal cells (cell bodies with pyramid shape) of the cerebral cortex and from neurons of nuclei in the brainstem. The fibers of the corticospinal tract originate in the cortex and terminate in the spinal cord. About one-third of the fibers arise from Brodmann's area 4, one-third from area 6 of the frontal lobe, and the remaining fibers from areas 3, 1, 2, and 5 of the parietal lobe. Most of these fibers terminate on neurons of the spinal circuits influencing the lower motoneurons. About 3% arise from giant pyramidal cells called Betz cells in area 4; the axons of these corticospinal neurons have monosynaptic contact with some alpha motoneurons and interneurons in lamina IX.

The axons of the somatotopically organized corticospinal tract descend through the ipsilateral posterior limb of the internal capsule (near the genu), the middle portion of the crus cerebri of the midbrain, the pons, and the pyramids of the medulla (**Fig. 11.2**). The corticospinal tract sends collateral branches from these long axons to some basal ganglia, thalamic nuclei, nucleus ruber and brainstem reticular nuclei, thereby exerting influences on nuclei within the brain as well as on lower motoneurons. (The corticospinal tract is also called the pyramidal tract because its fibers pass through the modullary pyramids.)

At the medulla-spinal cord junction, approximately 90% of the 1 million fibers in each tract cross as the pyramidal decussation and descend in the posterior half of the lateral funiculus as the *lateral corticospinal tract*, which terminates at all spinal levels in laminae IV through VII and IX (**Fig. 7.5**). About 8% of the fibers descend without crossing in the ipsilateral anterior funiculus as the *anterior corticospinal tract*, which terminates after crossing in the anterior white commissure in lamina VIII in cervical and upper thoracic cord levels. A few pyramidal fibers descend as uncrossed axons in the lateral corticospinal tract.

The functional roles of these pathways may be summarized as follows: (1) the lateral corticospinal tract is preferentially involved with movements of the limbs and has a key role in the execution of skilled movements; (2) the anterior corticospinal tract is preferentially involved with control of axial muscles (neck, shoulder, and trunk); and (3) the lateral corticospinal tract fibers originating from the parietal lobe form a reflected feedback pathway modulating sensory input in the dorsal horn of the spinal cord (Chap. 9).

The corticospinal tracts exert their influences on local spinal reflex circuits involving the interneurons and both alpha and gamma motoneurons. Glutamate is the likely neurotransmitter released by these tracts (Chap. 15). Acting through interneurons these tracts generally evoke EPSP's on the local circuits involved with the flexor limb musculature (agonists) and IPSP's on the circuits involved with the extensor musculature (antagonists).

Corticobulbar Fibers

The cerebral cortical (supranuclear, upper motoneuron) projections to the nuclei of the cranial nerves and nuclei of the ascending pathways are known as *corticobulbar fibers* (**Fig. 11.3**). This pathway has a role similar to the corticospinal pathway, particularly in the fractionation of movements (see subsequent discussion). There are three types of fibers:

1. *Indirect corticobulbar fibers* (often included with corticoreticular fibers) originate in the premotor, motor, and somesthetic areas (areas 6, 4, 3, 1, 2, and 5) of the cerebral cortex, descend in the genu of the internal capsule, and pass through both the ipsilateral and contralateral brainstem before synapsing directly with interneurons of the

brainstem reticular formation (see *pseudobulbar palsy*, page 249). These interneurons are integrated in circuits which innervate the cranial nerve motor nuclei including nerves III, IV, V, VI, VII, and XII and the nucleus ambiguus. The descending influences to the nucleus of the accessory nerve are probably conveyed via uncrossed indirect corticobulbar projects, which facilitate the contraction of the ipsilateral sternocleidomastoid and trapezius muscles.

2. *Direct corticobulbar fibers* from each hemisphere to the motor nuclei of the cranial nerves originate in the cerebral cortex, descend in the genu of the internal capsule, and pass as crossed and uncrossed fibers to and through both the ipsilateral and contralateral brainstem before synapsing with the lower motoneurons of the motor nuclei of cranial nerves V (muscles of mastication), VII (muscles of facial expression), and XII (tongue musculature) (**Fig. 11.3**). The lower motoneurons innervating the muscles of facial expression below the level of the eye (e.g., buccinator, labial muscles) are a clinically significant exception (Chap. 14); they are innervated only by corticobulbar fibers which have decussated (not innervated by descending uncrossed fibers; **Fig. 11.3**).

3. Fibers of reflected feedback pathways project influences from sensory cortical areas 3, 1, 2, and 5 (parietal lobe) to sensory relay nuclei of the ascending pathways including the nuclei gracilis and cuneatus of the posterior column-medial lemniscal pathway, principal sensory trigeminal nucleus, spinal trigeminal nucleus, and the nucleus of the solitary fasciculus. These fibers are involved with processing sensory influences in the nuclei of ascending pathways.

Extrapyramidal System

With the exception of the pyramidal system, the descending supraspinal tracts, together with their nuclei and feedback circuits influencing somatic motor activity of voluntary muscles, are incorporated into the so-called "extrapyramidal system." The term is loosely used, and many authorities have discarded it. The descending tracts, which convey influences to the lower motoneurons, are actually neuronal links in pathway systems of complex circuitry involving the cerebral cortex, basal ganglia, thalamus, cerebellum, brainstem reticular formation, and related structures. Such systems include the corticorubrospinal, cerebellorubrospinal, corticoreticulospinal, cerebelloreticulospinal, cerebellovestibulospinal, and vestibular nerve-vestibulospinal pathways. The extrapyramidal system is discussed in Chapter 24.

Corticoreticulospinal: Corticoreticular and Reticulospinal Tracts

The sequence of corticoreticular and reticulospinal tracts comprises the *corticoreticulospinal pathway* (Fig. 11.4). From their origin in the premotor cortex (area 6) of the frontal lobe, corticoreticular fibers descend along with the corticospinal tract and terminate in the pontine and medullary reticular nuclei of the brainstem reticular formation on both sides. The latter also receives input from ascending pathways and the cerebellum (Chap. 13).

The *reticulospinal tracts* include the *lateral (medullary) reticulospinal tract* and the *medial (pontine) reticulospinal tract* that extend throughout the spinal cord. These tracts are primarily uncrossed and are not somatotopically organized.

The *medial pontine reticulospinal tract* originates from the nuclei reticularis pontis oralis and caudalis (Chap. 13) and descends mainly as uncrossed fibers in the anterior funiculus (included in medial longitudinal fasciculus, see below) and terminates at all spinal levels in the medial parts of the ventral horn and intermediate zone (see subsequent discussion of its function).

The *lateral (medullary) reticulospinal tract* originates from the nucleus reticularis gigantocellularis (Fig. 13.10) and descends mainly as uncrossed fibers in the anterior region of the lateral funiculus. The fibers terminate at all spinal levels upon interneurons in the medial part of the ventral horn and intermediate zone. Its functional role is discussed in the section concerning functional groupings of descending pathways.

The fibers of both reticulospinal tracts terminate on interneurons in laminae VII, VIII, and IX and some on gamma motoneurons. They can facilitate and inhibit the local spinal circuits involved in both reflex and voluntary movements. These corticoreticulospinal pathways are involved in maintaining posture (upright position) for movements that orient the body toward the external stimuli and for crude stereotypic voluntary movements of the extremities, such as extending the limb toward an object.

This pathway acts as a link in the autonomic nervous system conveying influences to the sympathetic and parasympathetic centers in the spinal cord (Chap. 20). Descending fibers from the autonomic centers in the hypothalamus project their influences directly to spinal levels and to visceral centers in the reticular formation of the lower brainstem. This region, including the nucleus gigantocellularis, contains cardiovascular, respiratory, and other visceral centers. Their influences are conveyed to the spinal cord via the lateral reticulospinal tract. Expressions of this include the modulation of the heart beat, dilatation of the pupil, perspiration, shivering, and the activity of sphincters of the gastrointestinal and urinary systems.

Corticorubrospinal Pathway: Corticorubral and Rubrospinal Tracts

The corticorubral tract originates in areas 4 and 6 and terminates in the ipsilateral nucleus ruber (red nucleus) of the midbrain (Figs. 11.4 and 13.15). This nucleus is a processing center of the corticorubrospinal pathway. The rubrospinal tract originates in the magnocellular portion of the red nucleus and crosses over in the midbrain tegmentum as the ventral tegmental decussation. It descends in the lateral funiculus of the spinal cord and terminates in laminae V, VI, and VII at all spinal levels. This pathway facilitates the local circuitry and the alpha and gamma motoneurons involved with the flexor musculature and inhibits that involved with the extensor musculature, especially that of the upper extremity. In this respect, it is functionally similar to the lateral corticospinal pathway.

Vestibulospinal Tracts

The lateral vestibular nucleus gives rise to the lateral vestibulospinal tract, which descends as an uncrossed somatotopically organized tract throughout the entire length of the spinal cord in the anterior region of the lateral funiculus (**Figs. 11.4 and 16.7**). It terminates in the medial part of the anterior horn and intermediate zone and selectively excites motoneurons to the extensors. Fibers from the medial vestibular nucleus descend mainly, but not entirely, uncrossed as the medial vestibulospinal tract within the medial longitudinal fasciculus (MLF) of the anterior funiculus (**Fig. 16.7**). The vestibulospinal tracts terminate almost exclusively on interneurons of laminae VII and VIII, which, in turn, interact with the alpha and gamma motoneurons of lamina IX; some fibers terminate monosynaptically on alpha motoneurons in lamina IX. Both tracts exert facilitatory influences on muscle stretch (myotatic) reflexes. This reinforces the tonus of the extensor musculature of the trunk and extremities to maintain the upright posture.

Corticotectal, Tectobulbar, and Tectospinal Tracts

The corticotectal tract originates in the visual association areas 18 and 19 and terminates in the superior colliculus and other nuclei in the midbrain tectum. The tectobulbar tract terminates in the paramedian pontine reticular formation (PPRF). The PPRF is involved with the coordination of the conjugate movements of the eyes and their reflexive movements (Chaps. 14 and 16, **Fig. 16.7**).

The tectospinal tract from the superior colliculus decussates as the dorsal tegmental decussation in the midbrain tegmentum to join and descend in the ventral funiculus of the spinal cord as the MLF. Its fibers terminate in laminae VII and VIII of the cervical and upper thoracic levels. The corticotectospinal and corticotectobulbar pathways are involved with conveying influences via interneurons to the lower motoneurons innervating the extraocular, neck, and back musculature. In addition, the vestibular system is integrated into the activities of these muscles. These systems of pathways account for turning movements of the head, eyes, and trunk in response to visual and vestibular inputs (Chaps. 16 and 19). The eye movements are essentially reflexive and not volitional. The influences from visual area 19 are associated with

pursuit movements of the eyes (Chap. 16; **Fig. 16.6**). In essence, these pathways coordinate eye movements involving the axial (trunk) muscles as well as the vestibular influences on the muscles of the extremities during balancing activities.

Medial Longitudinal Fasciculus

The *medial longitudinal fasciculus* (MLF) is a composite bundle of fibers located in the brainstem (Chap. 13) and spinal cord (**Figs. 7.6 and 16.7**). It consists of a *"descending component"* and an *"ascending component."* The descending component extends from the midbrain throughout the spinal cord. It comprises the medial vestibulospinal tract, the medial reticulospinal tract (both described above), and the tectospinal tract originating from the superior colliculus. The latter tract descends through the MLF as far as upper cervical levels and terminates in laminae VII and VIII. The ascending component is the *vestibuloocular reflex pathway* in the pons and midbrain, extending from the level of the abducens nucleus to that of the oculomotor nuclei. This pathway originates from cell bodies located in the vestibular nuclei and in the paramedian pontine reticular formation (PPRF, Chap. 16). In addition, the MLF contains reciprocal fiber systems interconnecting the abducens and oculomotor nuclei (for conjugate eye movements) (Chap. 16).

Raphe-Spinal and Locus Ceruleus-Spinal Pathways (Aminergic Pathways)

The projections from certain brainstem nuclei to the spinal cord, called aminergic pathways, are characterized by the monoamine transmitters they release. Among these are serotonin (5-HT, 5-hydroxytryptamine) and norepinephrine (noradrenaline) (Chap. 15).

Serotonin is located in neurons of the nucleus raphe magnus, other raphe nuclei and some neurons of the brainstem reticular formation (Chaps. 13 and 15). Their axons descend in the dorsolateral funiculus of the spinal cord and terminate in laminae I, II, V, and the preganglionic sympathetic neurons of lamina VII. This reflected feedback pathway has a role in modulating noxious (pain) signals within the dorsal horn through endorphins (Chap. 9).

Norepinephrine is present in the neurons of the locus ceruleus and nucleus subceruleus (Chap. 13). The noradrenergic projection from these nuclei to the spinal cord descends in the ventrolateral funiculus and terminates in laminae I, II, V, VII, and IX.

These aminergic pathways have roles (1) in influencing preganglionic sympathetic neurons in the spinal cord, (2) in exerting facilitatory activity on the level of responsiveness of the lower motoneurons, (3) in modulating the relative intensity of various expressions of emotional states, and (4) modulating noxious stimuli associated with pain (Chap. 9).

Functional Groups of the Somatic Motor (Descending Pathways)

In a general way, each of the descending tracts of upper motoneurons can be placed into one of three functional groups: (1) the lateral group, (2) the anteromedial group, or (3) the aminergic group.

The *lateral group*, also called *lateral descending system*, comprises the lateral corticospinal and rubrospinal tracts. It terminates in the lateral portions of the ventral horn and intermediate zone of the spinal gray matter. Within the spinal gray matter are the anatomic linkages involved primarily in the control of voluntary movements associated with the limbs, especially with distal limb musculature. The corticospinal tract originates primarily from the primary motor cortex (area 4), supplementary motor cortex (area 6), and parietal lobe (areas 1, 2, 3, 5, and 7). The rubrospinal tract originates from the magnocellular portion of the nucleus ruber. Because these tracts decussate, they exert their influences on the side opposite from their sites of origin. Functionally, these lateral pathways have a critical role in the fine manipulative and independent movements of the extremities—especially of the hands and feet. They are involved in the *fractionation of movement* as is expressed in the ability to control and execute independent finger movements. More specifically, fractionation is the ability to control, for example, an individual muscle of the hand independently from other muscles involved with normal manual dexterity. The fibers of the lateral corticospinal tract that terminate

directly on the alpha motoneurons have a major role in effecting the expression of fractionation of movements. Following a lesion to this tract, there is a diminution or loss of fractionation. The rubrospinal tract may be clinically significant; it could account for certain residual motor function that persists after a lesion of the corticospinal tract. Those fibers of the corticospinal tract originating in the parietal lobe (areas 1, 2, 3, 5, and 7) are components of the *reflected feedback pathways*, noted previously; these fibers terminate in the dorsal horn, where they modulate sensory input.

The *anteromedial group*, also called *medial descending system*, comprises the anterior corticospinal tract, lateral and medial reticulospinal tracts, lateral and medial vestibulospinal tracts, and tectospinal tract. These tracts terminate in the medial part of the ventral horn and intermediate zone, which provides the anatomic linkages for the *coordinated activity of the axial and limb girdle musculature during postural movements*. These tracts exert bilateral control because (1) most contain both crossed and uncrossed fibers and (2) they terminate on interneurons that have axons that cross over to the opposite side. This may account for minimal loss of motor control of axial musculature following unilateral lesions to these tracts. In contrast, limb control is profoundly affected. Many of these descending tracts terminate in the cervical and upper thoracic levels; hence, these pathways preferentially control neck, upper trunk, and shoulder girdle musculature, rather than lower trunk and hip girdle musculature. The anterior corticospinal tract is involved with voluntary movements associated with axial muscles of the neck and trunk. The reticulospinal tracts, which receive a major input from the premotor cortex, are thought to be involved in the more automatic, involuntary movements of the axial and limb musculature involved with posture and locomotion. They may be significant in controlling girdle musculature. The lateral vestibulospinal tract that descends as an uncrossed tract throughout the entire length of the spinal cord is critical in the maintenance of balance (Chap. 16). The medial vestibulospinal tract, which is in the caudal extension of the MLF of the brainstem, descends bilaterally; it is involved with orienting head position through coordinating the activity of the neck and back musculature. The tectospinal tract originates from the deep layers of the superior colliculus, an important structure that receives input from the visual system. This tract is presumed to be involved with coordinating head and neck movements with eye movements.

These anteromedial pathways exert their influences on musculature bilaterally. Even such uncrossed tracts as the lateral vestibulospinal and reticulospinal tracts do so by terminating on interneurons some of which have axons that decussate in the anterior commissure to the opposite side.

The fibers of these upper motoneuron control pathways exert their effects (a) by direct synaptic connections with lower motoneurons and (b) by synaptic connections with interneurons that are integrated with local circuits influencing lower motoneurons. Thus, the activity of lower motoneurons is controlled by direct and indirect polysynaptic connections from the upper motoneurons and, in addition, from sensory input from spinal nerves to the reflex circuits (Chap. 8). The *aminergic pathways* have the role of modulating the excitability of the spinal neuronal circuits involved with regulating the activity of the lower motoneurons.

VOLUNTARY MOVEMENTS

Voluntary purposeful movements, such as the sequence of motions resulting in catching a ball, involve several cortical areas including: (1) primary motor cortex (area 4), (2) premotor cortex (area 6), (3) supplementary motor cortex (area 6), and (4) posterior parietal cortex (areas 5 and 7) (**Fig. 25.3**). The following is an outline of a current concept of the interrelation of these cortical areas involved in the initiation of complex volitional movements. The appreciation of the spatial coordinates of the object of interest (ball) involves the posterior parietal lobe (Chap. 25). This information is conveyed via axons terminating in the primary motor cortex, premotor cortex, and supplementary motor cortex, which process these inputs into their circuitry. These motor cortices have specific roles that interact to produce a sequence of coordinated movements that lead to catching the ball. Both the

premotor cortex and the supplementary motor cortex project somatotopically to the primary motor cortex. In turn, the supplementary motor cortex receives a critical input from the basal ganglia via a projection from certain neurons in the ventral lateral (VL) nucleus of the thalamus. The premotor cortex receives a major input from the cerebellum via a projection from another group of neurons in the VL nucleus. Details of the functional aspects of these inputs are presented in Chapters 18 and 24.

A motor program comprises the sequence of movements directed to a purposeful goal, e.g., a plan of action to catch a ball. This includes the selection and coordination of the muscles involved in the sequence of all the movements of the entire action. The *posterior parietal lobe* contributes processed sensory information that is essential for use to guide the movement to the goal. The *premotor cortex* and the *supplementary motor cortex* are involved in the planning and programming of the complex sequences and guidance of the movements and also contribute their influences to affect the output of area 4. The *premotor cortex* exercises its primary role in regulating the axial and proximal limb musculature essential in the initial phases of orientating the body and lower limb toward the goal and the upper limb in an appropriate position. The *supplementary motor cortex* exerts a role in the complex movements of the proximal limb musculature and, in addition, simultaneous movements of the limbs of both sides of the body. The *motor cortex (area 4)* has an essential role in the control of the distal muscles of the extremities especially in the dexterity, skill, and agility of finger movements. The precise control of individual fingers (and even toes in some individuals) is the result of the fractionation of muscle contractions.

The motor areas give rise to corticospinal and corticobulbar fibers to the brainstem and spinal cord. These areas also give rise to corticorubral fibers to the ipsilateral red nucleus and to corticoreticular fibers to the brainstem reticular nuclei of both sides.

SUGGESTED READINGS

Asanuma H. *The Motor Cortex.* New York, NY: Raven Press; 1989.

Brinkman C. Supplementary motor area of the monkey's cerebral cortex: short- and long-term deficits after unilateral ablation and the effects of subsequent callosal section. *J Neurosci.* 1984;4: 918–929.

Evarts E. Motor cortex output in primates. In: Jones E, Peters A, eds. *Cerebral Cortex, Sensory-Motor Areas, and Aspects of Cortical Connectivity.* New York, NY: Plenum Press; 1986;5:217–241.

Evarts E. Role of motor cortex in voluntary movements in primates. In: Brooks V. *Handbook of Physiology.* Bethesda, Md: American Physiological Society; 1981;II:1083–1120.

Grillner S. Neurobiological bases of rhythmic motor acts in vertebrates. *Science.* 1985;228:143–149.

Henneman E. Organization of the spinal cord and its reflexes. In: Mountcastle V, ed. *Medical Physiology.* 14th ed. St Louis, Mo: CV Mosby Co; 1980; 1:762–786.

Lacquanti F. Automatic control of limb movement and posture. *Curr Opin Neurobiol.* 1992;2: 807–814.

Murray E, Coulter J. Organization of corticospinal neurons in the monkey. *J Comp Neurol.* 1981; 195:339–365.

Pearson K. The control of walking. *Sci Am.* 1976; 235(6):72–86.

Phillips C. *Movements of the Hand.* Liverpool: Liverpool University Press; 1986.

Phillips C, Porter R. *Cortico Spinal Neurones: Their Role in Movement.* London: Academic Press; 1977.

Roland P, Larsen B, Lassen N, Skinhøj E. Supplementary motor area and other cortical areas in organization of voluntary movements in man. *J Neurophysiol.* 1980;43:118–136.

Tanji J, Evarts E. Anticipatory activity of motor cortex neurons in relation to direction of an intended movement. *J Neurophysiol.* 1976;39:1062–1068.

Wise S. The primate premotor cortex: past, present, and preparatory. *Annu Rev Neurosci.* 1985;8: 1–19.

Lesions of the Spinal Nerves and Spinal Cord 12

Injuries to the nervous system, as well as neurologic diseases, produce symptoms and clinical signs. This chapter outlines some effects of lesions of the spinal nerves and spinal cord. The term *lesion* refers to pathologic and traumatic damage of a tissue and includes the loss or modification of function related to the injury.

RELEASE PHENOMENON

The signs associated with a lesion of the nervous system are manifested by two types of abnormal functions or capacities, namely with (1) negative signs or (2) positive signs.

Negative signs are expressed as the loss of a function or capacity as the result of a lesion. Examples are the loss of strength of a muscle, or its inability to contract (motor), or the loss of a sensation such as touch or sight (sensory).

Positive signs are expressed as abnormal motor responses (motor) or bizarre sensations (sensory). Each positive sign is usually the expression of a *release phenomenon*. Each results from the withdrawal (release) of inhibitory influences from the normal neural circuitry that mediates the normal response or capacity. The inhibitory circuits act as governors that modulate, shape, and prevent the excitatory circuits from becoming overactive (see importance of inhibition, Chap. 3). The lesion incapacitates the regulating inhibitory influences that the injured regulator exerted on the released neural circuit. Release phenomena are expressed (1) in the abnormal movements in Parkinson's disease and Huntington's chorea, both of which are associated with biochemical lesions in the basal ganglia (Chap. 24), (2) in the distorted pain sensations of the thalamic syndrome (Chap. 23), or (3) in the phantom limb (Chap. 9).

LESIONS OF THE VENTRAL ROOTS

Depending on the specific spinal level, lesions of the ventral roots interrupt specific alpha and gamma motoneurons and preganglionic autonomic fibers (Fig. 12.1, Nos. 1 and 2A). The injury of all the lower motoneurons innervating a muscle or group of muscles results in a lower motoneuron paralysis or paresis of that muscle or muscles. This occurs in poliomyelitis—the polio virus may selectively affect lower moto-

neurons of the spinal cord and of the brainstem. When the preganglionic autonomic fibers are injured, trophic effects may accompany the lower motoneuron paralysis (see below).

Lower Motoneuron Paralysis (Flaccid Paralysis)

The signs of a *lower motoneuron (flaccid) paralysis* and associated trophic changes include the following:

1. All voluntary movements are abolished, and reflex contractions cannot be elicited when

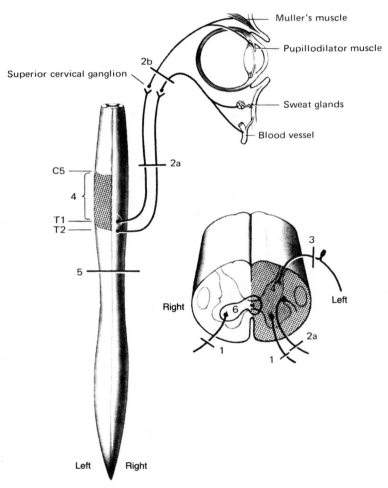

Figure 12.1: Schemata of the spinal cord to indicate the site of lesions noted in the text. The arabic numbers refer to specific lesions. C5 to T1 indicate the cervical enlargement, the region involved with the innervation of the upper extremity. 1, ventral roots of spinal nerves; 2a, preganglionic sympathetic fibers from T1 to T2 levels; 2b, postganglionic sympathetic fibers from the superior cervical ganglion; 3, dorsal roots of spinal nerves; 4, hemisection of the spinal cord (Brown-Séquard syndrome) extending through the cervical enlargement (stippled region); 5, transection of the spinal cord at a midthoracic level; and 6, lesion in region surrounding central canal throughout the cervical enlargement and extending into the anterior horn at the C8 and T1 level on one side.

all the lower motoneurons innervating a group of muscles are interrupted. The muscles are paralyzed. A *paresis* (partial paralysis, weakness) results when some, but not all, of the lower motoneurons normally innervating the muscle are functional.

2. The paralyzed muscles have lost their tone; therefore they are flaccid and offer little resistance to manipulation by the examiner. Because the myotatic reflex arcs are not intact, the deep tendon reflexes (DTRs) are absent (*areflexia*). If some of the lower motoneurons are functional, the tonus is reduced (*hypotonus*), and the DTRs are weak (*hyporeflexia*).

3. Reaching a peak about 2 to 3 weeks following denervation, muscles spontaneously contract. In time, the muscles atrophy. The spontaneous contractions of muscle fibers are known as fibrillation and fasciculation. *Fibrillation* is a single muscle fiber twitching, which can be seen only when the affected muscle is thinly covered as in the tongue and, rarely, in the hand. It can be detected by electromyographic examination. Fibrillation is a response associated with the hypersensitivity of a denervated muscle (Chap. 20). *Fasciculation* is the muscle twitching visibly through the skin resulting from the spontaneous discharge of a motor unit. As a lower motoneuron dies, it discharges repetitively to produce fasciculations of the muscle fibers it innervates.

4. The trophic changes include a dry, cyanotic skin which may be ulcerated (see below).

Trophic Functions and Changes

The autonomic nervous system is the motor system involved with influencing the activities of the involuntary (smooth) muscles, cardiac (heart) muscle, and glands (Chap. 20). In contrast, the somatic motor system is involved with influencing the voluntary (skeletal, striated) muscles. In addition to stimulating muscles to contract and glands to secrete, both the autonomic and somatic motor systems exert effects that initiate and regulate the molecular organization of other cells. These effects are expressions of the *trophic* (literally *nutritional*) functions of the nervous system.

Trophic influences by neurons are directed to different types of target tissues, including epithelium, nerve endings (e.g., taste buds), and muscle cells. Following lesions of fibers of the autonomic nervous system, trophic changes include a warm or cool, flushed or cyanotic skin, due to change in capillary circulation; abnormal brittleness of fingernails; loss of hair; dryness or ulceration of the skin; and lysis of the bones and joints.

The atrophy that occurs in voluntary muscles deprived of their lower (somatic) motoneuron innervation is more pronounced than the atrophy following disuse. Another profound effect on the voluntary muscle fibers in the former case is from the loss of trophic influences that are essential for the maintenance of the normal condition. Fibrillation is another expression of a change of the trophic influences.

Myasthenia Gravis—An Autoimmune Disease

Myasthenia gravis is a muscle weakness disability that is associated with defects of transmission at the motor end-plate junctions between nerve endings and the voluntary muscle acetylcholine receptors (ACh receptors). The defect is caused by an antibody-mediated attack which reduces the number of nicotinic acetylcholine receptors and is accompanied by sparse and shallow junctional folds and widened clefts of the postsynaptic membrane (sarcolemma) (Chap. 15; Fig. 2.4). As a consequence there is a reduction in the probability of evoking an action potential in the sarcolemma. This neuromuscular disease is characterized by a marked fatigability and weakness of the voluntary muscles that is improved by inhibitors of acetylcholinesterase such as physostigmine. Thus, by inhibiting the degradation of acetylcholine at the motor end-plate, the time is prolonged for the available transmitter to act on the remaining receptors.

The critical symptom of the affliction is weakness of voluntary muscles. Characteristic features include double vision due to decrease in the coordination of the extraocular muscles, drooping eyelids (weak levator palpebrae muscles), and weakness of the limb muscles. Intense activity of a muscle will rapidly lead to severe fatigue. In myasthenia gravis, lymphocyte T cells generated in the thymus gland become activated to react against the ACh receptors. The antibodies inactivate the ACh receptors as fast or faster than they can be synthesized for replacement. The normal turnover of ACh receptors is about 5 to 7 days. With the increased destruction of ACh receptors in myasthenia gravis the turnover rate is increased to 2 to 4 days. The therapeutic effects of thymectomy relates to the immunological role of the thymus. Following thymectomy about one half of patients with myasthenia gravis are "in remission" with no symptoms even when accompanied by no drug therapy.

Horner's Syndrome

Horner's syndrome occurs as a consequence of a lesion to certain fibers of the sympathetic division of the autonomic nervous system (Chap. 20). With regard to Horner's syndrome, the sympathetic division comprises fibers that emerge from T1 and T2 spinal cord segments and terminate in the superior cervical ganglion, which is located alongside the spinal column. Unmyelinated fibers arising from neurons in the ganglion follow arterial blood vessels and have synaptic terminals influencing sweat glands, smooth muscles that dilate the pupils of the eyes, smooth muscles of the cutaneous blood vessels, and smooth muscles (called Muller's muscle) that aid in elevation of the upper eyelid (**Fig. 12.1**). The sympathetic fibers from the spinal cord to the superior cervical ganglion are called *preganglionic fibers* and those from the superior cervical ganglion to the end organs are *postganglionic fibers* (Chap. 20).

Lesions of preganglionic sympathetic fibers from T1 and T2, or of the postganglionic sympathetic fibers from the superior cervical ganglion, will result in *Horner's syndrome* on the ipsilateral side of the face (**Fig. 12.1, Nos. 2A and B**). The affected pupil is smaller than the pupil of the opposite eye; it does not dilate (miosis) when the pupil is shaded (pupillodilator muscle unit is not stimulated to contract). The affected eyelid droops a bit (ptosis) because the superior palpebral smooth muscle (Muller's muscle) is denervated. The face is dry (denervated sweat glands), red, and warm (vasodilatation of cutaneous blood vessels).

LESIONS OF THE DORSAL ROOTS

The irritation of the fibers of one dorsal root (radix) by mechanical compression (tumor or slipped disk) or a local inflammation may produce pain with a radicular distribution (**Fig. 12.1, No. 3**). Because adjacent dermatomes overlap, the destruction of one dorsal root (e.g., by transection) may result in the slight diminution of all sensations (*hypesthesia*) in part of the dermatome innervated by that dorsal root. Destruction of several consecutive dorsal roots does result in the complete absence of all sensations (*anesthesia*) in all but the rostral and caudal dermatomes innervated by the sectioned roots. Irritation to the dorsal root fibers may result in *paresthesia* (abnormal spontaneous sensations such as numbness and prickling) or *hyperesthesia* (excessive sensibility to sensory stimuli in pain). The stimulation of a dorsal root may result in a *dermatomal vasodilatation* (due to reflex arc involving the autonomic nervous system).

If all dorsal roots innervating the upper extremity (C5 through T1) are transected (e.g., surgically by dorsal root rhizotomy), several symptoms may be additionally observed. Because the afferent limb of the reflex arcs is interrupted, reflex activity is absent (areflexia) and muscles are hypotonic. Although the limb muscles are not paralyzed (lower motoneurons are intact), motor activity is impaired. The deafferented limb hangs by the side and is generally not used. It can be volitionally moved when facilitatory influences from the descending supraspinal motor pathways stimulate the lower motoneurons. Because the lower motoneurons are intact and functional, there is little or no loss in muscle strength and no occurrence of fasciculations. There is some disuse atrophy, but because trophic influences are not lost, there is no trophic atrophy.

Lesions and irritations of the dorsal roots or posterior horn result in segmental (dermatomal) sensory disturbances. In dorsal root lesions all general senses in the region innervated by the root fibers (dermatome) are lost or diminished. In posterior horn lesions a *dissociated sensory loss* (loss of one sensation and the preservation of others) may occur in the dermatome, with, for example, pain and temperature sensibilities lost or reduced but touch and other associated general senses intact and normal. Dissociated sensory loss of pain and temperature also occurs in lesions in the vicinity of the central canal (see "Lesions in the Region of the Central Canal").

Following an injury restricted to one dorsal root, no area of anesthesia is revealed in the dermatome innervated, because of the overlap from fibers of adjacent dorsal roots. Such an injury, however, may produce so-called radicular (a root is a radix) pain, that is localized in the dermatome innervated by that root; such patients are aware of a tingling pain or even a diminished feeling of sensation.

LESIONS OF THE UPPER MOTONEURONS (UPPER MOTONEURON PARALYSIS, SPASTIC PARALYSIS)

Interruption of the upper motoneurons (UMNs) results in motor disturbances known as an *upper motoneuron paralysis*. The lesion in the genu and posterior limb of the internal capsule which results in the most typical constellation of UMN lesion signs involves the corticobulbar, corticospinal, corticorubrospinal, and corticoreticulospinal pathways. Often the symptoms of an UMN lesion are attributed to a lesion of the corticospinal tract; but actually the other UMN pathways also contribute to the symptoms because they too are within the lesion site. Apparently the only neurologic sign associated exclusively with a corticospinal tract lesion is the Babinski sign (see later).

Immediately after the onset of a lesion in the internal capsule (**Fig. 1.8**), the patient develops a paralysis of the lower muscles of facial expression (below level of the eye) and the upper and lower limb musculature (hemiplegia) on the opposite side of the body. The lower facial muscles are paralyzed if the lesion is in the genu and damages the corticobulbar fibers passing through (**Fig. 11.3**).

As a rule, following a unilateral corticobulbar lesion, all the voluntary muscles innervated by cranial nerves, except those of the lower face, are spared. This is because the lower motoneurons to upper facial muscles receive bilateral corticobulbar innervation, but the lower motoneurons to lower facial muscles receive corticobulbar innervation only from the contralateral side of the cortex (**Fig. 11.3**). Therefore, a unilateral lesion will lead to paralysis on the opposite side.

In the limbs, the deep tendon (stretch) reflexes are temporarily depressed and the muscles exhibit hypotonia. In time, from a few days to a few weeks, the stretch reflexes return and then become hyperactive. Muscle tone increases to hypertonia. The expression of hyperreflexia by the muscles is called spasticity and the muscles are said to be spastic. The basic cause for the spasticity is not fully understood. One explanation is that the UMN lesions reduce inhibitory influences upon both the gamma and alpha motoneurons more than they do excitatory influences. This is accompanied by hypersensitive dynamic gamma motoneurons, which stimulate the muscle spindles to increase their rate of discharge and thus increase the activity of the stretch reflex. Other evidence suggests that the spasticity is primarily due to hyperactive alpha motoneurons.

An upper motoneuron paralysis is called a *spastic paralysis*. Such a paralysis of the upper and lower limbs on one side is called a *hemiplegia*. The clinical signs of an UMN paralysis include increased muscle tone (hypertonia), increased deep tendon (stretch) reflexes (hyperreflexia), clonus, loss or diminution of cutaneous reflexes and the Babinski reflex (sign). Spasticity is thought to result from damage to upper motoneuron pathways other than the corticospinal tract; selective damage to the pyramids in the medulla of laboratory animals produces decreased, and not increased, muscle tone.

Hypertonus is expressed in the firmness and stiffness of muscle—primarily in the flexors of the upper limb and in the extensors of the lower limb. These are antigravity muscles; the upper limbs hold themselves up and the lower limbs support the body. This increased resistance (hypertonus) to passive movement is expressed as the examiner tries to flex or extend each limb. The brisk knee jerk following the tapping of the quadriceps muscle tendon is an example of *hyperreflexia*. The spastic body parts exhibit increased resistance to manipulation, especially the flexors of the upper limbs and the extensors of the lower limbs. However, if the force exerted by an examiner persists, the resisting muscles yield suddenly in a *clasp knife* fashion. The sudden yielding of resistance is apparently due to the surge of afferent input from group II fibers from the muscle spindles and also possibly from C pain fibers from low-threshold pain receptors and, according to some, from the Ib fibers from the Golgi tendon organs.

Clonus is the rhythmic oscillation of a joint (e.g., ankle or knee) which occurs when a second party suddenly dorsiflexes the foot (light pressure on the sole of foot pushes toes toward knee) and maintains the dorsiflexion attitude under continuous light pressure. The dorsiflexion actually puts the gastrocnemius muscle, its muscle spindles, and its Achilles tendon under moderate stretch. The resulting stretch reflex contraction of the gastrocnemius produces plantar flexion of the foot. This is accompanied by the stretch of the tibialis anterior and other dorsiflexor muscles of the foot and their muscle spindles. The resulting stretch reflex contraction of the tibialis anterior produces a dorsiflexion of the foot. The cycle repeats. Clonus persists as long as the gastrocnemius is kept in a moderate state of contraction by passively applied elastic pressure.

There is also loss or diminution of cutaneous or superficial reflexes. Stimulation of the skin of the thorax, abdomen, or extremities evokes weak or no reflex responses.

The *Babinski reflex* (sign) can be elicited. When the lateral aspect of the sole of the foot is stroked with a blunt point, the big toe dorsiflexes (hyperextension), the tip of the toe points to the knee, and the other toes spread (fan)—called extensor plantar response.

SYMPTOMS OF VALUE IN LOCALIZING LESIONS TO SPINAL LEVELS

Some symptoms which occur with a dermatomal distribution are associated with a specific dorsal root or roots. Furthermore, symptoms which show signs of lower motoneuron paralysis are associated with specific ventral root or roots.

For example: (1) A band of anesthesia with a dermatomal distribution results from the destruction of specific dorsal root fibers. (2) Paresthesias or radicular (root) pain with a dermatomal distribution results from irritation of fibers in specific dorsal root fibers. (3) Flaccid paralysis and other lower motoneuron signs result from the destruction of motoneuron cells and fibers in the anterior horn or ventral roots.

SPINAL CORD HEMISECTION (BROWN-SÉQUARD SYNDROME)

A hemisection (unilateral transverse lesion) of the spinal cord results in a number of changes in the body at that level or caudal to it (**Fig. 12.1, No. 4**). For instructional purposes, assume that the lesion is a hemisection extending from C5 through T1 spinal levels; the peripheral nerves associated with these spinal levels innervate the upper extremity. In relating the side of a lesion (right or left) to the side of the body where signs are expressed in the nervous system, one must relate the site of the pathway's crossing over to the location of the lesion. (1) Symptoms occur on the same side (ipsilateral) and below the level of the lesion when the damaged neurons are those which normally convey influences from the same side of the body (ascending sensory tracts) or to the same side of the body (descending motor tracts). In the spinal cord, structures involved with ipsilateral functions include the posterior column, dorsal roots, lateral corticospinal tract, rubrospinal tract, reticulospinal tracts, and ventral roots. (2) Symptoms occur on the opposite (contralateral) side below the level of the lesion when the damaged neurons convey information from or to the opposite side of the body. In the spinal cord, this includes the decussated fibers of the anterolateral pathway, the lateral and anterior spinothalamic tracts. In the brainstem this includes the spinothalamic tract, medial lemniscus, and corticospinal tract.

The fiber tracts injured and resultant symptoms and signs include:

1. At the spinal levels of transection (C5 through T1), the entering fibers of the dorsal roots and the emerging fibers of the lower

motoneurons and preganglionic sympathetic fibers (C8 and T1) are interrupted. The result is the complete absence of all sensations in the upper extremity on the side of lesion. Pain and temperature are lost on the contralateral upper extremity due to interruption of the lateral spinothalamic tract on the side of lesion. Paresthesias and radicular pain may be sensed over the ipsilateral C5 and T1 dermatomes from the irritation of some intact dorsal root fibers; because of dermatome overlap from C4 and T2, the C5 and T1 dermatomes have a hypesthesia. The entire ipsilateral limb is flaccid; it exhibits all the signs of a lower motoneuron paralysis. Horner's syndrome on the ipsilateral side of the face, and trophic changes in the ipsilateral upper extremity are due to the interruption of the preganglionic sympathetic neurons.

2. *Posterior column (fasciculi gracilis and cuneatus)*. Loss of position sense, appreciation of passive movement, vibratory sense, and two-point discrimination on the same side at and below the spinal levels of the lesion. These modalities are unaffected from the neck because the fibers conveying them are located wholly above the level of the lesion. Ataxia of the gait (stumbling and staggering gait) associated with injury of the posterior column cannot be observed because of the paralysis.

3. *Lateral spinothalamic tract*. Loss of pain and temperature on the opposite side at and below the spinal levels of the lesion. This includes the contralateral upper extremity because lateral spinothalamic fibers decussate within one or two levels of the spinal root origin.

4. *Anterior spinothalamic tract*. Touch sensibility is probably little affected on the opposite side below the spinal level of the lesion because this modality is also conveyed in the uncrossed fasciculi gracilis and cuneatus.

5. *Corticospinal tract and other descending supraspinal tracts*. The spastic syndrome following the interruption of these fibers results in an upper motoneuron paralysis including spasticity, hyperactive deep tendon reflexes (hyperreflexia), diminution or loss of superficial reflexes, a Babinski sign, and muscle clonus below (but not at level of) the site of the lesion on the ipsilateral side. The hyperactive DTRs are illustrated by a brisk knee jerk or ankle jerk.

INTRINSIC ARTERIAL SUPPLY TO THE SPINAL CORD

In general, two arteries and their branches supply the spinal cord (**Fig. 12.2**). Branches of the unpaired anterior spinal artery vascularize the anterior two thirds of each spinal segment. The branches of the paired posterior spinal arteries supply the remainder of the spinal cord.

The *anterior spinal artery syndrome* results in signs due to bilateral injury to the anterior

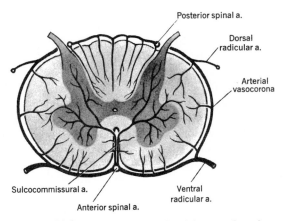

Figure 12.2: The arterial supply of the spinal cord.

horns, anterolateral pathways, and lateral corticospinal (pyramidal) tracts. The symptoms occur suddenly and are often associated with severe pain. Flaccid paralysis, fasciculations, and atrophy bilaterally at the segments involved are due to lesions in the anterior horns (lower motoneuron paralysis). Spastic paralysis below the level of the lesion results from bilateral lesions of the descending motor tracts (upper motoneuron paralysis). Pain and temperature sensibilities may be lost bilaterally below the level of a thrombosis because of involvement of the anterolateral pathways. These sensations may be spared because adequate blood may be supplied by the posterior spinal arteries.

SPINAL CORD TRANSECTION (PARAPLEGIA)

Immediately after the complete transection of the spinal cord at a midthoracic level (**Fig. 12.1, No. 5**), paraplegia associated with the loss of detectable neural activity caudal to the lesion site results. *Paraplegia* is the paralysis of both lower limbs resulting from the sectioning of the UMNs on both sides of the spinal cord.

All voluntary movements and somatic and visceral reflex activities are abolished. Sensations from the body below the transection level are absent. This period of extremely depressed activity, called *spinal shock* lasts about 2 to 3 weeks in humans (it varies in duration from 4 days to 6 weeks). Spinal shock is apparently due to the sudden withdrawal of facilitatory influences from the descending pathways, especially the corticospinal tract.

The isolated spinal cord and its spinal nerves gradually exhibit autonomous neural activity which is divided into a sequence of phases of variable lengths: (1) minimal reflex activity, (2) flexor spasm activity (superficial reflexes), (3) alternation between flexor and extensor spasm activities, and (4) predominant extensor spasm activity (deep reflexes). After a year or two, paraplegic patients may be placed in one of several categories: (1) that in which extensor spasms predominate over flexor spasms, called *paraplegia-in-extension* (observed in about two thirds of paraplegics); (2) that in which flexor spasms predominate, called *paraplegia-in-flexion*; and

(3) that in which a flaccid paralysis persists (less than 20%). The absence of autonomic nervous system influences from the brain is accompanied by a variety of disturbances in the control of automatic activities of the urinary, genital, and anorectal systems.

Loss of thermoregulatory control below the level of the lesion is expressed with a cool, dry skin with no evidence of sweating (Chap. 20). However, reflex sweating can occur when a noxious stimulus is applied (e.g., response to the insertion of the needle during a spinal tap). There is loss of voluntary control of the urinary bladder. The urinary bladder can be evacuated by reflex activity such as by appropriate cutaneous stimulation.

Quadriplegia is the paralysis of all four limbs and is associated with a transection of the spinal cord in the region of the cervical enlargement. *Monoplegia* involves the paralysis of one limb.

LESION IN THE REGION OF THE CENTRAL CANAL (SYRINGOMYELIA)

A syrinx (cavity) may develop in the region of the central canal; from there cavitation may extend to other sites (**Fig. 12.1, No. 6**). Assuming that the lesion is located in the cervical enlargement (from C5 to T1 spinal cord levels), the initial clinical signs are the loss of pain and temperature sensibility in both upper limbs. The loss is due to the interruption of the decussating pain and temperature fibers passing through the anterior white commissure, conveying information from both upper limbs. Proprioception and light touch are not affected in either the upper and lower limbs or body because the posterior columns are intact. There is no loss of pain and temperature sensation in the body and lower limbs because the anterolateral pathways (except for fibers from the upper limb) are functional.

The extension of the lesion into the anterior horn of C8 and T1 spinal levels on one side produces, on the side of the lesion, lower motoneuron disturbances and trophic changes on the ulnar side of the arm, forearm, hand, and fourth and fifth fingers, as well as possible Horner's syndrome, because the ulnar nerve originates from C8 to T1 levels as do the preganglionic sympathetic fibers to the superior cervical ganglion.

TABES DORSALIS

Tabes dorsalis is a form of neurosyphilis in which the primary pathology of the dorsal root ganglia is accompanied by secondary degenerative changes in the posterior columns, especially in the fasciculi gracilis bilaterally. The pain fibers are also involved. In the initial stages, the irritation of dorsal root fibers produces paresthesias and intermittent attacks of sharp pain. In time, the symptoms include: diminished sensitivity to pain; loss of kinesthetic sense; diminished-to-absent deep tendon reflexes (ankle and knee jerks); loss of muscle tone; and marked impairment of muscle, joint, and vibratory senses accompanied by an ataxic gait. Patients walk with legs held apart, head bent and eyes looking down, raising their knees high and slapping their feet on the ground. The eyes stare at the ground to pick up cues which substitute for the lost kinesthetic senses.

As in ataxia, the patient with tabes dorsalis exhibits Romberg's sign, i.e., the inability to stand with eyes closed and feet together without swaying or actually falling. With the eyes open, an afflicted person may be able to keep upright by using visual cues to compensate for loss of proprioception.

AMYOTROPHIC LATERAL SCLEROSIS

Amyotrophic lateral sclerosis (ALS) is a progressive degenerative motor tract disease with bilateral involvement of the pyramidal tracts and anterior horns. Because there is degeneration of both upper and lower motoneurons, signs of both upper and lower motoneuron paralysis are expressed. Most of the affected muscles show evidence of the degeneration of lower motoneurons, including paralysis, atrophy, fasciculations and weakness; these signs often are initially expressed by the muscles of the hands and arms. Some muscles exhibit signs of upper motoneuron paralysis, hyperreflexia and, at times, Babinski signs. The lower motoneurons of cranial nerves may also exhibit signs of de-

generation. Sensory changes do not usually occur.

COMBINED SYSTEM DEGENERATION

Combined system degeneration is a complication of pernicious anemia (a disease due to lack of intrinsic factor for absorption of vitamin B_{12}) in which there is subacute degeneration bilaterally of the fibers of the posterior columns and lateral columns, especially those involved with the lumbosacral cord. The clinical symptoms include: (1) loss of position and vibratory senses, numbness, and dysesthesia in the lower extremities and (2) such upper motoneuron signs as spasticity, muscle weakness, hyperactive deep tendon reflexes, Babinski reflexes, and Romberg's sign.

DEGENERATION, REGENERATION, AND SPROUTING

An injured neuron reacts to an insult, whether it is a transection, a crush, a toxic substance, or a deprivation of blood supply. The entire neuron responds and may reconstitute itself (**Fig. 2.10**).

Degeneration

The degenerative reactions following transection include changes in (1) the cell body (chromatolysis), (2) the nerve fiber between the cell body and the trauma (primary degeneration), and (3) the nerve fiber distal to the trauma (secondary, anterograde, or Wallerian degeneration). The cell body swells, Nissl bodies undergo "dissolution" or chromatolysis, and the nucleus is displaced to the side of the cell body. These are manifestations of metabolic activities which can ultimately lead to the regeneration of the severed fiber. The chromatolysis is indicative of the enhanced protein synthesis. The few degenerative changes in the nerve proximal to the cut include the breakdown of the myelin sheath and axon in the vicinity of the injury. The axon and myelin sheath of the fiber distal to the trauma become fragmented and are removed by macrophages, usually over a period of weeks.

Nerve Regeneration in Peripheral Nervous System

Regeneration is essentially a process of differentiation and growth (Fig. 2.10). The neurolemma (Schwann) cells in the proximal stump near the trauma and in the distal stump divide mitotically to form continuous cords of the neurolemma cells. These cords extend from the proximal stump, through the small gap between the stumps into the distal stump, and up to the sites of the sensory receptors and motor endings. The cell bodies synthesize proteins and other metabolites which flow distally into the regenerating and lengthening axons. In nerve *regeneration*, the ends of the proximal axons branch into numerous sprouts which grow distally at about 4 mm per day into the gap and distal stump along the neurolemmal cords (which act as guidelines) to the sites of the nerve endings. Each regenerating axon of the proximal stump may divide to form as many as 50 terminal sprouts. In turn, each neurolemmal cord may act as the guiding scaffold for numerous regenerating axons. The regenerating axons that survive are those that terminate in the proper nerve endings. The potential of each neurolemmal cord to act as a guide for many regenerating axons increases the possibility of reinnervating the receptor associated with its cord. When fully myelinated, each regenerating branch tends to have a conduction velocity of about 80% of that of the original fiber. The superfluous axonal branches eventually degenerate.

Collateral Sprouting

A denervated neurolemmal cord is presumed to exert trophic influences upon a nearby normal nerve fiber; the latter responds by sprouting new collateral branches from its nodes of Ranvier. This is known as *preterminal axonal sprouting* or *collateral nerve sprouting*. The collateral branch joins the axonless neurolemmal cord, grows down the cord, and reinnervates the nerve ending. Collateral nerve sprouting occurs in both the peripheral nervous system and central nervous system (CNS) (the latter does not have neurolemmal cords) (Fig. 2.10).

Regeneration in the Central Nervous System

Loss of neurons is a normal consequence throughout life. This neuronal loss is generally accompanied by a compensatory sprouting of axonal branches by other CNS neurons in the vicinity. Many of these axonal sprouts invade the territory previously innervated by the dead neuron and form new synapses. This activity, known as *reactive synaptogenesis*, is an attempt to replace lost synapses. The molecular and trophic factors (such as a brain-derived neurotrophic factor; Chap. 2) involved to enhance the sprouting and synapse formation are not known.

The cut ends of axons of neurons of the peripheral nervous system sprout and grow along the cords of Schwann cell-basal lamina and eventually may form, as previously noted, new functional synaptic connections. The release of a neurotrophic factor by the Schwann cells may be the critical factor that promotes this growth and regeneration.

In contrast, the cut ends of axons of mature neurons of the CNS may initially sprout and regenerate some fibers, possibly in response to a nerve growth factor. This regeneration, however, is soon aborted. It is possible that this inability to sustain axonal outgrowth may be due to (1) absence of basal laminae in the CNS and (2) blockage by polypeptides released by glial cells. As yet, the formation of functional synapses following this form of regeneration has yet to be established.

The young neurons of fetal and neonatal mammals have a great capacity for regeneration. This is the logic of transplanting young neurons into the brains of adult mammals to attain some degree of functional recovery following damage in the brain. For example, the transplantation of dopaminergic neurons into the striatum in patients with Parkinson's disease is being carried out in an attempt to obtain some clinical recovery (Chap. 24).

SUGGESTED READINGS

Adams R, Victor M. *Principles of Neurology.* 5th ed. New York, NY: McGraw-Hill; 1993.

Brodal A. Self-observations and neuro-anatomical considerations after a stroke. *Brain.* 1973;96: 675–694.

Gilman S, Newman S. *Manter and Gatz's Essentials of Clinical Neuroanatomy and Neurophysiology.* 8th ed. Philadelphia, Pa: FA Davis Co; 1992.

Haines D. *Correlative Neuroanatomy: The Anatomical Basis of Some Common Neurological Deficits.* Baltimore, Md: Urban & Schwartzenberg; 1985.

Lance J, McLeod J. *A Physiological Approach to Clinical Neurology.* London: Butterworth; 1981.

Nathan P, Smith M, Cook A. Sensory effects in man of lesions of the posterior columns and of some other afferent pathways. *Brain.* 1986;109: 1003–1041.

Rowland L, ed. *Merritt's Textbook of Neurology.* 9th ed. Philadelphia, Pa: Williams & Wilkins; 1995.

Rowland L. Diseases of chemical transmission at the nerve-muscle synapse: myasthenia gravis. In: Kandel E, Schwartz J, Jessell T, eds. *Principles of Neural Science.* 3rd ed. New York, NY: Elsevier; 1991:235–243.

Rowland L. Diseases of the motor unit. In: Kandel E, Schwartz J, Jessell T, eds. *Principles of Neural Science.* 3rd ed. New York, NY: Elsevier; 1991: 244–257.

Sunderland S. *Nerves and Nerve Injuries.* 2nd ed. Edinburgh: Churchill Livingstone, 1978.

Brainstem: Medulla, Pons, and Midbrain 13

The roles of the brainstem may be divided into three broad categories. The first is to provide transit and processing nuclei for ascending and descending pathways that convey influences to and from the cerebrum, cerebellum, and spinal cord. The second is to play a part in a range of activities such as consciousness, the sleep-wake cycle, and respiratory and cardiovascular control. The third relates to actions of the cranial nerves, which are comprised of sensory neurons terminating in brainstem nuclei and motoneurons originating in brainstem nuclei.

LONGITUDINAL ORGANIZATION OF THE BRAINSTEM

The brainstem is longitudinally organized into four regions: (1) the roof posteriorly; (2) the base or basilar portion anteriorly; (3) the tegmentum in the center; and (4) the ventricular cavity, between the tegmentum and the roof (Fig. 13.1).

Roof

The posterior boundary of the brainstem is known as the *roof*. In the midbrain the roof is called the *tectum* (quadrigeminal plate). The cerebellum (not itself a brainstem structure) serves as the roof of the pons, and the tela choro-

idea and its choroid plexus are the roof of the medulla. The tectum includes the pretectum (light reflex; Chap. 19), superior colliculus (optic reflexes; Chap. 19), inferior colliculus (auditory system; Chap. 16), and the emerging trochlear nerve (n. IV) caudally (Figs. 13.2 and 13.3).

Basilar Portion

The basilar portion is called the *crus cerebri* in the midbrain, *ventral portion* or *pons proper* in the pons, and *pyramids* in the medulla (Figs. 13.1 and 13.4). The basilar portion consists of descending pathways originating in the cerebral cortex. These include (1) corticobulbar and corticoreticular fibers, which terminate in the tegmentum, and the corticospinal tract which terminates in the spinal cord (Figs. 11.2 and 11.4), and (2) the corticopontine fibers (to pontine nuclei of the pons proper) and pontocerebellar fibers (Chap. 18).

Tegmentum

The tegmentum extends throughout the entire length of the brainstem (Fig. 13.1). Major structures within the tegmentum include (1) the reticular formation (RF), which forms the central core of the tegmentum; (2) such pathways as the posterior column-medial lemniscus path-

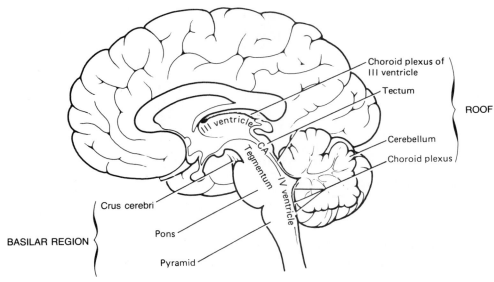

Figure 13.1: Median sagittal section of the cerebrum and brainstem to illustrate the longitudinal stratification of the latter into: (1) roof, (2) ventricular portion, (3) tegmentum, and (4) basilar portion. The *roof* consists of the tectum (including superior and inferior colliculi), superior and inferior medullary velum, cerebellum, and choroid plexus of the fourth (IVth) ventricle. The *ventricular portion* comprises the cerebral aqueduct (CA), IVth ventricle, and the central canal in the caudal medulla. The *tegmentum* occupies the core of the three brainstem subdivisions and includes the reticular formation with its nuclei and pathways, cranial nerves and their nuclei, sensory and cerebellar relay nuclei, the ascending lemniscal pathways, etc. The *basilar portion* comprises the crus cerebri, the basilar portion of the pons, and the medullary pyramid. (Refer to Figs. 1.1 and 1.5.)

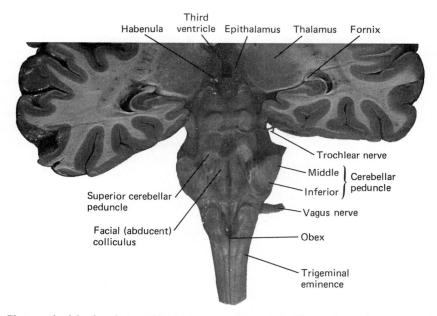

Figure 13.2: Photograph of the dorsal view of the brainstem and a section of the cerebrum. Structures in the brainstem section can be identified by referring to Fig. 13.3. (Courtesy of Dr. Howard A. Matzke, University of Kansas Medical Center.)

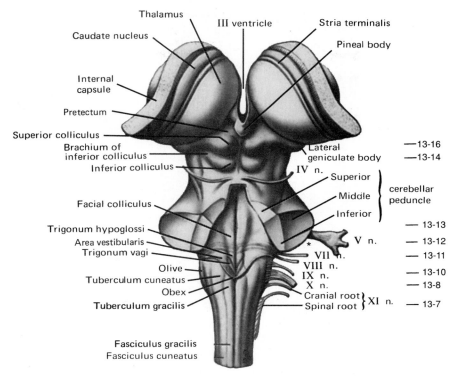

Figure 13.3: Posterior surface of the brainstem. Lines adjacent to the figure indicate the levels of the transverse sections illustrated in Figs. 13.7 through 13.16. Roman numerals represent some cranial nerves (Chap. 14). Asterisk (*) represents location of cerebellopontine angle.

way, anterolateral pathway (spinothalamic tract), trigeminal pathways, medial longitudinal fasciculus (MLF), and auditory pathways; and (3) cranial nerve nuclei and roots of 10 cranial nerves (**Fig. 13.4**). The intrinsic tract of the tegmentum conveying influences rostrally and caudally is the *central tegmental tract*—it is equivalent to the spinospinalis tract of the spinal cord.

Ventricular Cavity

The ventricular cavity includes the cerebral aqueduct (of Sylvius) in the midbrain and the fourth ventricle in the pons and medulla.

SURFACE BRAINSTEM LANDMARKS

The cerebral structures illustrated in **Figures 13.2 to 13.5** include the *third ventricle, thalamus* (Chap. 23), *pineal body* (Chap. 21) of the

diencephalon, the *internal capsule, corona radiata, lentiform nucleus, caudate nucleus, olfactory bulb* and *tract*, and *optic nerve* and *tract* of the *cerebrum* (**Fig. 1.9**). The locations of the emergence of the cranial nerves from the brain are discussed in Chapter 14.

Posterior Surface

The roof of the midbrain consists of the *lamina quadrigemina (tectum)* that comprise the paired *superior colliculi (optic system)* and the paired *inferior colliculi (auditory system)*. The superior colliculus and the *pretectum* are associated with visual guidance and tracking activities related to eye and head movements, as well as the light reflex and accommodation (Chap. 19). The inferior colliculi are involved with acoustic and acousticomotor activities. The brachium of the inferior colliculus consists of fibers of the auditory pathway connecting the inferior colliculus and the medial geniculate body of the thalamus

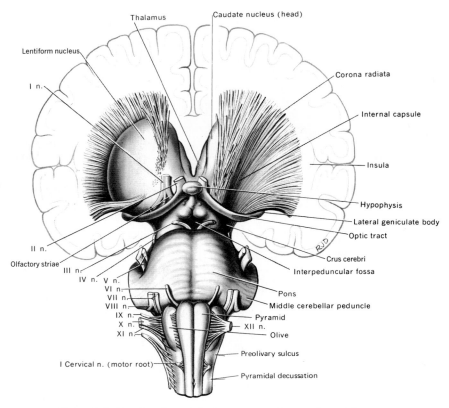

Figure 13.4: Basal surface of the brainstem and roots of cranial nerves.

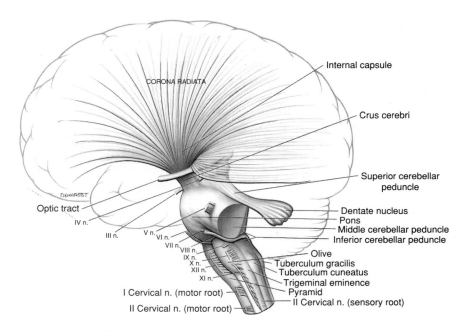

Figure 13.5: Lateral surface of the brainstem and roots of cranial nerves.

(Chap. 16). The lateral geniculate body is a thalamic nucleus of the visual pathways (Chap. 19). The trochlear nerve (n. IV) emerges caudal to the inferior colliculi.

The roof (cerebellum and tela choroidea of the IVth ventricle) of the pons and medulla has been removed (Figs. 13.2 and 13.3). The laterally located cut cerebellar peduncles comprise the *inferior, middle,* and *superior cerebellar peduncles* (Chap. 18). The floor of the IVth ventricle (and roof of tegmentum) contains the *facial colliculus (abducent colliculus)* formed by the underlying abducens nucleus and genu of the facial nerve (Fig. 13.12). The area vestibularis, trigonum vagi, and trigonum hypoglossi (Fig. 13.3) are eminences formed by the underlying vestibular nuclei, dorsal vagal nucleus, and hypoglossal nucleus, respectively (Figs. 13.10 and 13.11). The tuberculum cuneatus, tuberculum gracilis, and olive (Fig. 13.3) are eminences formed by the nucleus cuneatus, nucleus gracilis, and inferior olivary nucleus of the medulla, respectively (Figs. 13.8 and 13.9). The obex is a fold of tissue dorsal to the site where the IVth ventricle funnels into the central canal; it is used as a landmark by neurosurgeons.

Basal Surface

The oculomotor nerve (n. III) emerges from the interpeduncular fossa located between the crus cerebri of the cerebral peduncles of the midbrain (Figs. 13.4 and 13.15). Note that (1) the cranial nerve V emerges laterally from the midpons, (2) cranial nerves VI, VII, and VIII emerge from medial to lateral along the junction of the pons and medulla, (3) cranial nerves IX, X, and XI emerge in a rostral to caudal sequence from the postolivary sulcus dorsal to the olive, and (4) cranial nerve XII emerges from the preolivary sulcus between the olive and a pyramid. The pyramids are paired columns formed by the pyramidal (corticospinal) tracts.

Lateral Surface (Fig. 13.5)

Most of the structures labeled in this view are noted above and in the text. Most of the fibers of the superior cerebellar peduncle originate in the dentate nucleus of the cerebellum. The olive

is formed by the underlying inferior olivary nucleus.

BRAINSTEM CRANIAL NERVES

Cranial nerves III through XII emerge from the brainstem (Fig. 13.4). Arising from the basal surface slightly lateral to the midline are n. III (oculomotor nerve) from the interpeduncular fossa, n. VI (abducent nerve) at the pons-medulla junction, and n. XII (hypoglossal nerve) as filaments from the preolivary sulcus located between an olive and a pyramid. Cranial nerve IV (trochlear nerve) emerges from the posterior surface of the caudal midbrain (Fig. 13.3).

The remaining cranial nerves arise from the lateral surface of the brain stem (Figs. 13.4 and 13.5). They include n. V (trigeminal nerve) from the midpons; n. VII (facial nerve) and n. VIII (vestibulocochlear nerve) from the pons-medulla junction; and n. IX (glossopharyngeal nerve), n. X (vagus nerve), and n. XI (cranial root of spinal accessory nerve) as nerve filaments from the postolivary sulcus. The spinal roots of n. XI arise from filaments emerging laterally from between the dorsal and ventral roots of spinal cord levels C1 to C6 (Fig. 13.5).

BRAINSTEM LANDMARKS OF FUNCTIONAL SIGNIFICANCE

The internal anatomy of the brainstem can be visualized by appreciating the topographic relations of some major tracts and the cranial nerves.

Corticopontine, Corticobulbar, and Corticospinal Tracts

These tracts, originating from the cerebral cortex, descend successively through the internal capsule, crus cerebri of the midbrain, and basilar pons (Figs. 11.2 and 13.5). The corticopontine fibers terminate in the pontine nuclei. Along their course, corticobulbar fibers terminate in neuronal pools influencing both the motor and sensory cranial nerve nuclei located within the tegmentum (Figs. 13.7 to 13.16). The corticospinal tracts continue as the pyramids of the medulla. They cross over as the decussation of the pyramidal tracts at the junction between the brainstem and spinal cord (Fig. 13.8) and enter the lateral columns of the spinal cord (Fig. 11.2).

Posterior Column-Medial Lemniscus Pathway (see Chap. 10)

The fasciculi gracilis and cuneatus terminate in the nucleus gracilis (forming the tuberculum gracilis) and nucleus cuneatus (forming the tuberculum cuneatus)(Figs. 13.2, 13.3, 13.8, and 13.9). Fibers from these nuclei decussate as the internal arcuate fibers in the lower medulla to form the medial lemniscus (Fig. 13.9), which ascends through the tegmentum and terminates in the ventral posterolateral nucleus of the thalamus (Fig. 10.3). As the medial lemniscus ascends, it gradually shifts from an anteromedial location in the medulla to a posterolateral location in the midbrain (Figs. 13.9 to 13.16).

Anterolateral Pathway (see Chap. 9)

This pathway ascends from the spinal cord and continues within the lateral aspect of the tegmentum as the spinothalamic tract until it terminates in the ventral posterolateral nucleus of the thalamus (Figs. 13.8, 13.9, 13.12 to 13.16).

Trigeminal Pathways

The trigeminal nerve enters the brainstem in the lateral midpons (Figs. 10.5 and 13.4). Some of its fibers descend as the spinal tract of n. V that forms a ridge called the *trigeminal eminence* (Fig. 13.5). Some fibers from the principal sensory nucleus and spinal nucleus of n. V decussate to form the anterior trigeminothalamic tract, which is located between the medial lemniscus and the spinothalamic tract in the pons and midbrain (Fig. 13.15). Nondecussating fibers form the posterior trigeminothalamic tract (Figs. 10.5 and 13.14), located posterolaterally in the tegmentum. The trigeminothalamic fibers terminate in the ventral posteromedial nucleus of the thalamus (Figs. 9.5 and 10.5).

Medial Longitudinal Fasciculus (MLF)

This fiber bundle extends from the midbrain through the spinal cord. In the brainstem, the MLF is located anterior to the cerebral aqueduct and the fourth ventricle and on either side of the midline (Figs. 13.8 to 13.16). Its fibers have a critical role in coordinating the two eyes with each other (conjugate movements; Chap. 16) and with adjustments for alterations in head position.

Auditory Pathways (see Chap. 16)

Auditory pathways receive their input from the cochlear nerve and nuclei located on the surface of the inferior cerebellar peduncle in the rostral medulla (Fig. 13.11). The auditory pathways ascend as the *lateral lemniscus*, located in the lateral tegmentum just dorsolateral to the spinothalamic tract (Fig. 13.13). The fibers of the lateral lemniscus terminate in the *inferior colliculus* (Fig. 13.14), which gives rise to the *brachium of the inferior colliculus*. The brachium terminates in the medial geniculate body of the thalamus (Figs. 13.15 and 13.16).

Spinocerebellar and Pontocerebellar Tracts

The spinocerebellar pathways are located in the lateral tegmentum of the brainstem (Fig. 10.6). The posterior spinocerebellar tract and the cuneocerebellar tract from the accessory cuneate nucleus pass through the inferior cerebellar peduncle (Figs. 13.10 to 13.12). The anterior spinocerebellar tract ascends to the lower midbrain and passes through the superior cerebellar peduncle (Fig. 13.13). Fibers from the pontine nuclei decussate as pontocerebellar fibers and pass through the middle cerebellar peduncle (Figs. 13.14 and 18.3). The three cerebellar peduncles on each side (Figs. 13.2 and 13.3) give access to the entire cerebellum.

Reticular Formation (RF)

The brainstem tegmentum consists of the (1) nuclei and fibers of cranial nerves (Chap. 14), (2) long tracts of sensory and motor pathways (Chaps. 9, 10 and 11), and (3) the RF (Fig. 13.6).

The RF is the central or reticular core of the tegmentum. It is an intricate neural network composed of reticular nuclei (Fig. 13.6), ascending reticular pathways, descending reticular pathways, and local reflex circuits of cranial

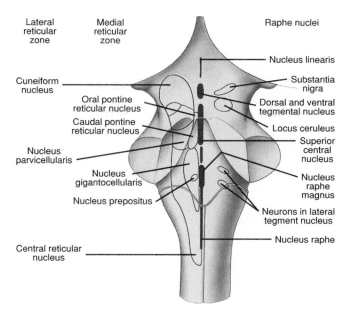

Figure 13.6: Posterior view of the brainstem illustrating some of the nuclei of the reticular formation. Nuclei of the lateral and medial reticular zones are noted on the left; and the raphe nuclei, locus ceruleus, and noradrenergic lateral tegmental nuclei on the right, together with the substantia nigra. Refer to Figs. 13.8 through 13.16. The reticular nuclei projecting to the cerebellum (e.g., lateral reticular nucleus and pontine reticulotegmental nucleus) are not included. (Adapted from DeMyer.)

nerves. Phylogenetically older than most of the other surrounding structures, the RF consists of a diffuse yet organized network of nuclei and tracts—hence the term reticular. The RF network consists of multipolar neurons with long ascending and descending axons with highly collateralized branches synaptically linked with interneurons into complex loops of circuits (Chap. 22, **Fig. 22.1**). The brainstem RF is an anatomical component of the *reticular system* (Chap. 22).

The brainstem component of the reticular system exerts significant modulatory effects on the activities of the spinal cord, brainstem, and cerebrum including the cerebral cortex. The ascending reticular pathways include the reticular activating system which is involved with sleep-wake cycles and in modulating awareness. The descending reticular pathways display their roles in motor activities as expressed in behavioral performances. The nuclei of the RF are organized in three longitudinal zones (1) median raphe zone, (2) medial reticular zone, and (3) lateral reticular zone (**Fig. 22.1**).

Some of the brainstem reticular nuclei are arranged in distinctive groups. On the basis of their neural connections and the biochemical nature of their neurotransmitters, they form three major aminergic (monoaminergic) systems or pathways called the (1) noradrenergic (transmitter is norepinephrine), (2) dopaminergic (transmitter is dopamine), and (3) serotonergic (transmitter is serotonin) systems (**Figs. 15.1, 15.2**).

Noradrenergic System

The two locations of noradrenergic neurons are the locus ceruleus (LC, a nucleus located in the upper pons) and scattered groups of neurons in the lateral tegmentum of the pons and medulla (**Figs. 13.6 and 15.2**).

The LC (cerulean blue color in the fresh human brainstem) receives its major input from nuclei in the vicinity of the nucleus gigantocellularis. The axon of each LC neuron has a T-like bifurcation forming ascending and descending fibers (**Fig. 22.1**). These output branches are more widely distributed than those of any other known nucleus. The axons collateralize profusely into fibers which sprout thousands of branches. These are distributed directly to the thalamus, hypothalamus, hippocampus, cerebral cortex, cerebellum, and the dorsal and ventral horns of the spinal cord (Fig. 15.2). The tegmental adrenergic neurons have a primary distribution to the brainstem and spinal cord and lesser projections to the thalamus, cerebral cortex, and cerebellum. These catecholamine pathways with their diffuse connections exert modulating influences on numerous functions, rather than initiating or mediating specific functions. Such a role in phases of the sleep-wake cycle are probable. The LC has a coordination role in preparing for the appropriate responses when activated by novel or intense sensory stimuli. The lateral tegmental neurons exert their roles in the autonomic nervous system by evoking a decrease in arterial pressure and heart rate. To be specific about functions evoked can be complicated for the following reason. The modulatory activity of the circuits can produce differences and nuances in the physiological and behavioral expressions because of the variety of ways input can be biased, depending upon the degree of stimulation (or inhibition) of excitatory (or inhibitory) neurons in the complex circuitry.

Serotonergic System

The quantity of serotonergic neurons in the brainstem outnumber those of the adrenergic and dopaminergic systems. The cell bodies of the neurons of this extensive system are located in the raphe nuclei (Figs. 13.6 and 15.1). The neurons of the raphe nuclei in the upper pons and midbrain project via the median forebrain bundle to the oculomotor nuclei, substantia nigra, striatum, hypothalamus, limbic structures such as the hippocampus, and the cerebral cortex. The neurons of the raphe magnus have fibers projecting locally to the facial nucleus and caudally to the sensory dorsal horn and the motor ventral horn of the spinal cord.

The widespread connections of this system are expressed by its modulatory and augmenting role, rather than by a specific behavior. It functions in enhancing learning of avoidance behavior and in increasing the excitability of lower motoneurons. Inhibitory roles are expressed in the dorsal horn of the spinal cord by modulating and repressing pain, producing analgesia, and increasing the pain threshold (Chap. 9). This system may have a role in initiating sleep. This is consistent with the insomnia that occurs following the experimental destruction of the raphe nuclei.

Dopaminergic System

The dopaminergic nuclei are present in the substantia nigra (pars compacta) (Figs. 13.6, 13.15, and 15.1) and ventral tegmental area (VTA medial to substantia nigra) of the midbrain. Their neurons project rostrally as the mesostriatal, mesolimbic, and mesocortical pathways to the cerebrum (meso for mesencephalon or midbrain).

The mesostriatal system from the substantia nigra to the striatum (caudate nucleus and putamen) of the basal ganglia has a significant role in motor function (Chap. 24). The loss of these fiber projections following damage to the nigral neurons results in Parkinsonism (Chap. 24). The mesolimbic system from the VTA are connected to such limbic structures as the nucleus accumbens, amygdala, septal region, and ventral striatum (Chaps. 22, 24). The mesocortical projections are from the VTA to frontal and cingulate gyri of the cortex (Chaps. 22, 25). The latter two systems have been linked to the affliction known as schizophrenia (*dopamine hypothesis of schizophrenia*). The concept is that this affliction may be related to the relative excess of dopaminergic neuronal activity. Those antipsychotic drugs that have therapeutic effects are presumed to block dopamine receptors and, thus, reduce dopaminergic transmission.

Sensory Nerves, Their Sensory Ganglia, and Nuclei of Termination

The sensory cranial nerves and their ganglia (equivalent to the dorsal root ganglia) include the trigeminal nerve (n. V) with its trigeminal (Gasserian, semilunar) ganglion, facial nerve (n. VII) with its geniculate ganglion, vestibulocochlear (acoustic or auditory) nerve (n. VIII) with its vestibular and spiral ganglia, the glossopharyngeal nerve (n. IX) with its superior and inferior ganglia, and the vagus nerve (n. X) with its superior and inferior ganglia (Fig. 14.2).

The brainstem nuclei of the sensory cranial nerves are arranged in continuous columns (Fig. 14.2) as follows:

1. A *general somatic column* associated with cranial nerves V, VII, IX, and X. It comprises the *mesencephalic nucleus of n. V*, which is located lateral to the ventricular canal in the upper pons and midbrain (Fig. 13.13); the *principal sensory nucleus of n. V*, which is located in the lateral tegmentum in the midpons (Fig. 13.13); and the *spinal nucleus of n. V*, which is located in the lateral tegmentum in the lower pons, medulla, and first two cervical spinal levels (Figs. 13.7 to 13.12).

2. A *visceral column* associated with the cranial nerves VII, IX, and X. This column, known as the *nucleus solitarius*, is located in the posterior tegmentum of the medulla (Figs. 13.9 to 13.11).

3. A *special somatic column* associated with cranial nerve VIII (Fig. 14.2). The four *vestibular nuclei* are located in the posterolateral tegmentum of the lower pons and upper medulla (Figs. 13.10 and 13.11); the two *cochlear nuclei* are located on the outer surface of the inferior cerebellar peduncle (Fig. 13.11).

Motor Nerves and Their Nuclei of Origin Within the Brainstem

The brainstem nuclei of the motor cranial nerves are arranged in three discontinuous columns (Fig. 14.3):

1. A *general somatic column* associated with cranial nerves III, IV, VI, and XII. These motor nuclei are located in the posteromedial tegmentum. Those of nerves III and IV are in the midbrain (Figs. 13.14 to 13.16), that of n. VI in the lower pons (Fig. 13.12), and that of n. XII through the length of the medulla (Figs. 13.9 and 13.10).

2. A *special visceral column* consists of three nuclei associated with cranial nerves V, VII, IX, X, and XI. The *motor nucleus of n. V* is located in the lateral tegmentum of the midpons (Fig. 13.13); the *motor nucleus of n. VII* is in the caudal pontine tegmentum

(Fig. 13.12); and that of IX, X, and XI, known as the *nucleus ambiguus*, is within the central tegmentum through the length of the medulla (Figs. 13.9 to 13.11).

3. A *general visceral (parasympathetic) column* associated with cranial nerves III, VII, IX, and X (Fig. 14.3). The parasympathetic nucleus associated with n. III is the accessory nucleus of n. III (nucleus of Edinger-Westphal) in the midbrain (Fig. 13.15); the nucleus with n. VII is the superior salivatory nucleus in the posterolateral tegmentum of the lower pons (Fig. 13.12); the nucleus with n. IX is the inferior salivatory nucleus located in the posterior tegmentum of the rostral medulla (Fig. 13.11); and the nucleus with n. X is the dorsal vagal nucleus located in the posterior tegmentum of the medulla (Figs. 13.9 and 13.10).

TRANSVERSE SECTIONS THROUGH THE BRAINSTEM

In the following account, the anatomic relations of the intrinsic structures of the brainstem are briefly described in a representative series of transverse sections moving successively higher from the upper cervical segment through the upper midbrain.

First Cervical Segment of the Spinal Cord

The first cervical segment has several distinctive features (Fig. 13.7). The fibers of the lateral corticospinal tract are located more medially than in the other spinal levels. Its location, abutting the gray matter, indicates that the tract has not completed its decussation. The myelinated fibers of the *spinal tract of n. V* and the large *spinal nucleus of n. V*, which extend to the C2 level, are the equivalents of the posterolateral tract and substantia gelatinosa of the spinal cord. The fibers of the *spinal root of cranial nerve XI* originate in the anterolateral aspect of the anterior horn and pass posteriorly and then laterally before emerging from the lateral side of the spinal cord. Although the dorsal root is absent at C1, the ventral root of the first cervical nerve is present.

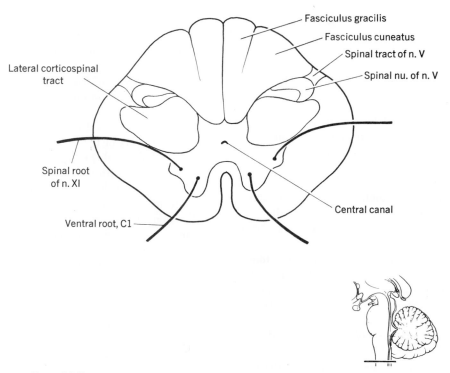

Figure 13.7: Transverse section of the upper portion of the first cervical segment.

Level of the Pyramidal Decussation

This level is within the medulla (**Fig. 13.8**). The most distinguishing feature is the crossing of 85 to 90% of the corticospinal fibers as the *pyramidal decussation*. It is composed of inter-digitating descending fibers which decussate and course in a caudal and posterior direction to the dorsal aspect of the lateral funiculus of the spinal cord. Dorsal spinal roots are absent. The spinal tract of n. V is composed of fibers from cranial nerves V, VII, IX and X which descend as far as C2 to terminate throughout the length of the spinal nucleus of n. V (**Fig. 9.5**). The fasciculus gracilis is smaller than the fasciculus cuneatus; both fasciculi are in the same location as in the spinal cord. The *nucleus gracilis* is present; it is the nucleus of termina-tion for the fibers of the fasciculus gracilis. The posterior and anterior spinocerebellar, spino-thalamic, and spinotectal tracts have a rela-tively similar position as in the spinal cord. The MLF passes on the ventrolateral side of the decussating pyramidal fibers. The *central*

reticular nucleus of the medulla occupies the bulk of the RF from the spinal cord-medulla junction to the midolivary level. In the medial part of the ventral gray matter of the caudal medulla is a rostral extension of the anterior horn (lamina IX) of the spinal cord; this nu-cleus, which gives rise to ventral root fibers of the first cervical nerves, is called the *supra-spinal nucleus*.

Level of Decussation of the Medial Lemniscus

The distinguishing feature of this level is the curve of the *internal arcuate fibers*, which, after arising from cells in the enlarged nuclei gracilis and cuneatus, sweep anteriorly in an arc and decussate across the midline to form the medial lemniscus of the opposite side (**Fig. 13.9**). Upon entering the medial lemniscus, these fi-bers bend and ascend rostrally through the brainstem to the ventral posterolateral nucleus of the thalamus. The fasciculi gracilis and cu-neatus are small because their ascending fibers terminate within the nuclei gracilis and cunea-

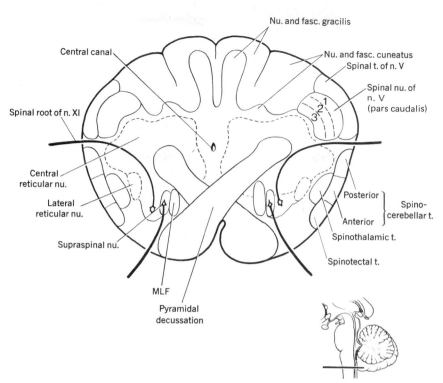

Figure 13.8: Transverse section of the lower medulla at the level of the pyramidal (corticospinal) decussation. The pars caudalis of the spinal trigeminal nucleus is called the posterior horn of the medulla because it is divisible into a (1) marginal lamina, (2) substantia gelatinosa, and (3) magnocellular layer.

tus. The *spinal tract and nucleus of the trigeminal nerve* are displaced anteriorly. Some fibers arise from this nucleus and, with the internal arcuate fibers, cross to the opposite side, ascending as the *anterior trigeminothalamic tract* to the ventral posteromedial nucleus of the thalamus (**Fig. 9.5**). They are second-order neurons, conveying pain and temperature information derived from the trigeminal nerve; nervus intermedius (VII); glossopharyngeal; and vagus nerves.

In addition to the spinal nucleus of n. V, four other cranial nerve nuclei are present at this level. The sensory *nucleus solitarius* (GVA and SVA) and the parasympathetic motor *dorsal vagal nucleus* (GVE) and the *motor nucleus ambiguus* (SVE) are involved with the vagus nerve, which emerges through the dorsolateral sulcus of the medulla. The former two nuclei are located anterior to the nucleus gracilis and medial to the internal arcuate fibers; the latter (nucleus ambiguus) is located in the middle of the teg-

mentum just lateral to the internal arcuate fibers. Many of the fibers of the nucleus ambiguus from this level form the cranial root of the accessory nerve.

Anterior to the central canal on either side of the midline is the pair of *hypoglossal nuclei* (GSE); from each nucleus arises a hypoglossal nerve which passes through the medial tegmentum and emerges from the medulla between a pyramid and the olive (inferior olivary nuclear complex) at the preolivary sulcus.

The ascending tracts located in the lateral medulla—comprising the posterior and anterior spinocerebellar, spinothalamic, and spinotectal tracts—occupy the same general location as in the more caudal levels.

Three prominent cerebellar relay nuclei of the medulla are the source of fibers which pass through the inferior cerebellar peduncle before terminating in the cerebellum. The first, the *accessory cuneate nucleus* of the lower medulla, located lateral to the cuneate nucleus, is the

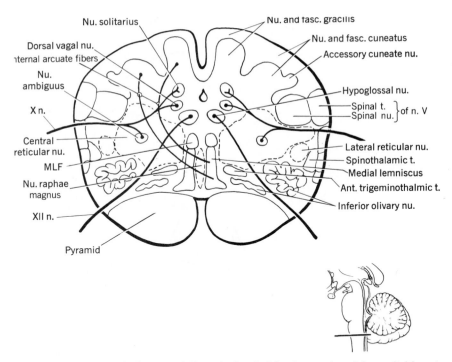

Figure 13.9: Transverse section of the lower medulla at the level of the decussation of the medial lemniscus (internal arcuate fibers).

homologue of the dorsal nucleus of Clarke in the spinal cord; it receives proprioceptive input from the cervical and upper thoracic regions, especially the upper extremities, via uncrossed fibers ascending in the fasciculus cuneatus. The ipsilaterally projecting cuneocerebellar fibers from the accessory cuneate nucleus are the pathway from the upper extremity that is equivalent to the posterior spinocerebellar tract from the lower extremity. The second relay nucleus, the *lateral reticular nucleus*, is located in the vicinity of the spinothalamic tract at the level of the caudal two thirds of the inferior olivary nuclei. This nucleus receives afferent input from the spinal cord via spinoreticular and collateral branches of spinothalamic fibers and from fibers from the red nucleus of the midbrain. The third cerebellar relay group, the *inferior olivary complex*, is discussed in the next section.

Of the descending tracts and fibers, only the pyramids, composed of corticospinal fibers, are clearly demarcated. The anterior border of the MLF is not clearly defined because its fibers

overlap with those of the medial lemniscus. At this level the MLF is composed of (1) the pontine reticulospinal tract from the pars oralis and pars caudalis of the pontine reticular nuclei, (2) the interstitiospinal tract from the interstitial nucleus of Cajal, (3) the tectospinal tract from the midbrain tectum, and (4) vestibulospinal fibers from the medial vestibular nucleus.

Just posterior to the inferior olivary nuclear complex within the RF are the fibers of the rubrospinal tract from the red nucleus in the midbrain, the medullary reticulospinal tract from the nucleus reticularis gigantocellularis of the medulla, and the vestibulospinal tract from the lateral vestibular nucleus. The fibers of these tracts are intermingled with other fibers; hence, they are not clearly delineated.

The *reticular nuclei* include the nucleus raphe magnus, central reticular nucleus and lateral reticular nucleus; these belong to the raphe, central and lateral nuclear groups, respectively. Just rostral to this level is the obex **(Fig. 13.3)**, located at the most caudal extent of the fourth ventricle.

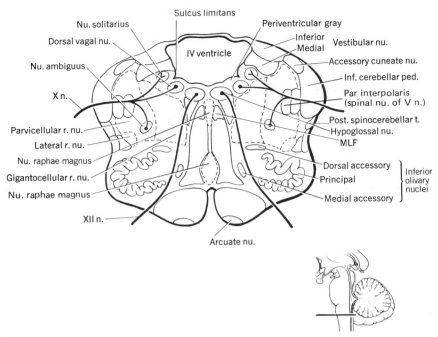

Figure 13.10: Transverse section of the medulla at the level of the middle of the olive. The arcuate nuclei are minor nuclei projecting to the cerebellum.

Level of the Middle Third of the Inferior Olivary Complex

The distinguishing features of this level (**Fig. 13.10**) are the nuclei of the inferior olivary complex, fourth ventricle, inferior cerebellar peduncle, and cranial nerve nuclei. The *olivary complex* comprises the phylogenetically new *principal inferior olivary nucleus* and the phylogenetically old *dorsal* and *medial accessory olivary nuclei*. The fibers from the inferior olivary complex decussate and pass successively through the medial lemnisci, the vicinity of the contralateral olivary complex, and the inferior cerebellar peduncle before terminating in the cerebellum. The accessory olivary nuclei have fibers which project primarily to the vermis of the cerebellum. The fibers from the principal olivary nucleus terminate in the contralateral cerebellar hemisphere. The olivocerebellar fibers convey excitatory influences to the deep cerebellar nuclei and to the entire cerebellar cortex. The input to the inferior olivary nuclei is derived from the spinal cord, cerebral cortex, red nucleus, periaqueductal gray of the mid-

brain, and deep cerebellar nuclei. The spino-olivary fibers ascend in the anterior funiculus. Originating from the frontal, parietal, temporal, and occipital lobes, the cortico-olivary fibers course with the corticospinal fibers before terminating bilaterally. The fibers from the red nucleus and periaqueductal gray descend in the central tegmental tract. From the deep cerebellar nuclei, fibers pass through the superior cerebellar peduncle, cross in the lower midbrain, and descend in the central tegmental tract.

In the tegmentum anterior to the floor of the IVth ventricle is a row of cranial nerve nuclei. Two motor nuclei, located medial to the fovea (sulcus limitans), are the hypoglossal (GSE) and dorsal vagal (GVE) nuclei. Two sensory nuclear groups, located lateral to the fovea, are the nucleus solitarius (GVA, SVA) and the medial and inferior vestibular (SSA) nuclei. The nucleus ambiguus (SVE) is a motor nucleus located in the middle of the tegmentum. The spinal nucleus of n. V is a sensory nucleus in the dorsolateral tegmentum. The vagus nerve is associated with the nucleus ambiguus, dorsal vagal nucleus, nucleus solitarius, and the spinal nucleus of n. V.

The *paramedian reticular nuclei* (nuclei lateral to medial lemniscus in vicinity of inferior olivary nucleus) and the nearby *arcuate nucleus* relay influences via the inferior cerebellar peduncles to the cerebellum. The cells of the *raphe nuclei*—the *nucleus raphe magnus*—contain serotonin (5-hydroxytryptamine). Fibers from these cells project to the spinal cord (Chap. 9).

The *central reticular nuclear group* in the upper medullary levels is the *gigantocellular reticular nucleus*, which is located posterior to the inferior olivary complex. This large-celled nucleus occupies the medial two-thirds of the RF as far rostral as the medullary-pontine junction. Input to this nucleus is derived largely from (1) widespread areas of the cerebral cortex via crossed and uncrossed corticoreticular fibers, (2) higher brainstem levels via the central tegmental tract, (3) neurons from the parvicellular nucleus of the lateral nuclear group, and (4) spinoreticular fibers ascending in the anterolateral funiculus of the spinal cord. The output from this nucleus is projected (1) rostrally via the central tegmental tract to higher brainstem levels and the intralaminar nuclei of the thalamus, and via the median forebrain bundle to the hypothalamus, and (2) caudally via the medullary (lateral) reticulospinal tract to the spinal cord.

The *lateral reticular zone* comprises the *lateral reticular nucleus* and *parvicellular reticular nucleus*. Input to the parvicellular reticular nucleus is derived from (1) widespread areas of the cerebral cortex via crossed and uncrossed corticoreticular fibers; (2) collateral fibers conveying influences from the auditory, vestibular, trigeminal, and visceral pathways; and (3) spinoreticular fibers from the spinal cord. The output from the parvicellular reticular nucleus is directed medially to the gigantocellular reticular nucleus. Except for possible minor changes, the locations of the ascending and descending tracts and pathways are similar to those described under "Level of Decussation of the Medial Lemniscus." The posterior spinocerebellar tract is close to the inferior cerebellar peduncle, which it is about to join.

Tangential Section at the Levels of the Glossopharyngeal and Vestibulocochlear Nerves

This medullary level is in the vicinity of the medullopontine junction (**Fig. 13.11**). It is different from the midolivary level in several respects. Among these are the absence of the hypoglossal and dorsal vagal nuclei; presence of cranial nerve nuclei associated with the glossopharyngeal, cochlear, and vestibular nerves; and the presence of the inferior cerebellar peduncle, which can be seen extending from the medulla into the cerebellum.

The nuclei associated with the glossopharyngeal nerve include the nucleus solitarius, spinal nucleus of n. V, inferior salivatory nucleus, and nucleus ambiguus. These nuclei are discussed in Chapter 14.

On the outer surface of the inferior cerebellar peduncle are the dorsal and ventral cochlear nuclei. The fibers of the cochlear nerve branch in an organized sequence so that each fiber is distributed in a precise topographic pattern to both the dorsal and ventral cochlear nuclei. At a slightly higher level (right side of **Fig. 13.11**), the fibers of the vestibular nerve pass at right angles among the fibers of the inferior cerebellar peduncle on their way to the four vestibular nuclei (the medial, inferior, and lateral vestibular nuclei are illustrated).

In **Figure 13.11**, the large inferior cerebellar peduncle (left side) is illustrated as it passes (right side) into the cerebellum. The peduncle comprises the following fibers passing to the cerebellum: posterior spinocerebellar, cuneocerebellar and olivocerebellar tracts, along with fibers from such nuclei as the lateral reticular and paramedian reticular nuclei. A portion of the inferior cerebellar peduncle, called the *juxtarestiform body*, is composed of fibers associated with the vestibular system conveying influences to and from the vestibulocerebellum and the fastigial nuclei of the cerebellum (Chap. 16).

The reticular nuclei at this level include the raphe magnus, gigantocellularis, and parvicellularis.

The four deep cerebellar nuclei, oriented in order from medial to lateral, are the fastigial, globose, emboliform, and dentate nuclei. The globose and emboliform nuclei are collectively

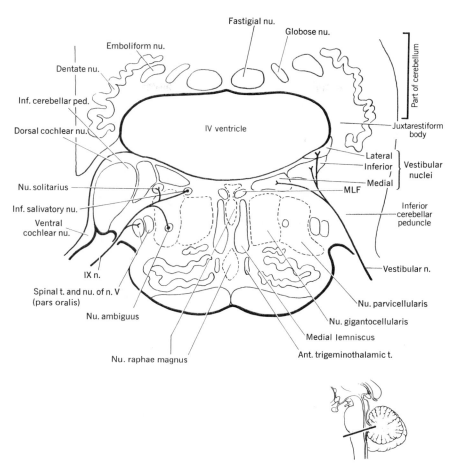

Figure 13.11: Transverse section (slightly oblique) of the upper medulla at the level of the cochlear and glossopharyngeal nerves (left) and the vestibular nerve (right). Section includes the cerebellum and its deep cerebellar nuclei.

called the *nucleus interpositus*. The fibers of the inferior cerebellar peduncle pass lateral to the dentate nucleus. The juxtarestiform body is located between the deep cerebellar nuclei and the lateral border of the fourth ventricle.

Level of Nuclei of Sixth and Seventh Cranial Nerves

The general pattern of organization at this level (Fig. 13.12) differs from that of the levels of the medulla primarily because of the massive size of the ventral or basilar pons relative to the dorsal or tegmental pons. The *ventral pons* represents a modified, rostral continuation of the pyramids of the medulla. The *tegmental pons* represents the rostral continuation of the medulla exclusive of the pyramids. The boundary between the dorsal andventral pons is a

plane located just anterior to the medial lemniscus. The IVth ventricle is large.

The *basilar pons* consists of the pontine nuclei, the terminal branches of the descending corticopontine fibers to the pontine nuclei, and the pontocerebellar fibers; the latter fibers pass from the pontine nuclei through the middle cerebellar peduncle to the cerebellum (**Fig. 18.3**).

Except for a few significant modifications, the dorsal pons resembles the medulla. The MLF is still located anterior to the IVth ventricle and just lateral to the midline, while the spinal tract and nucleus of the trigeminal nerve are in the dorsolateral tegmentum. However, the medial lemniscus has shifted from a ventromedial tegmental location (vertical orientation) in the

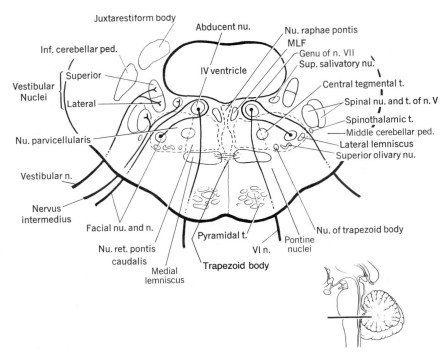

Figure 13.12: Transverse section of the lower pons at the level of the sixth and seventh cranial nerves.

medulla to a ventral tegmental location (horizontal orientation) in the pons. The central tegmental tract is prominent in the middle of the RF.

The cranial nerve nuclei present at this level have their equivalents in the medulla. The *abducent nucleus, motor nucleus of the facial nerve,* and the *superior salivatory nucleus* are located within the tegmentum in sites similar to those occupied within the medulla by the hypoglossal nucleus, nucleus ambiguus, and dorsal vagal nucleus, respectively. The *superior vestibular nucleus* is found in the posterolateral tegmentum. The course of the fibers of the abducent and facial nerves is characteristic and significant. The lower motoneurons of the sixth nerve emerge from the abducent nucleus and pass ventrally through the medial tegmentum and basal pons lateral to the pyramidal tract before emerging medially at the pontomedullary junction. After leaving from the facial nucleus, the lower motoneurons form a bundle that follows a circuitous course. The facial nerve passes posteromedially, ascends for a short distance medial to the abducent nucleus, and then, as the

genu of n. VII, passes posterior to the abducent nucleus; finally, it turns laterally before continuing anterolaterally and caudally through the lateral tegmentum to emerge from the brainstem at the *cerebellopontine angle* (**Fig. 13.3**). The hillock in the floor of the fourth ventricle at the site of the abducent nucleus and the internal genu is called the *facial* or *abducent colliculus*. The *nervus intermedius* is a part of n. VII (Chap. 14); some of its fibers originate in the superior salivatory nucleus and others terminate in the spinal nucleus of n. V and the nucleus solitarius.

The superior and inferior salivatory nuclei are actually diffuse and confluent groups of cells located within and close to the parvicellular reticular nucleus (**Figs. 13.11 and 13.12**). Nuclei and tracts of the auditory pathways are found at this level. They are the *superior olivary complex* and nuclei of the *trapezoid body*; the tract is the *lateral lemniscus,* which is located in the ventrolateral tegmentum. Auditory fibers decussating between the olives constitute the trapezoid body (**Figs. 13.12 and 16.5**).

The reticular nuclei at this level, and those

of the lower pons caudal to the principal nucleus of the trigeminal nerve, are the *nucleus raphe pontis* (a raphe nucleus), the *nucleus reticularis pontis caudalis* (a central reticular group nucleus), and the *nucleus parvicellularis* (a lateral reticular nucleus). The paramedian reticular nuclei, extending rostrally from a level near the abducent nucleus, form the so-called paramedian pontine reticular formation (PPRF) or pontine gaze center involved in control of synergistic horizontal eye movements (Chaps. 16 and 19).

Level of the Trigeminal Nerve

The characteristic features at this midpontine level (**Fig. 13.13**) are (1) the *principal sensory nucleus* and *motor nucleus of the trigeminal nerve* and (2) the *superior cerebellar peduncle* on the lateral aspect of the narrowing fourth ventricle.

The *principal nucleus of n. V* is a nucleus of termination of the sensory root of the trigeminal nerve; other fibers of this root have their cell bodies in the *mesencephalic nucleus of n. V*, which is located lateral to the ventricle. The *motor nucleus of n. V*, located medial to the prin-

cipal nucleus, contains the cell bodies of origin of the lower motoneurons of the motor root of the trigeminal nerve.

The *superior cerebellar peduncle* is primarily composed of cerebellar efferent fibers originating in the dentate, emboliform, and globose nuclei; these fibers decussate in the lower midbrain tegmentum and (1) ascend to the nucleus ruber and to the rostral intralaminar and ventrolateral thalamic nuclei and (2) descend in the brainstem tegmentum to the reticulotegmental nucleus of the pons and the inferior olivary and paramedian nuclei of the medulla. The anterior spinocerebellar tract courses posteriorly in the superior cerebellar peduncle; its fibers terminate in the anterior vermal cortex.

The medial lemniscus has shifted somewhat laterally, and the spinothalamic tract and lateral lemniscus have shifted slightly dorsolaterally along the outer margin of the RF. The MLF, central tegmental tract, rubrospinal tract, and the structures of the basilar pons have the same topographic relations to one another as described in the last section. The lateral lemniscus contains a small diffuse aggregation of neurons called the nucleus of the lateral lemniscus.

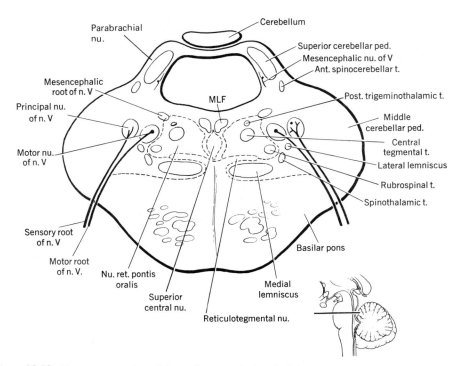

Figure 13.13: Transverse section of the midpons at the level of the entrance of the trigeminal nerve.

The reticular nuclei extending from this level up to the lower midbrain are (1) the *superior central nucleus* (a raphe nucleus), (2) the *reticulotegmental nucleus* (actually an extension of the pontine nucleus of the basilar pons into the tegmentum; as do the pontine nuclei, the reticulotegmental nucleus projects its fibers to the cerebellum), and (3) the *nucleus reticularis pontis oralis* and *LC* (**Figs. 13.13** and **13.14**) (central reticular nuclei). The cells of the LC are noradrenergic neurons whose axons are distributed to the (1) cerebellum; (2) cerebrum, including directly to the cerebral cortex; (3) brainstem; and (4) spinal cord. The LC appears cerulean blue in the "fresh" gross brain.

Level of the Inferior Colliculus

The distinguishing features at this level (**Fig. 13.14**) include the inferior colliculus and the decussation of the superior cerebellar peduncle.

The ventricular system is represented by the narrow *cerebral aqueduct* that is surrounded by the periaqueductal gray, which is involved in pain control (Chap. 9, **Fig. 9.4**).

The large *nucleus of the inferior colliculus* is a major processing station in the auditory pathways. It receives input from ascending auditory fibers of the lateral lemniscus and descending fibers from the medial geniculate body; it projects influences (1) rostrally to the medial geniculate body, via the brachium of the inferior colliculus, and to the superior colliculus and (2) caudally to auditory nuclei via the lateral lemniscus. The bilateral nuclei of the inferior colliculi are interconnected by fibers in the commissure of the inferior colliculus. As a group, the medial lemniscus, spinothalamic tract, and lateral lemniscus have shifted laterally and dorsally along the outer margin of the RF of the tegmentum. In this shift, the lateral lemniscus approaches the inferior colliculus; its

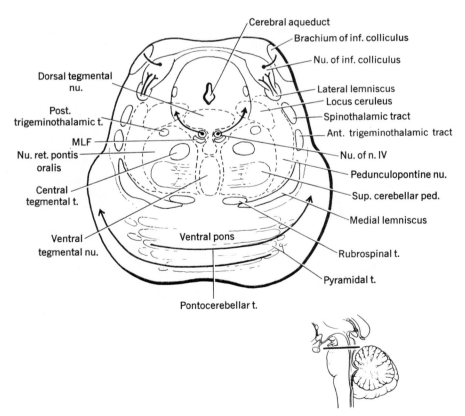

Figure 13.14: Transverse section of the lower midbrain at the level of the inferior colliculus and nucleus of the fourth cranial nerve.

fibers enter and terminate in the nucleus of the inferior colliculus. The rostrally projecting fibers from the latter form the brachium of the inferior colliculus, which is located in the dorsolateral tegmentum of the upper midbrain.

The *posterior trigeminothalamic tract*, from the ipsilateral principal nucleus of n. V, is located in the tegmentum posterior to the central tegmental tract. The anterior trigeminothalamic tract, from the contralateral spinal and principal nuclei of n. V, is located between the medial lemniscus and spinothalamic tract. The MLF is notched posteriorly by the nucleus of the trochlear nerve. The fibers of the trochlear nerve (IV) pass as a dorsocaudally directed arc from this nucleus along the outer edge of the periaqueductal gray matter; they decussate completely in the superior medullary velum and emerge from the posterior tectum caudal to the inferior colliculus. The LC is located deep to the inferior colliculus.

The reticular nuclei at this level include (1) the *dorsal* and *ventral raphe tegmental nuclei* (raphe nuclei), (2) the rostral portion of the *nucleus reticularis pontis oralis* and *LC* (central reticular nuclei), and (3) *pedunculopontine* and *cuneiform nuclei* (lateral reticular group nuclei). The dorsal tegmental nucleus (supratrochlear nucleus) is located dorsal to the trochlear nucleus in the periaqueductal gray matter; it receives input from the mammillary body. The ventral tegmental nucleus is present ventral to the MLF; it is apparently a rostral extension of the superior central nucleus. The pedunculopontine nucleus lies in the caudal midbrain lateral to the superior cerebellar peduncle and medial to the medial lemniscus. It is the only brainstem nucleus which receives direct input from the globus pallidus (Fig. 24.3).

Section Through Midbrain at Level of Superior Colliculus

The major characteristic features at this level (Fig. 13.15) are the *superior colliculus, nucleus of the oculomotor nerve, red nucleus, substantia nigra,* and *crus cerebri*. The medial geniculate body, marking the most caudal nucleus of the diencephalon (or thalamus), is present.

The laminated superior colliculus and the

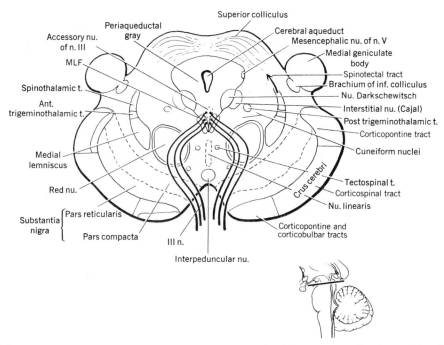

Figure 13.15: Transverse section of the upper midbrain at the level of the superior colliculus and the third cranial nerve.

rostrally located pretectum (**Fig. 13.16**) are complex reflex centers. The superficial layers of the superior colliculus receive direct input from the retina and the visual cortex. The deep layers receive inputs from the auditory and somatosensory systems. The superior colliculus has roles in orienting the head and eyes toward a visual stimulus. The pretectum is involved in the direct light and the consensual light reflexes (Chap. 19).

The *red nucleus* is a large oval nucleus in the medial tegmentum. It is composed of a caudal magnocellular part and a rostral parvicellular part. Some fibers of the superior cerebellar peduncle terminate within the nucleus, while others pass through it, and along its outer margins as a "capsule," on their way to the ventral lateral, ventral anterior, and some intralaminar thalamic nuclei.

The rubrospinal tract originates from cells in the caudal one-fourth of the red nucleus; its fibers cross as the ventral tegmental decussation before descending as the rubrospinal tract in the anterior tegmentum.

The *oculomotor nuclear complex* is located

in a V-shaped region formed by the paired MLF. The fibers of the oculomotor nerve (III) arise in this nucleus and course anteriorly through the medial tegmentum, including the red nucleus, on their way to emerge as rootlets from the interpeduncular fossa.

The *substantia nigra* is located between the tegmentum and the crus cerebri. It is divided into a pars compacta and a pars reticularis. The large cells of the compact (or black) part contain melanin pigment and primary catecholamines; these cells synthesize and convey dopamine, via nigrostriatal fibers, to the neostriatum (caudate nucleus and putamen). The cells of the reddish brown pars reticularis contain iron, but no melanin pigment.

The *crus cerebri* is the basilar part of the midbrain. It is composed of descending corticofugal fibers which originate in the cerebral cortex. The corticospinal and corticobulbar fibers are located in the middle two-thirds (**Fig. 13.15**). They are said to be somatotopically organized at this level with the head, upper-extremity and lower-extremity musculature influenced by nerve fibers arranged from medial to lateral

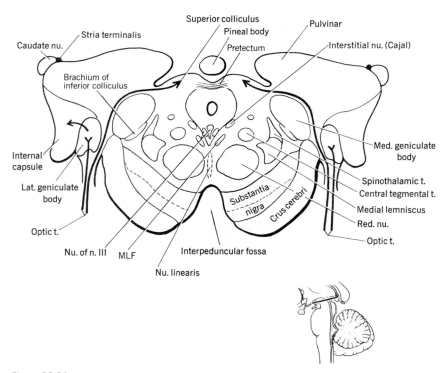

Figure 13.16: Transverse section at the junction of the upper midbrain and diencephalon.

within the crus. Frontopontine fibers are located in the medial portion, and the corticopontine fibers from the parietal, temporal, and occipital cortical areas are located in the lateral portion of the crus. The most medial and lateral portions of the crus may contain some corticobulbar fibers.

The medial lemniscus, anterior trigeminothalamic tract, and spinothalamic tract have shifted to a slightly more dorsal location in the tegmentum. The brachium of the inferior colliculus (auditory tract) is located dorsolateral to the spinothalamic tract; it is heading to the medial geniculate body. The posterior trigeminothalamic tract is located in the dorsomedial tegmentum. The interpeduncular nucleus is located at the midline just dorsal to the interpeduncular fossa. Dorsal to this nucleus is the VTA (not labeled) (Chap. 15). Neurons of VTA have been implicated with the reward properties of cocaine addiction (Chap. 22).

Reticular nuclei at this level include nuclei linearis (raphe nuclei); *nucleus ruber*, which is considered to be a specialized central reticular nucleus; and *cuneiform nuclei* (lateral reticular nuclear group). Nonreticular nuclei include the *interpeduncular nucleus, mesencephalic nucleus of the trigeminal nerve, interstitial nucleus of Cajal*, and the *nucleus of Darkschewitsch*.

Transverse Section Through Junction of Midbrain and Thalamus

Structures of the upper midbrain and the adjoining cerebrum are located in this section (**Fig. 13.16**). The midbrain is only slightly changed from the previous section. The pulvinar and medial and lateral geniculate bodies belong to the thalamus (Chap. 23). Also illustrated are the caudate nucleus (a basal ganglion; Chap. 24), stria terminalis (a tract of the limbic system; Chap. 22), internal capsule (fibers of the cerebrum; Chap. 23), and pineal body (Chap. 21).

The brachium of the inferior colliculus (auditory pathways) terminates in the medial geniculate body of the thalamus. Note that the fibers in the optic tract end either in the lateral genic-

ulate body of the thalamus or in the superior colliculus and pretectum (Chap. 19). The ascending reticular pathway fibers of the central tegmental tract terminate in the intralaminar nuclei of the thalamus (**Fig. 22.1**).

Refer to the previous section for a discussion of the superior colliculus, pretectum (pretectal area), oculomotor nerve (n. III), substantia nigra, and crus cerebri.

SUGGESTED READINGS

Brodal A. *The Reticular Formation of the Brain Stem: Anatomical Aspects and Functional Correlations.* London: Oliver & Boyd; 1957.

Burton H, Craig A Jr. Distribution of trigeminothalamic projection cells in cat and monkey. *Brain Res.* 1979;161:515–521.

Foote S, Bloom F, Aston-Jones G. Nucleus locus ceruleus. New evidence of anatomical and physiological specificity. *Physiol Rev.* 1983;63:844–914.

Garver D, Sladek J Jr. Monoamine distribution in primate brain. I. Catecholamine-containing perikarya in the brain stem of Macaca speciosa. *J Comp Neurol.* 1975;159:289–304.

Hobson J, Brazier M, eds. *The Reticular Formation Revisited: Specifying Function for a Nonspecific System.* IBRO Mono. New York, NY: Raven Press; 1980;6:1–552.

Jacobowitz D, MacLean P. A brainstem atlas of catecholaminergic neurons and serotonergic perikarya in a pygmy primate (Cebuella pygmaea). *J Comp Neurol.* 1978;177:397–416.

Moore R, Bloom F. Central catecholamine neuron systems: anatomy and physiology of the norepinephrine and epinephrine systems. *Annu Rev Neurosci.* 1979;2:113–168.

Peterson B, ed. The reticulospinal system and its role in the control of movement. In: Barnes C, ed. *Brainstem Control of Spinal Cord Function.* Orlando, Fla: Academic Press; 1984.

Steriade M, McCarley R. *Brainstem Control of Wake-Sleep States.* New York, NY: Plenum; 1990.

Snyder S. Opiate receptors and internal opiates. *Sci Am.* 1977;236:44–56.

Cranial Nerves

14

Classification of cranial nerves
Ganglia in the head
Cranial nerve nuclei within the brainstem
Some functional and clinical considerations

The twelve pair of cranial nerves are the peripheral nerves of brain (Fig. 14.1). The olfactory and optic nerves are nerves of the cerebrum (telencephalon). The other ten pair are nerves of the brainstem (and, to a slight extent, of the cervical spinal cord). They supply structures of the head and neck and, in the case of the vagus nerve, structures of the trunk. Some cranial nerves contain only afferent fibers, others only efferent fibers, and some both afferent and efferent fibers (Table 14.1). The afferent fibers arise from cell bodies located in peripheral ganglia; their central processes enter the brainstem and end in sensory nuclei of termination (Fig. 14.2). Efferent fibers arise from cell bodies located in the brainstem motor nuclei of origin (Fig. 14.3). Cranial nerves pass to and from the brain through foramina, canals, and fissures in the skull.

CLASSIFICATION OF CRANIAL NERVES

Many of the cranial nerves have the same general functional components as those found in the spinal nerves: general somatic afferent (GSA), general visceral afferent (GVA), general somatic efferent (GSE), and general visceral efferent (GVE) components. In addition, many cranial nerves have special components: special somatic afferent (SSA), special visceral afferent (SVA), and special visceral (branchial) efferent (SVE) components. The terms defining the components are used as follows: *somatic* refers to

head, body wall, and extremities; *visceral* to viscera; *afferent* to sensory (input); *efferent* to motor (output); *general* to wide areas of the head and body; and *special* to the specialized functions of olfaction (smell), gustation (taste), vision, audition, equilibrium (vestibular system), and branchiomeric (gill arch) muscles. There are no important differences between visceral and somatic afferent fibers.

Special Afferent Nerves

These sensory nerves serve the special senses, i.e., smell, sight, hearing, and balance (equilibrium). Included are two SSA nerves:

optic (II)
vestibulocochlear (VIII)
and an SVA nerve:
olfactory (I)

Taste fibers (also SVA) are present as components of three of the branchiomeric nerves (see below).

General Somatic Efferent Nerves

These are motor nerves that contain (1) fibers that innervate voluntary muscles derived from embryonic somites, specifically skeletal muscles, except branchiomeric ones, and (2) parasympathetic fibers that innervate the involuntary muscles of the eye, i.e., general *visceral* efferents (GVEs). In the first category, general *somatic* efferent (GSE), are:

oculomotor (III)
trochlear (IV)

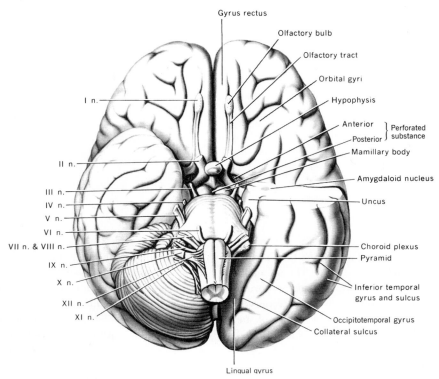

Gyrus rectus

Olfactory bulb

Olfactory tract

Orbital gyri

Hypophysis

I n.

Anterior } Perforated
Posterior } substance

Mamillary body

II n.

Amygdaloid nucleus

III n.
IV n.   Uncus
V n.
VI n.

VII n. & VIII n.   Choroid plexus

IX n.   Pyramid

X n.

Inferior temporal
gyrus and sulcus

XII n.

XI n.

Occipitotemporal gyrus

Collateral sulcus

Lingual gyrus

Figure 14.1: Basal surface of the brain and roots of the cranial nerves. The cerebellum and rostral portion of the temporal lobe are removed on the right side of figure.

abducent (VI)

hypoglossal (XII)

They are responsible for innervating the voluntary somatic (extraocular) muscles of the eye and tongue. In addition to its GSE fibers, the oculomotor nerve contains parasympathetic (GVE) fibers to the involuntary muscles of the eye (Chap. 19).

Special Visceral Nerves

In this category are motor nerves that innervate branchiomeric muscles, i.e., striated muscles that arise from branchial arches of the embryo. (Branchial arches are a series of elevations, separated by clefts, on the walls of the primitive pharynx. The clefts are so clearly homologous to those found in lower vertebrates, such as fish, that they are believed to be phylogenetically related to gills. In embryonic development muscle-forming cells called *myoblasts* congregate in the branchial arches, and from them much of the head and neck musculature develops.)

The nerves in this category are mixed in function. The fibers innervating the branchiomeric muscles are known as visceral components, not because they are part of the autonomic nervous system, but because of their association with the visceral functions of eating and breathing. The nerves with SVE components are:

trigeminal (V)

facial (VII)

glossopharyngeal (IX)

vagus (X)

spinal accessory (XI)

The SVE components of these nerves are distributed among the branchial arches as follows: the first arch (jaw) by n. V, the second (hyoid) arch by n. VII, the third arch by n. IX, and the remaining arches by nerves X and XI. Three of the nerves—facial, glossopharyngeal, and vagus—also contain SVA fibers subserving taste, parasympathetic fibers (GVE), and GVA fibers **(Table 14.1).**

Table 14-1: Cranial Nerves and Their Functional Components

Name	Components	Functions (Major)
I. Olfactory nerve	Special visceral afferent	Smell
II. Optic nerve	Special somatic afferent	Vision
III. Oculomotor nerve*	General somatic efferent	Movement of eyes
	General visceral efferent (parasympathetic)	Pupillary constriction and accommodation
IV. Trochlear nerve*	General somatic efferent	Movements of eyes
V. Trigeminal nerve	Special visceral efferent	Muscles of mastication and eardrum tension
	General somatic afferent	General sensations from anterior half of head including face, nose, mouth, and meninges
VI. Abducent nerve*	General somatic efferent	Movements of eyes
VII. Facial nerve†	Special visceral efferent	Muscles of facial expression and tension on ear bones
	General visceral efferent (parasympathetic)	Lacrimation and salivation
	Special visceral afferent	Taste
	General visceral afferent	Visceral sensory
VIII. Vestibulocochlear nerve	Special somatic afferent	Hearing and equilibrium reception
IX. Glossopharyngeal nerve†	Special visceral efferent	Swallowing movements
	General visceral efferent (parasympathetic)	Salivation
	Special visceral afferent	Taste
	General visceral afferent	Visceral sensory
X. Vagus nerve† and cranial root of XI	Special visceral efferent	Swallowing movements and laryngeal control
	General visceral efferent (parasympathetic)	Parasympathetics to thoracic and abdominal viscera
	Special visceral afferent	Taste
	General visceral afferent	Visceral sensory
XI. Spinal accessory nerve (spinal root)	Special visceral efferent	Movements of shoulder and head
XII. Hypoglossal nerve*	General somatic efferent	Movements of tongue

* In addition, there are GSA fibers for proprioception from the muscles of the eye (III, IV, VI) and tongue (XII).
† In addition, there are GSA fibers for cutaneous sense from just behind the external ear (VII, IX, and X).

GANGLIA IN THE HEAD

The named ganglia in the head are of two types: (1) sensory ganglia containing the cell bodies of neurons of the first order (equivalent to the dorsal root ganglia of the spinal cord), and (2) parasympathetic ganglia. The *sensory ganglia*, including their associated cranial nerves and functional components, are: trigeminal (Gasserian, semilunar) ganglion and mesencephalic nucleus of n. V (GSA); geniculate ganglion of n. VII (GVA, SVA, and GSA); vestibular and spiral ganglia of n. VIII (SSA); superior (GSA) and inferior (SVA) ganglia of n. IX; and superior (GSA) and inferior (SVA) ganglia of n. X (Fig. 14.2). The mesencephalic nucleus of n. V is unique; it consists of cell bodies of the trigeminal ganglion which are displaced to the brainstem.

The *parasympathetic* ganglia (GVE), where preganglionic fibers synapse with postganglionic fibers, include the ciliary ganglion of n. III; pterygopalatine (sphenopalatine) and submandibular ganglia of n. VII; and the otic ganglion of n. IX (Fig. 14.3). The ganglia of the vagus nerve (n. X) are located in or near organs of the body (e.g., heart and gastrointestinal tract; Fig. 20.3).

CRANIAL NERVE NUCLEI WITHIN THE BRAINSTEM

The sensory nuclei of termination of the afferent fibers and the nuclei of origin of the motor fibers of the cranial nerves are organized in discontinuous nuclear "columns" within the brainstem. The olfactory nerve (n. I, SVA) and the optic

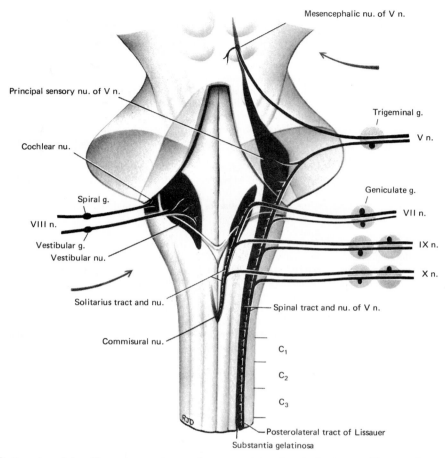

Figure 14.2: Location of the afferent (sensory) cranial nerve nuclei within the brainstem. These nuclei are organized into three columns. The superior (medial) and inferior (lateral) ganglia of the ninth and tenth cranial nerves are not labeled.

nerve (n. II, SSA) are telencephalic and not brainstem cranial nerves.

Sensory Nuclei of Termination (Fig. 14.2)

The *SSA column* includes the *vestibular and cochlear nuclei* (n. VIII), which are located in the posterolateral tegmentum of the upper medulla and lower pons. The *GSA column* includes the *mesencephalic nucleus of n. V* (proprioception), located in the posterointermediate midbrain tegmentum; the *principal (chief* or *main) sensory nucleus of n. V* (touch), located in the lateral midpontine tegmentum; and the *spinal trigeminal nucleus* (pain and temperature), located in the lateral tegmentum of the lower pons, medulla, and the upper two cervical spinal levels

(fibers from nerves V, VII, IX, and X terminate in these nuclei). The mesencephalic nucleus of n. V is actually composed of cell bodies of neurons of the first order; it is a displaced portion of the trigeminal ganglion. The *visceral afferent column* consists of the *nucleus solitarius* located in the midposterior tegmentum of the medulla; its components include taste (SVA) and other visceral influences (GVA) which are conveyed via fibers in three cranial nerves: nerves VII, IX, and X.

Motor Nuclei of Origin (Fig. 14.3)

The *GSE column* includes *nuclei of the oculomotor nerve* (midbrain), *trochlear nerve* (lower midbrain), *abducent nerve* (lower pons), and *hypo-*

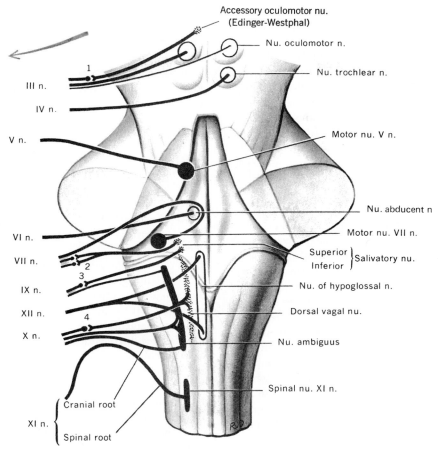

Figure 14.3: Location of the efferent (motor) cranial nerve nuclei within the brainstem. These nuclei are organized into three columns. Arabic numerals indicate parasympathetic ganglia: (1) ciliary ganglion, (2) pterygopalatine and submandibular ganglia, (3) otic ganglion, and (4) terminal ganglia.

glossal nerve (medulla). These nuclei, located in the posteromedial tegmentum, are composed of lower motoneurons innervating the voluntary muscles of the eye and tongue. The *GVE column* includes the *accessory oculomotor nucleus of Edinger-Westphal* (midbrain, n. III), the *superior salivatory nucleus* (posterior tegmentum of lower pons, n. VII), the *inferior salivatory nucleus* (posterior tegmentum of upper medulla, n. IX), and the *dorsal motor nucleus of the vagus nerve* (posterior tegmentum of medulla, n. X). These nuclei are composed of the cell bodies of preganglionic parasympathetic neurons of the autonomic nervous system. The salivatory nuclei are identifiable only by physiologic effects. The *special visceral (branchial) efferent column* includes the *motor nucleus (masticatory nucleus)*

of the fifth nerve (midpons, n. V), *motor nucleus of the seventh nerve* (lower pons, n. VII), and *nucleus ambiguus* (medulla, nerves IX, X, and XI). These nuclei of the lower motoneurons to the branchiomeric muscles are located in the middle of the tegmentum. The spinal nucleus of n. XI is the SVE component in the spinal cord.

SOME FUNCTIONAL AND CLINICAL CONSIDERATIONS

Olfactory (n. I)

The olfactory nerve is composed of bipolar SVA neurons whose cell bodies are located in the nasal mucosa of the nasal cavity. These neurons are most unusual in that each acts as a chemoreceptor, a transducer, and a first-order neuron. As a receptor it responds directly to environmental chemicals producing odors, as a transducer it evokes graded potentials, and as a transmitter of nerve impulses it communicates with neuronal complexes within the olfactory bulb (Figs. 1.9 and 22.2). Each olfactory neuron has a lifetime limited to about 30 days: it is replaced by "basal cells" in the olfactory mucosa. These basal cells are continuously differentiating throughout life into new neurons that form new synaptic connections in the olfactory bulb.

Neurons of the olfactory bulb project to several neural structures including the uncus and the amygdala (Chap. 22). The perception of smell is associated with the cortex of the uncus (area 28; Figs. 1.7 and 25.6). The olfactory system is more than just a perceiver of odors; it is also an activator and a sensitizer of other neural systems—those which are substrates for many emotional responses and behavioral patterns (Chap. 22). Odors can evoke such reflexes as salivation and secretions of digestive juices. Odors are described only in subjective terms, as there are no basic odors comparable to the primary colors. The loss of the sense of smell has minor significance to humans, as indicated by the lack of vernacular synonym for the technical term anosmia. An impaired sense of smell, as experienced during a cold, is expressed by the bland taste of food.

Optic (n. II)

The bipolar cells of the retina are the SSA first-order neurons of the visual pathway. The optic nerve is actually a tract of the brain composed of axons of the ganglion cells of the retina (Chap. 19).

Oculomotor (n. III), Trochlear (n. IV), and Abducent (n. VI)

These cranial nerves have lower motoneurons (GSE) which innervate the extraocular voluntary muscles and the levator palpebrae muscle (eyelid). The integrated actions of these nerves are responsible for the *conjugate movements of the eye* (called gaze; simultaneous movement of the two eyes in the same direction). Each nerve has proprioceptive (GSA) fibers, which may have their cell bodies along the nerve, in the trigeminal ganglion, or in the mesencephalic nucleus of n. V. The third nerve has preganglionic parasympathetic (GVE) fibers synapsing with postganglionic neurons in the ciliary ganglion. They have a role in accommodation and pupillary constriction (Chap. 19).

Functional Role of the Extraocular Muscles

The precise role of these muscles in eye movements is complex, the action of an individual muscle varying with the position of the eyeball within the orbit. The following account is schematic. Nerve III innervates the levator palpebrae, superior rectus, inferior rectus, medial rectus, and inferior oblique muscles. Nerve IV innervates the superior oblique muscle, and nerve VI innervates the lateral rectus muscle. The integrated activity of these muscles results in horizontal, vertical, oblique, and convergence movements. The levator palpebrae muscle elevates the eyelid. The medial rectus is an *adductor* of the eye (pupil directed to nose), and the lateral rectus is an *abductor* (pupil directed to temple). These horizontal recti move the eyeball in the horizontal plane. In lateral gaze, the medial rectus of one eye and the lateral rectus of the other eye contract synergistically (Chap. 16). During convergence, both medial recti contract. In contrast, the action of the muscles responsible for vertical movements—superior and inferior recti and superior and inferior oblique muscles—are influenced by the position of the eyeball in the orbit. The superior rectus elevates the eye (pupil up); the elevation increases with abduction. The inferior rectus depresses (pupil down); the depression increases with abduction. The superior oblique intorts (rotates the upper part medially) the abducted eye and depresses (moves pupil down) the adducted eye. Intorsion increases with greater abduction, and depression increases with greater adduction. The inferior oblique elevates the adducted eye and extorts the abducted eye.

Lesion of the Oculomotor Nerve

Convergence of the eyes occurs when viewing a close object; it keeps the image precisely aligned on the fovea of both eyes (Chap. 19).

Except for convergence, all normal eye movements are conjugate movements, i.e., the two eyes turn so that their visual axes remain parallel. The paralysis of one or more extraocular muscles results in *diplopia* (double vision) due to the faulty conjugate movements. A complete lesion of an oculomotor nerve produces the following: (1) *ptosis* or drooping of the eyelid and inability to elevate the eyelid because of unopposed action of the orbicularis muscle, which closes the eyelid (innervated by n. VII); (2) dilated pupil (*mydriasis*) and unresponsiveness of eye reflexes to light (pupillary constrictor and ciliary muscle paralysis from IIIrd nerve injury and the unopposed action of the pupillary dilator muscle which is innervated by the intact sympathetic fibers); (3) pupils of unequal size (anisocoria); (4) ophthalmoplegia with the eye permanently abducted, slightly depressed, and unable to move inward or upward. This crossed horizontal diplopia is due to the unopposed action of the lateral rectus and the superior oblique muscles. The eye cannot be adducted or elevated.

Lesion of the Trochlear Nerve

A complete lesion of the trochlear nerve results in a vertical diplopia, head tilt, and limitation of ocular movement on looking down and in. Diplopia is maximal when the eyes are turned down; this makes it difficult for the subject to descend stairs or read. To align the eyes in order to minimize or eliminate the diplopia, the patient tilts his head to the shoulder of the side opposite the paralyzed muscle. Because the trochlear nerve decussates within the brainstem, the nucleus of the trochlear nerve is located on the side opposite to that of the nerve itself; hence a lesion of a nucleus of the trochlear nerve is expressed in the contralateral eye.

Lesion of the Abducent Nerve

A complete lesion of the abducent nerve results in a horizontal diplopia with the ipsilateral eye adducted because of the unopposed action of the normal medial rectus muscle. Abduction is limited. The diplopia is maximal when the subject attempts to gaze to the side of the lesion (because the eye with the paralyzed lateral rectus muscle cannot be adequately abducted). It

is minimal with gaze to the normal side because the visual axis of the normal eye can be made to parallel that of the affected eye.

Trigeminal (n. V)

The trigeminal nerve branches into three divisions: ophthalmic, maxillary, and mandibular. Each division supplies a distinct region; there is no overlap in the regions innervated by each of the three divisions (this contrasts with dermatomal overlap of spinal root distribution).

The sensory fibers enter at the midpons level as the *sensory root (portio major)*, while the *motor fibers* emerge through the adjacent *motor root (portio minor)*.

Sensory Root

The sensory input (GSA) is conveyed via first-order fibers (with cell bodies in the trigeminal ganglion) from the skin of the scalp anterior to the coronal plane through the ears. The innervated region comprises the face, orbit, mucous membranes of the nasal cavity, nasal sinuses and oral cavities, teeth, and most of the dura mater. These first-order neurons terminate in the principal sensory nucleus and the spinal trigeminal nucleus of n. V (**Figs. 9.5 and 10.5**).

Some first-order neurons have their cell bodies in the mesencephalic nucleus of n. V. These proprioceptive neurons receive input via the mandibular nerve from the muscles of mastication and pressure receptors in the periodontal ligaments of the teeth. These inputs are relayed monosynaptically to the lower motoneurons of the motor nucleus of n. V to complete two neuron jaw reflexes (similar to the knee-jerk reflex). The mesencephalic nucleus also receives proprioceptive input from the extraocular muscles (**Fig. 10.5**).

Motor Root

The lower motoneuron fibers from the motor nucleus of n. V (SVE) pass through the motor root and the mandibular division before innervating the jaw muscles of mastication (masseter, pterygoids, and temporalis muscles), tensor tympani, and some other muscles. The jaw jerk can be evoked by tapping the chin of the slightly opened mouth with a reflex hammer (**Fig. 10.5**).

Lesion of the Trigeminal Nerve

The interruption of all trigeminal nerve fibers unilaterally results in (1) anesthesia and loss of general senses in the regions innervated by n. V, and (2) a lower motoneuron paralysis (loss of jaw reflex and fibrillations, weakness, and atrophy of jaw muscles). The sensory changes include the loss of sensitivity of the nasal mucosa to ammonia and other volatile chemicals (smarting effect) in the ipsilateral nostril and the loss of corneal sensation on the same side. The interruption of sensory fibers from the cornea (ophthalmic division) results in loss of the ipsilateral and contralateral (consensual) corneal reflex (Chap. 19). The afferent limb of the corneal reflex terminates in the spinal trigeminal nucleus, pars oralis (Fig. 9.5). This nucleus activates both efferent limbs through influences projected to both facial motor nuclei (n. VII), whose motor fibers innervate the orbicularis oculi muscles of both eyes (both eyes blink). The loss of proprioceptive input may result in the relaxation of the ipsilateral muscles of facial expression (innervated by n. VII). The loss of the jaw jerk results from the interruption of both the afferent and efferent limbs of the arc. Because of the action of the contracting pterygoid muscles on the normal side, the jaw, when protruded, will deviate and point to the paralyzed side.

Sharp, agonizing pain localized over the distribution of one or more branches of the trigeminal nerve is known as *trigeminal neuralgia* or *tic douloureux*. This condition (of unknown cause) may be accompanied by muscle twitchings (tic) and disturbances in salivary secretion. The stimulation of a region, called a *trigger zone*, may initiate an attack.

The supranuclear influences upon the motor nucleus of n. V are outlined in Chapter 11. Because the motor nucleus of n. V is influenced by both crossed and uncrossed corticobulbar and corticoreticular pathways, unilateral supranuclear (upper motoneuron) lesions usually do not impair trigeminal motor activity.

Facial Nerve (n. VII)

The facial nerve consists of (1) the *facial nerve proper* or *motor division* comprised of lower motoneurons (SVE), and (2) the *nervus intermedius*

with its sensory (GSA, SVA, and GSA) and parasympathetic divisions (GVE). All sensory neurons of the first-order have their cell bodies in the *geniculate ganglion*. The GVA input from the viscera in the soft palate and tonsillar region and the SVA (taste) input from the anterior two thirds of the tongue terminate in the nucleus solitarius (see later). Fibers from the motor nucleus of n. VII (SVE) take a hairpin course through the lower pons (they recurve as the internal genu around the nucleus of n. VI) before emerging into and passing through the cerebellopontine angle. These fibers innervate the muscles of facial expression, including the orbicularis oculi (closes eyelid and protects eye), buccinator (manipulates cheek), and stapedius (moves stapes bone [Chap. 16]) muscles. The parasympathetic preganglionic fibers from the superior salivatory nucleus have synaptic connections with postganglionic neurons in the pterygopalatine and submandibular ganglia; these fibers stimulate the lacrimal, nasal, oral, submaxillary and sublingual glands, and blood vessels (Fig. 13.12).

Lesion of the Facial Nerve

A lesion interrupting the facial nerve (e.g., *Bell's palsy*) is primarily expressed as a lower motoneuron paralysis of the muscles of facial expression. The paralysis of Bell's palsy may occur suddenly and be followed within a few months by a spontaneous recovery. On the ipsilateral side, the forehead is immobile, the corner of the mouth sags, the nasolabial folds of the face are flattened, facial lines are lost, and saliva may drip from the corner of the mouth. The patient is unable to whistle or puff the cheek because the buccinator muscle is paralyzed. When the patient is smiling, the normal muscles draw the contralateral corner of the mouth up while the paralyzed corner continues to sag. Corneal sensitivity remains (n. V), but the patient is unable to blink or close the eyelid (n. VII). To protect the cornea from damage (e.g., drying) therapeutic closure of eyelids or other measures are taken (e.g., patient wears an eye mask, or lids are closed by sutures). Lacrimation and salivation on the lesion side may be impaired. Taste will be lost on the ipsilateral anterior two thirds of the tongue. An increased acuity to sounds (*hyperacusis*), especially to low tones, results from the paralysis of the stapedius muscle, which normally dampens the amplitude of the vibrations of the ear ossicles.

When the cornea is touched, the eyelid is immediately closed. In this *corneal reflex*, the trigeminal nerve is the sensory limb from the cornea of the eye, and the facial nerve is the motor limb causing the orbicularis oculi muscle to close the eyelid. The closure of the eyelid on the same side as that stimulated is known as the *direct corneal reflex*, while the closure of the contralateral eyelid is known as the *consensual corneal reflex*. Stated otherwise, if the facial nerve on one side is completely destroyed, the sensitive cornea cannot evoke a direct corneal reflex but can evoke a consensual corneal reflex. If the fibers of the nervus intermedius on both sides are intact and motor fibers of the facial nerve are destroyed on one side, then the direct corneal reflex is absent on that side; however, lacrimal secretion may increase on both sides because of parasympathetic activity.

Upper Motoneurons

A unilateral supranuclear lesion of the upper motoneurons (corticobulbar and corticoreticular fibers) to the facial nucleus results in a marked weakness of the muscles of expression of the face below the eye on the side contralateral to the lesion. The frontalis muscle (wrinkles forehead) and the orbicularis oculi muscle (closes eyelid) are unaffected. The accepted explanation states that (1) bilateral upper motoneuron projections from the cerebral cortex influence the lower motoneurons innervating the frontalis muscle and orbicularis oculi, and (2) only unilateral, crossed upper motoneuron projections influence the lower motoneurons innervating the muscles of facial expression of the lower face. Hence, the contralateral muscles are deprived of upper motoneuron influences (**Fig. 11.3**).

In some patients with supranuclear lesions, the weak, lower facial muscles will remain paralyzed to volitional influences but will respond to emotional or mimetic influences (joke, distress). The influences that evoke this involuntary response are not known.

Note the distinction between a lower moto-neuron lesion and an upper motoneuron lesion involving the muscles of facial expression (**Fig. 11.3**). In a lower motoneuron paralysis, all the muscles of facial expression on the same side as the lesion are paralyzed. In an upper motoneuron paralysis following a lesion of the corticobulbar fibers in, for example, the internal capsule, *the muscles of facial expression in the lower face below the angle of the eye on the side opposite the lesion are paralyzed.*

Taste

In humans, taste sensations can be obtained following appropriate stimulation of the taste receptors in the tongue, palate, and pharynx. Four taste modalities are generally recognized: salt, sweet, sour, and bitter. Actually, a truly objective classification of the tastes has not been developed, probably because there are no primary taste qualities. All are chemically induced sensations. It is normally impossible to perceive pure taste without sensing an overlay of smell because taste thresholds are significantly higher than smell thresholds.

The true taste qualities in humans are derived from the stimulation of chemoreceptors called *taste buds*. Each taste bud contains upward of 25 *neuroepithelial taste cells*. In addition, other less-differentiated cells, called *sustentacular cells*, act as reserve cells to replenish the taste cells when they die out. Each mature taste cell is replaced every 200 to 300 hours.

The taste cells of the taste buds are in synaptic contact with afferent taste fibers, with each taste bud receiving branches from several trunk axons. In turn, each axon sends branches to several taste buds. The fibers of the facial, glossopharyngeal, and vagal nerves pass into the medulla and terminate in the rostral and lateral areas of the nucleus solitarius; this portion is called the *gustatory nucleus*.

The axons from the gustatory nucleus ascend within the tegmentum without crossing and terminate in the medial portion of the ventral posteromedial nucleus of the thalamus. Fibers from cell bodies there pass through the posterior limb of the internal capsule and terminate in the lower end of the postcentral gyrus and possibly in the cortex of the insula and superior temporal gyrus.

Vestibulocochlear (n. VIII)

The cochlear nerve, an exteroceptive nerve concerned with hearing, consists of nerve fibers of bipolar neurons with cell bodies in the spiral ganglion (Chap. 16). Its peripheral fibers receive their input from the hair cells in the spiral organ of Corti. Its central processes terminate in the dorsal and ventral cochlear nuclei. The vestibular nerve, a proprioceptive nerve concerned with equilibrium and orientation of the head in space, consists of nerve fibers of bipolar neurons with cell bodies in the vestibular ganglion (Chap. 16). Its peripheral processes receive their input from hair cells in the cristae (in ampullae of the semicircular ducts) and in the maculae (of the utricle and saccule). Its central processes terminate in the four vestibular nuclei in the brainstem and uniquely in the cerebellum (Chap. 18).

Glossopharyngeal (n. IX)

The GVA input of n. IX from the palatine, tonsillar, and pharyngeal regions and from the *carotid sinus* (pressoreceptor, arterial pressure) and *carotid body* (chemoreceptor, CO_2 and O_2 concentration in blood) is conveyed via first-order fibers (cell bodies in inferior ganglion) to the gustatory portion of the nucleus solitarius. The SVA input (taste) from the posterior third of the tongue is relayed via first-order neurons (cell bodies in inferior ganglion) to the nucleus solitarius. Some GSA afferents from the tympanic cavity and external auditory meatus with cell bodies in the superior ganglion terminate in the spinal trigeminal nucleus. The sensory fibers innervating the fauces trigger the gag reflex and swallowing. The SVE lower motoneurons from the nucleus ambiguus innervate pharyngeal and palatine muscles (effect swallowing) and the stylopharyngeal muscle (elevates upper pharynx). The preganglionic parasympathetic (GVE) influences from the inferior salivatory nucleus are relayed via the otic ganglion to the parotid gland.

Interruption of all fibers of n. IX results in the following symptoms: (1) loss of sensation, including taste, in the posterior third of the tongue and adjacent area; (2) unilateral loss of the *gag (pharyngeal)* and *palatal, uvular* and *carotid reflexes*; and (3) difficulty in swallowing

(*dysphagia*) and deviation of palate and uvula to the normal side (unopposed by paralyzed muscles). Glossopharyngeal neuralgia (similar to trigeminal neuralgia) may be triggered by chewing or swallowing.

Vagus (n. X)

The vagus nerve has not only general and SVA components but general and SVE components as well (Table 14.1). In addition, there is a GSA component. The GVA input is from the respiratory system (larynx, trachea, and lungs), cardiovascular system (carotid sinus and body, heart, and various blood vessels), gastrointestinal tract, and dura mater in the posterior fossa. The peripheral processes extend from the organs to the cell bodies located in the inferior ganglion adjacent to the medulla; their central processes terminate in the nucleus solitarius. The SVA fibers sense "taste" from receptors in the epiglottis part of the pharynx. Their peripheral processes extend to cell bodies in the inferior ganglion; central processes terminate in the gustatory portion of the nucleus solitarius.

The GVE component consists of preganglionic parasympathetic fibers from the dorsal vagal nucleus that project to terminal ganglia close to their target structures (Chap. 20). From there, postganglionic neurons extend to the cardiovascular, respiratory, and gastrointestinal systems of the thorax and abdomen. A GVE influence to the heart itself is conveyed over preganglionic parasympathetic neurons from cells which may be located close to the nucleus ambiguus. The SVE output is by lower motoneurons from the nucleus ambiguus that innervate the voluntary muscles of the soft palate, pharynx, and intrinsic laryngeal muscles (some of the fibers from the nucleus ambiguus course via n. XI before joining the vagus nerve).

The GSA component consists of fibers from the ear's tympanic cavity and external auditory meatus (with cell bodies in the superior ganglion) that terminate in the spinal trigeminal nucleus.

Lesion of the Vagus Nerve

A complete unilateral lesion of the vagus nerve results in the following symptoms: (1) the flaccid soft palate produces a voice with a twang;

(2) swallowing is difficult (*dysphagia*) because of the unilateral paralysis of pharyngeal constrictors; the pharynx is shifted slightly to the normally innervated side. A transient *tachycardia* (increased heartbeat) is a consequence of the interruption of some parasympathetic stimulation. (See below regarding lesion of the recurrent laryngeal nerve.) Bilateral lesions of the vagus nerve may be rapidly fatal because of laryngeal paralysis of the adducted vocal folds.

Accessory (Spinal Accessory) (n. XI)

The accessory nerve consists of two roots, spinal and cranial (bulbar) (Fig. 14.3). (1) The fibers of the spinal root originate from anterior horn cells of cervical levels 1 through 5, emerge, and ascend on the side of the spinal cord (dorsal to the denticulate ligament) and medulla, and join the cranial root in the jugular foramen; the spinal root innervates the ipsilateral sternomastoid and the upper half of the trapezius muscles. (2) The fibers of the cranial root originate from the nucleus ambiguus, course with n. XI a short distance before branching and joining n. X, and eventually form the recurrent laryngeal nerve which innervates the intrinsic laryngeal muscles.

Lesion of the Accessory Nerve

The lower motoneuron paralysis of the spinal root fibers is indicated by a weakness in the ability to rotate the head so that the chin points to the side opposite the lesion (paralyzed sternomastoid muscle) and in a downward and outward rotation of the upper scapula (paralyzed upper trapezius muscle). After a unilateral lesion of the cranial root fibers (or recurrent laryngeal nerve), the ipsilateral vocal cord becomes fixed and partially adducted; the voice is hoarse (*dysphonia*) and reduced to a whisper.

Reflexes Involving Nerves VII, IX, X, and XI

Taste—Salivary Gland Reflex

Following stimulation of the taste receptors, gustatory impulses are conveyed to the rostral end of the nucleus solitarius (gustatory nucleus) as follows: from the anterior two thirds of the tongue, via the facial nerve; from the posterior third of the tongue, via the glossopharyngeal nerve; and from the epiglottis via the vagus nerve. Projections from the nucleus solitarius terminate in the parasympathetic neurons of the superior and inferior salivatory nuclei. From these nuclei, preganglionic fibers course through the facial and glossopharyngeal nerves to the sphenopalatine, submandibular, and otic ganglia. From these ganglia, postganglionic fibers travel to the salivary glands and stimulate secretion (Chap. 20).

Carotid Sinus Reflex

Baroreceptors in the wall of the carotid sinus (located at the bifurcation of the common carotid artery into the external and internal carotid arteries) respond to an increase in blood pressure by producing more nerve impulses in the visceral afferent fibers of the glossopharyngeal nerve to the nucleus solitarius. From this nucleus, influences are conveyed to (1) the dorsal vagal (parasympathetic) nucleus and (2) the "vasomotor center" in the rostral ventrolateral reticular formation of the medulla.

The stimulated motor limb of the reflex arc, acting through the inhibitory efferent fibers of the vagus nerve, decreases the heart rate and the cardiac output. In contrast, the stimulated "vasomotor center" projects influences via the reticulospinal tract to the sympathetic preganglionic neurons of the intermediolateral cell columns of the spinal cord (Chap. 20). The sympathetic influences result (1) in an increase in the heart rate and cardiac output and (2) in the decrease in blood pressure by lowering peripheral resistance through the vasodilation of the peripheral blood vessels.

Attacks of *syncope* (fainting) occur in individuals with hypersensitive carotid sinus reflexes when light external pressure (tight collar) is applied to the sinus.

Carotid Body Reflex

The carotid body (located near the carotid sinus) can initiate a sequence of neural events affecting the respiratory cycle. The activation of the chemoreceptors of the carotid body (responding to CO_2, O_2, and pH levels in the blood) increases the frequency of the action potentials conveyed via the glossopharyngeal nerve to the nucleus solitarius. From this nucleus, interneurons project to the "respiratory center complex" within the brainstem reticular formation. From this "center," influences are transmitted via reticulospinal fibers to the lower motoneuron of the phrenic and intercostal nerves. This results in inspiratory movements. The accompanying inflation of the lungs stimulates the stretch receptors in the bronchiolar walls to increase the frequency of impulses conveyed via the vagus nerve to the nucleus solitarius. Inhibitory influences from this nucleus to the "respiratory center complex" finally end the inspiratory phase of respiration.

Gag (Pharyngeal) Reflex

Stimulation of the pharyngeal region activates the contraction and elevation of the pharynx. The afferent limb of this reflex is in the glossopharyngeal nerve to the nucleus solitarius. Interneuronal connections to the nucleus ambiguus stimulate the efferent limb of lower motoneurons, traveling over fibers of the glossopharyngeal and vagus nerves to the voluntary muscles of the palate and pharynx.

Cough Reflex

Generally, coughing occurs following the irritation of the larynx, trachea, and/or bronchial tree. The afferent limb conveys impulses via the vagus nerve to the nucleus solitarius. Interneuronal connections are made with the "respiratory center complex" and with the nucleus ambiguus. The "center" activates the rest of the arc, resulting in forced expiration. The nucleus ambiguus and its lower motoneuron axons stimulate the pharyngeal and laryngeal musculature to participate in the act of coughing.

Hypoglossal (n. XII)

The lower motoneuron fibers originate in the nucleus of the hypoglossal nerve and innervate the ipsilateral tongue musculature, including its intrinsic muscles and the genioglossus, styloglossus, and hypoglossus. Interruption of the fibers of n. XII produces an ipsilateral lower motoneuron paralysis of the tongue. The fibrillations of the early stages are followed by atrophy of muscles, which results in a wrinkled tongue surface on the side of the lesion. When

protruded, the tongue deviates to the paralyzed side. The deviation is due to the unopposed contraction of the contralateral genioglossus, which pulls the root of the tongue forward while the paralyzed ipsilateral muscle acts as a pivot. The proprioceptive fibers (GSA) from the tongue muscles are presumed to have cell bodies scattered along the nerve.

SUGGESTED READINGS

Agur A. *Grant's Atlas of Anatomy*. 9th ed. Baltimore, Md: Williams & Wilkins; 1991.

Beckstead R, Morse J, Norgren R. The nucleus of the solitary tract in the monkey: projections to the thalamus and brain stem nuclei. *J Comp Neurol.* 1980;190:259–282.

Brodal A. *The Cranial Nerves: Anatomy and Anatomicoclinical Correlations*. Oxford: Blackwell; 1959.

Brunjes P, Frazier L. Maturation and plasticity in the olfactory system of vertebrates. *Brain Res Rev.* 1986;11:1–45.

Büttner-EnNever J, ed. *Neuroanatomy of the Oculomotor System*. New York, NY: Elsevier; 1989.

Finger T, Silver W, eds. *Neurobiology of Taste and Smell*. New York, NY: Wiley; 1987.

Fromm G, Terrence C, Maroon J. Trigeminal neuralgia. Current concepts regarding etiology and pathogenesis. *Arch Neurol.* 1984;41:1204–1207.

Graziadei P, Graziadei M. Neurogenesis and plasticity of the olfactory sensory neurons. *Ann N Y Acad Sci.* 1985;457:127–142.

Kinnamon S. Taste transduction: a diversity of mechanisms. *Trends Neurosci.* 1988;11:491–496.

Leigh R, Zea D. *The Neurology of Eye Movements*. 2nd ed. Philadelphia, Pa: FA Davis Co; 1991.

Margolis F, Getshell T, eds. Molecular Biology of the Olfactory System. New York, NY: Plenum; 1988.

May M, ed. *The Facial Nerve*. New York, NY: Thieme; 1985.

Norgren R. Central neural mechanisms of taste. In: Darian-Smith I, ed. *Handbook of Physiology*. Section I: The Nervous System. Bethesda, Md: American Physiological Society; 1984;3:1087–1128.

Porter J. Brainstem terminations of extraocular muscle primary afferent neurons in the monkey. *J Comp Neurol.* 1986;247:133–143.

Role L, Kelly J. The brain stem: cranial nerve nuclei and the monoaminergic systems. In: Kandel E, Schwartz J, Jessell T, eds. *Principles of Neural*

Science. 3rd ed. New York, NY: Elsevier; 1991: 683–699.

Roper S. The cell biology of vertebrate taste receptors. *Annu Rev Neurosci*. 1989;12:329–353.

Scott T, Yaxley S, Sienkiewicz Z, Rolls E. Gustatory responses in the nucleus tractus solitarius of the alert cynomolgus monkey. *J Neurophysiol*. 1986; 55:182–200.

Shirley S, Persaud K. The biochemistry of vertebrate olfaction and taste. *Seminars in Neuroscience*. 1990;2:49–68.

Travers J, Travers S, Norgren R. Gustatory neural processing in the hindbrain. *Annu Rev Neurosci*. 1987;10:595–632.

Wilson D, Leon M. Information processing in the olfaction system. In: Lund J, ed. *Sensory Processing in the Mammalian Brain*. New York, NY: Oxford University Press; 1989.

Wilson-Pauwels L, Akesson E, Stewart P. *Cranial Nerves: Anatomy and Clinical Comments*. Toronto: Decker; 1988.

Neurotransmitters as the Chemical Messengers of Certain Circuits and Pathways

15

Acetylcholine

Amino acid transmitters

Biogenic amines (monoamines)

Neuropeptides (neuroactive peptides)

Nitric oxide, carbon monoxide, and adenosine

Communication among neurons of neural circuits and pathways occurs *primarily* by the release of neuroactive chemical messengers called *neurotransmitters (transmitters)* or *neuromodulators* (Chap. 3). For a chemical agent to be called a neurotransmitter (transmitter), it must be synthesized in the neuron, become localized in a presynaptic terminal, be released into a synaptic cleft, bind to a receptor site (binding site) on the postsynaptic membrane of another neuron or effector (muscle fiber or gland cell) where it regulates ion channels, and lastly, be removed by a specific mechanism from its site of action. Those neuroactive substances that have not been demonstrated to fulfill all these requirements are often called *putative neurotransmitters*. *Transmitters* have been designated by some as those chemical messengers that interact with receptors directly linked to channel proteins. *Neuromodulators* are those chemical messengers that interact with a receptor frequently linked to a G-protein and a second messenger system (Chap. 3). The term neurotransmitter (transmitter) is commonly used to include neuromodulators.

Whether a neuroactive agent elicits an excitatory or an inhibitory response, or whether it acts as a neurotransmitter or a neuromodulator,

is dependent upon the receptor protein to which it binds on the postsynaptic membrane. The agent acts as a neurotransmitter when the receptor protein is directly linked to an ion channel protein. Then, the ion selected by the channel determines whether the response is excitatory or inhibitory. Thus, it is possible for a specific transmitter to elicit an excitatory effect on one neuron and an inhibitory effect on another neuron. The agent acts as a neuromodulator when the receptor protein to which it binds on the postsynaptic membrane is linked to a G-protein. The subsequent interactions of the G-protein and the second messenger system with the ion channels will then designate the response (Chap. 3).

The chemical messengers that are presumed to be neurotransmitters or neuromodulators comprise more than 50 neuroactive substances. They have been classified as (1) small molecule transmitters and (2) neuropeptides (neuroactive peptides). The former are of three types: (1) *acetylcholine* is the only low-molecular weight transmitter not derived from an amino acid; (2) the four amino acids are *gamma amino butyric acid (GABA)*, *glycine*, *glutamate*, and *aspartate*; and (3) the four biogenic amines (monoamines) include the three catecholamines *norepineph-*

rine (noradrenalin), epinephrine (adrenalin), and dopamine, all derived from the amino acid tyrosine (catecholamines are amino acids without the carboxyl group), and serotonin, derived from the amino acid tryptophan. The numerous neuropeptides include such putative neuromodulators as (1) opioid peptides, (2) gastrointestinal (gut-brain) peptides, (3) hypothalamic releasing peptides (hormones), and (4) neurohypophyseal (pituitary) peptides (hormones).

The neurotransmitters, neuromodulators, and receptors have been categorized in several ways. In one classification, the neuroactive messengers that usually act (1) as neurotransmitters are acetylcholine and the four amino acids just noted, and (2) as neuromodulators are the biogenic amines and neuropeptides. In another classification, the receptors are divided into Class 1 and Class 2 receptors. Class 1 (fast) receptors are those that are directly linked to an ion receptor and mediate millisecond responses when activated by a transmitter. Class 2 (slow) receptors are those that are coupled to G-proteins which, in turn, are linked to ion channels or to second messenger systems. These receptors are generally modulatory, either dampening or enhancing the signal that acts on Class 1 receptors. In the former schema, acetylcholine and the four amino acids noted above may be designated as neurotransmitters, and the biogenic amines and neuropeptides as neuromodulators; however, some chemical messengers may be placed in both classes, depending upon the receptor. For example, acetylcholine acts as a neurotransmitter interacting with nicotinic ACh receptors that elicit (fast, Class 1) excitatory responses through the neuromuscular junction upon voluntary muscles. In contrast, acetylcholine acts as a neuromodulator interacting with muscarinic ACh receptors that elicit (slow, Class 2) inhibitory responses on cardiac muscle.

Some mature neurons release only one transmitter or modulator at all of its synapses. Other neurons may release two chemical messengers from their presynaptic terminals, one being a small molecule transmitter and the other a neuroactive peptide (see p. 46). The full significance of coexistence of two messengers in different vesicles in an axon terminal is still a matter of considerable discussion. In a broad context, this dual presence expands the means by which each neuron can convey complex messages with subtle signal content. The neuropeptide may act to augment what the primary transmitter is programmed to accomplish, as for example, by strengthening or prolonging the action of the transmitter. The responses of the common target cell to the combination of transmitter signals may be varied by increasing or decreasing the amounts and proportions of the agents (messengers) released.

Chemical synapses are characterized both by their agents and by the receptor type (or subtypes, e.g., 14 serotonergic receptor subtypes have been described) on the postsynaptic membrane interacting with the agent. Some axon terminals can have their own receptors, called autoreceptors, that respond to the chemical messenger released at the terminals; they have a role in regulating the release of transmitter (**Fig. 3.9**). Transmitters and modulators identify chemical systems that comprise pathway complexes (**Figs. 15.1 and 15.2**).

ACETYLCHOLINE

Acetylcholine (ACh) is a small molecule transmitter synthesized from choline and acetyl coenzyme A (acetyl CoA), catalyzed by the enzyme choline acetyltransferase (ChAT). It is degraded into choline and acetate in the synaptic cleft by the enzyme ACh esterase. Neurons that release ACh are known as cholinergic neurons. Both enzymes are synthesized in the cell body of the neuron and conveyed by fast axoplasmic transport to the axon terminal, where the formation of ACh takes place (Chap. 3). Some choline is recycled in the terminal after being returned from the synaptic cleft following the degrading of released ACh (Chap. 3).

Subtypes of ACh receptors have been identified. (1) Those in the sarcolemma of a neuromuscular junction are called nicotinic receptors because the action of ACh on muscle fibers can be mimicked by nicotine. Their responses can be blocked by curare. The ACh exerts excitatory influences through receptors that directly gate the Na^+ and K^+ channels to open. (2) Those in sympathetic neurons and some cerebral cortical neurons are called muscarinic receptors, be-

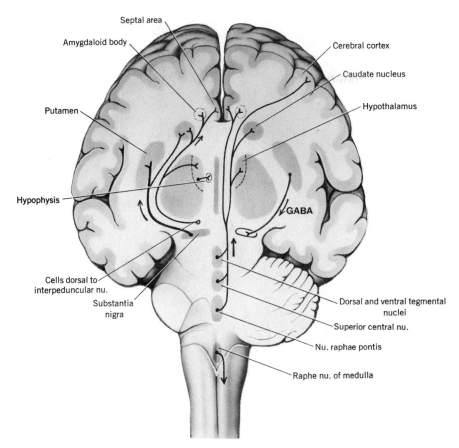

Figure 15.1: The dopaminergic pathways (left) and the serotonergic (5-HT) pathway (right). These pathways are described in the text. The raphe nucleus of the medulla is called the nucleus magnus. The cells dorsal to the interpeduncular nucleus are neurons of the ventral tegmental area (VTA).

cause the action of ACh on these postsynaptic cells can be blocked by muscarine (also blocked by atropine). These receptors activate a sequence of G-proteins and other components of a second messenger system that close certain K^+ channels (Chap. 3).

The "decision" as to whether the response to a neuroactive agent is excitatory or inhibitory, or as to whether the agent acts as a neurotransmitter or as a neuromodulator, depends upon receptor protein in the postsynaptic membrane to which it binds. If the receptor is directly associated with the channel, the agent acts as a neurotransmitter. As previously stated, the nature of the effect—excitatory or inhibitory—is determined by whether or not the ion channels selected are opened or closed. Thus, one transmitter can have an excitatory effect upon one

neuron and an inhibitory effect on another neuron. If the receptor is linked through a G-protein, then the agent acts as a neuromodulator and the nature of the response by the channels is affected by the second messenger system (Chap. 3; **Fig. 3.9**).

AMINO ACID TRANSMITTERS

Whereas the other neurotransmitters are the products of biochemical pathways within specific neurons, the amino acid transmitters are ubiquitous cellular components. Of the known putative transmitters, they are the most numerous and act on the greatest number of synapses.

The four designated amino acid transmitters are GABA, glycine, glutamate, and aspartate.

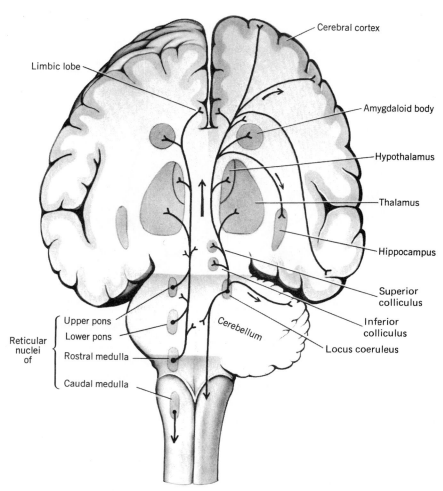

Figure 15.2: Noradrenergic pathways. The ascending pathway on the left originates from the medullary and pontine reticular nuclei and terminates in the cerebrum. The descending pathway on the left originates from medullary reticular nuclei and terminates in the spinal cord. The projections from the locus ceruleus on the right course (1) via the lateral pathway to the cerebrum, (2) via the ascending pathway to the midbrain and cerebrum, and (3) via the descending pathway to the spinal cord.

On the basis of their chemical structure alone, these four are related. GABA acts by opening the chloride channels and thus produces hyperpolarizing currents and inhibitory postsynaptic potentials (IPSPs). Glycine usually exerts inhibitory, but can produce excitatory effects. Glutamate and possibly aspartate act by producing excitatory (depolarizing) postsynaptic potentials (EPSPs).

Gamma Amino Butyric Acid (GABA)

This widely distributed CNS transmitter, derived from glutamate, is released at inhibitory synapses. GABAergic neurons comprise the granule cells of the olfactory bulb (Chap. 14), amacrine cells of the retina (Chap. 19), Purkinje cells and basket cells of the cerebellum (Chap. 18), basket cells of the hippocampus (Chap. 22), many striatal cells of the basal ganglia (Chap. 24), and interneurons in numerous CNS centers.

The Purkinje cells of the cerebellar cortex exert inhibitory influences upon the deep cerebellar nuclei (Chap. 18). The GABAergic neurons of the striatum (caudate nucleus and putamen) project to the substantia nigra and to the globus pallidus (Chap. 24). Reduction in GABA in these neurons in patients with Huntington's chorea contributes to the presence of uncontrolled involuntary movements (Chap. 24).

Benzodiazepines (e.g., librium and valium) are drugs used for alleviating such generalized anxiety disorders as restlessness, difficulty in concentration, and feeling on edge. The effect on specific neurons produced by these drugs results from the enhancement of the action of GABA. The benzodiazepines bind to GABA receptors and, by so doing, enhance the inhibitory effects of GABA by increasing the affinity of the receptors for GABA. The resulting increase in Cl^- influx through Cl^- channels acts to reduce the anxiety and provides for muscle relaxation.

Glycine

This transmitter, with a restricted distribution in the CNS, is present in the interneurons of the spinal cord (Renshaw cells) (**Fig. 3.10**). The neurons exert inhibitory effects by opening the Cl^- channels of the lower motor neurons (Chaps. 3 and 6). In the cerebral cortex, however, the small amounts of glycine have excitatory effects at glutamatergic synapses.

By inhibiting the release of glycine, the tetanus toxin evokes violent muscle spasms. The blocking of glycine receptors is the likely explanation for the production of the muscle spasms following strychnine poisoning.

Glutamate (Glutamic Acid)

Glutamate (glutamic acid) is the most common excitatory transmitter in the CNS. Among its many locations are the cerebral cortex, dentate gyrus of the hippocampus, striatum of the basal ganglia, and spinal cord. Essentially all the major efferent projections from the cerebral cortex are components of glutamatergic systems. These comprise the corticobulbar, corticothalamic, corticostriate, and corticopontine pathways. The mossy fibers projecting to the cerebellum are thought to be glutamatergic. Glutamate, synthesized from glucose, exerts its role by opening Na^+ and K^+ channels.

The glutamate receptors comprise several major types as well as some subtypes. They have been classified into two general categories: (1) those that directly gate ion channels and (2) those that indirectly gate ion channels through second messengers. Those receptors that directly gate include two groups called (a) N-methyl-D-aspartate (NMDA) receptors and (b) non-NMDA receptors. They are named and characterized according to the agonists that activate them (or according to the antagonists that inhibit them). The NMDA receptor is one that is activated by its agonist—the amino acid NMDA. The non-NMDA receptors can be activated by drugs such as *kainate (K)* and *quisqualate (Q)*; hence K or Q NMDA receptors.

Non-NMDA receptors are permeable to both Na^+ and K^+ ions, but most are not permeable to Ca^{++} ions. Since a non-NMDA receptor type is closely linked to voltage-gated Ca^{++} channels, it differs in that it results in a relatively prolonged depolarization by sustaining open Ca^{++} channels longer than is produced by stimulating the other receptors. This extended depolarization, linked to the increased influx of Ca^{++} into the neuron, may be integrated with intracellular changes associated with long-term signal transmission. This has been proposed to have relevance as a phenomenon in the quest for a cellular basis of learning and memory.

The NMDA receptor is also inhibited by the hallucinogenic drug called "angel dust" (phencyclidine hydrochloride—PCP).

All areas of the cerebral cortex project excitatory glutamatergic input to the striatum (caudate nucleus and putamen) of the basal ganglia (Chap 24). Alterations in the nature of the corticostriatal pathway may be the initial functional changes in the development of Huntington's chorea and some other neurodegenerative diseases.

Aspartate

Aspartate occurs in abundance in the CNS and it has many functions; however, its role as a major excitatory amino acid transmitter currently is considered doubtful. According to in vivo studies, it activates NMDA and other excitatory amino acid receptors, but evidence is lacking for its presence in presynaptic vesicles.

BIOGENIC AMINES (MONOAMINES)

The biogenic amines comprise (1) the catecholamines *norepinephrine, epinephrine, dopa-*

mine, and (2) *serotonin (5-hydroxytryptamine)*. They are chemical messengers used by neurons as well as by endocrine and other cells. A catecholamine is an organic compound that contains a catechol nucleus and an amino group. The monoamines are synthesized within each neuron from the amino acid tyrosine in the presence of appropriate enzymes. The sequence of enzymatic steps from tyrosine are dopamine to norepinephrine to epinephrine. Serotonin is synthesized within the neuron from the amino acid tryptophan.

The monoamine transmitters are released into the synaptic cleft. The recovery of the released transmitter occurs by uptake into the presynaptic ending where it is recycled for future use. Neurons releasing norepinephrine and epinephrine are *adrenergic*, those releasing dopamine, *dopaminergic*, and those releasing serotonin, *serotonergic*. The activity of these monoamine transmitters is limited by their reuptake by transporters (**Fig. 3.9**) into the presynaptic ending, where they are recycled into vesicles for future release.

Monoamines may have different specific effects on the postsynaptic cell depending on the type or subtype of receptor protein. Several varieties of subtypes of receptors are present for each monoamine. These receptors have different properties and are differentially distributed in the nervous system with the result that they have a variety of effects and even opposite responses. Thus, it is not possible to state that a specific neurotransmitter is either excitatory or inhibitory in its action; it can be both depending on the postsynaptic receptor type.

The three *biogenic pathways* in the brainstem are (1) the dopaminergic pathways (system) which originate in the midbrain; (2) the noradrenergic pathways (system) which originate in two nuclear groups called the locus ceruleus (LC) and lateral tegmental nucleus; and (3) the serotonergic pathways (system) which originate in the raphe nuclei (**Figs. 15.1 and 15.2**).

Norepinephrine and Epinephrine

Norepinephrine and epinephrine are released by the adrenal medulla, postganglionic sympathetic neurons, and CNS. Both act through a common set of subtypes of receptors (alpha-1, alpha-2, beta-1, and beta-2), and then via sec-

ond messengers. The beta receptors are found in the brain, with a high density of beta-1 receptors in the cerebral cortex and beta-2 in the cerebellum. When activated, the alpha-1 receptors, acting through a second messenger, elicit muscle contractions or glandular secretions. The alpha-1 receptors are mainly located presynaptically and act to modulate transmitter release. This accounts to some degree for the slow-acting and long-lasting effects following transmitter release. Some of these influences modify neuronal activity in the neuropil by enhancing the signal-to-noise ratio through lateral inhibition (Chap. 3).

Neurons with cell bodies in certain reticular nuclei in the brainstem tegmentum contain large quantities of norepinephrine; these are the *locus ceruleus* (LC) and the *lateral tegmental nucleus* (**Fig. 13.6**; Chap. 13). Axons from these nuclei are remarkable in that they are extensively branched and project directly without interruption until each branch makes synaptic connections through varicosities and synapses in practically every major region of the CNS. Axons of the LC extend (a) rostrally via the central tegmental tract, dorsal longitudinal fasciculus, and medial forebrain bundle to the tectum, thalamus, hippocampus, and the cerebral cortex; (b) via the superior cerebellar peduncle to the cerebellar cortex; (c) to many regions of the brainstem; and (d) caudally to the spinal cord (**Fig. 15.2**).

The "almost universal" distribution from the LC is consistent with the suggested function that the LC acts as a modulator setting (brain tone) background. Stimulation of the LC does not yield any well-defined specific effect. Rather, the LC is conceived as having the role of suppressing irrelevant stimuli (background neural noise) and in enhancing relevant stimuli. LC projections apparently modify behavioral arousal, the degree of alertness, electroencephalographic activity, and sleep.

The tegmental nuclei have axons with a more limited distribution to the base of the cerebrum and the spinal cord. These projections are thought to be involved in processing associated with lateral inhibition. Through its extensive distribution, the noradrenergic system may have a role in mood (connections with limbic system), memory (connections with cerebral cortex), and

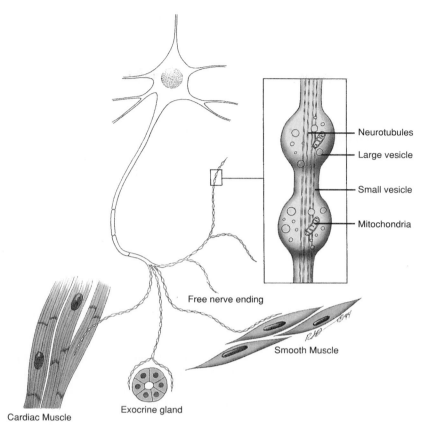

Figure 15.3: Composite illustration of a postganglionic noradrenergic neuron of the sympathetic nervous system. Each varicosity (enlargement) of the axon, called a bouton, contains both large and small vesicles. Neuropeptides are localized in the large and norepinephrine in the small vesicles. These transmitters, when released, influence the nearby effectors (Chap. 20). The linear array of varicosities along the axon are called *boutons en passage*, and those at the end of an axon, *terminal boutons*. Some of the structures innervated are illustrated. Often smooth muscle cells are joined by gap junctions (nexus) to form multicellular functionally integrated units. (Adapted from Dahlstrom.)

hormone regulation and homeostasis (projections to the hypothalamus and the autonomic nervous system).

Norepinephrine is the transmitter associated with the postganglionic neurons of the sympathetic nervous system, except for those innervating the sweat glands (**Fig. 15.3**; Chap. 20).

Epinephrine (Adrenalin)

This monoamine is present in the adrenal medulla from which it is released in response to physiologic and psychologic stresses. It is also a transmitter released by neurons located in the tegmentum of the lower brainstem. Some are located in the LC. Some axons containing epinephrine project rostrally to the hypothalamus

and others caudally to the intermediolateral cell column in the spinal cord where preganglionic sympathetic neurons are located (Chap. 20). These neurons may exert inhibitory effects.

Dopamine

Dopaminergic neurons, primarily located in several sites within the brainstem, exceed the number of adrenergic neurons within the CNS by several fold. They and their projections form several dopaminergic systems, which can be classified by the length of their efferent dopamine fibers.

Short Systems

Dopaminergic interneurons within the retina and olfactory bulb, through their inhibitory synapses, enhance the signal-to-noise ratio through lateral inhibition (Chap. 3).

Intermediate-Length Systems

(a) The tuberohypophysial dopaminergic projections from the hypothalamus to the anterior and intermediate lobes of the pituitary gland are involved in the inhibition of the release of prolactin and melanocyte-stimulating hormone (Chap. 21). (b) The incertohypothalamic dopaminergic projections link the zona incerta (rostral extension of the brainstem reticular formation in the diencephalon) to the hypothalamus. (c) Dopaminergic neurons are present in the periaqueductal and periventricular gray of the brainstem tegmentum in the vicinity of the nucleus solitarius and dorsal motor nucleus of the vagus nerve. These neurons project into the brainstem tegmentum. The latter two (b and c) are presumed to have roles in the reticular system (Chap. 22).

Serotonin (5-hydroxytryptamine, 5-HT)

Serotonin is present in the cell bodies of neurons located primarily in the raphe nuclei of the brainstem (Chap. 13; **Figs. 9.4 and 15.1**). It is also found in mast cells (associated with nociception, Chap. 9), platelets, and enterochromaffin cells of the gut (Chap. 20). Axons from the raphe nuclei are distributed diffusely throughout the brain and spinal cord. Neurons of the rostral (midbrain) raphe nuclei have axons that join the median forebrain bundle and terminate in the diencephalon, striatum, cerebral cortex, and the ependyma lining the ventricles. Those in the middle nuclei (pons) have axons that terminate in the cerebellum and reticular formation, and those from the caudal nuclei (medulla) have axons that project to the spinal nucleus of the trigeminal nerve and to the gray matter of the spinal cord.

Following its release from mast cells and other damaged cells, serotonin is the agent that activates and sensitizes the nociceptors of the primary "pain" fibers (A-delta and C fibers) (Chap. 9). In the nervous system, serotonin is involved with second messenger systems as a modulator. The projections to the spinal trigeminal nucleus and dorsal horn of the spinal cord act to inhibit the pain fibers, and those to the

ventral horn act to activate by facilitation (Chap. 9). In addition, serotonin has roles in a complex of physiologic activities including changes in blood pressure, body temperature, the sleep-wake cycle, certain psychological and psychotic states, and responses to certain drugs.

The drug fluoxetine (Prozac) is widely used to help people cope with a range of behavioral symptoms including degrees of mild to severe depression, deficiency in the ability to experience pleasure, fear of rejection, and lack of self confidence. It acts by blocking the serotonin transporter in the axon terminal and the reuptake of serotonin from the synaptic cleft. The result is an increase in the level and duration of the action of serotonin, which is translated in a few weeks into the therapeutic effect.

NEUROPEPTIDES (NEUROACTIVE PEPTIDES)

The *neuropeptides* comprise the largest class of neuroactive substances, functioning primarily as neuromodulators. They are proteins composed of short chains of 5 to 50 amino acids. Many were first discovered in non-neural tissues, such as the gastrointestinal (GI) tract, and then were later found to be messengers in the nervous system. The proteins, from which peptides are derived, are synthesized in the cell body of the neuron through the sequence of ribosomes, endoplasmic reticulum, and Golgi apparatus. From the large precursors, the active neuropeptides are cleaved by enzyme pepsidases. The active neuropeptides are then packaged within the cell body into large vesicles which are transported by fast axoplasmic flow through an axon to the nerve terminals. Unlike the vesicles that contain small molecule transmitters, the neuropeptide vesicles are not refilled with transmitter in the axon terminals. Neuropeptides (peptidergic transmitters) are produced in cells derived from embryonic neural precursor structures (neural plate and neural crest); these include neurons, chromaffin cells of the adrenal medulla, enterochromaffin cells of the gut (Chap. 20), and islet cells of the pancreas. Peptides act exclusively on the G-protein linked receptors to mediate slow postsynaptic responses (Chap. 3).

The neuropeptides found in the brain may be grouped as several families. Among these are (1) *opioid peptides (opiates)* such as enkephalins, endorphins, and dynorphins; (2) *gastrointestinal (gut-brain) peptides* such as vasoactive intestinal polypeptide (VIP), substance P, and neurotensin; and (3) *hypothalamic releasing peptides (hormones)* such as vasopressin and oxytocin (Chap. 21).

Vesicles of small molecule (classical) transmitters are frequently co-localized with vesicles of neuropeptides in the axon terminals of numerous neurons (**Fig. 15.3**). Two neuropeptides, each in its own vesicles, may also coexist in the same terminal. Some examples of co-localization are ACh with enkephalins, ACh with VIP, GABA with somatostatin, glutamate with substance P, serotonin with substance P, and norepinephrine with enkephalins. The co-release of a fast acting transmitter with a neuromodulator peptide having a long lasting effect increases the versatility of synaptic activity. The significance of co-release on the functional activity of the nervous system has yet to be fully evaluated and understood. Evidence indicates that neuropeptides have a role in some aspects of sensing and of emotion. They seem to modulate the perception of pain and such aspects of emotion as pleasure and response to stress (Chap. 21).

The co-release of ACh and VIP by the postganglionic parasympathetic fibers innervating the salivary glands illustrates the dual role of these two chemical messengers. Each agent acts on a different target cell. Stimulation of the parasympathetic nerves, which release ACh (contained in small synaptic vesicles), causes increased secretion from the gland and VIP (contained in large vesicles) relaxes smooth muscles of the blood vessels, resulting in vasodilation and increased blood flow through the organ.

Opioid Peptides

Opioid denotes to being opiate-like in terms of a functional similarity to morphine (a compound extracted from opium). *Opioid peptides* are endogenous (originating within the body) or synthetic agents that exhibit pharmacological activity similar to morphine. Since the opioid peptides bind with morphine receptors of CNS neurons, they are also called morphinomimetic peptides. Several subtypes of opiate receptors exist, all of which are linked to G-proteins. The endogenous opioids do not cross the blood-brain barrier. Chemical groups of opioid peptides include the *endorphins* and *enkephalins*. *Opiates* are drugs that are derived from the opium poppy. They are used therapeutically as powerful analgesics by binding to opiate receptors.

Endorphins (endogenous morphine)

The endorphin neurons have cell bodies that are located in the ventral (arcuate area) hypothalamus. Long axons project from these endorphin neurons to the amygdala and to the periventricular region of the thalamus and brain stem including the raphe nuclei, adjoining reticular formation, and LC. The endorphins bind to opioid receptors which produces analgesia, sedation, and miosis (pupillary constriction). These agents have a central role in controlling the drives for food, water, and sexual activity—all associated with the limbic system (Chap. 22). The effects of opiates in humans is not so much as a specific blunting of pain, but rather it is an induced state of indifference or emotional detachment from the experience of distress.

Enkephalins

The enkephalin neurons are widely distributed in the CNS. Each neuron has short axon projections. They are located in the hypothalamus, basal ganglia (globus pallidus and substantia nigra), amygdala and some limbic structures, periaqueductal gray of the midbrain, raphe nuclei, and reticular formation of the brain. Their presence in the spinal nucleus of the trigeminal nerve and the dorsal horn (substantia gelatinosa) of the spinal cord is in regions associated with neurons in the pain pathways (Chap. 9). In some regions, such as the cerebral cortex, there are interneurons containing enkephalins. The *dynorphins* are enkephalins that are concentrated in the structures of the limbic system and hypothalamus (Chaps. 21 and 22).

Enkephalin opioids are believed to modulate pain impulses by acting to reduce sensitivity to pain peripherally (PNS) as well as centrally (CNS) by activating opiate receptors in the periaqueductal gray of the midbrain (release of en-kephalins) (Chap. 9). Morphine induced eu-phoria and the euphoric effects of opiates are presumed to be generated by activating the re-ceptor sites of the enkephalin neurons of the amygdala and structures of the limbic system.

The relief of pain associated with acupunc-ture treatment results from the release of enke-phalins by the brain, which bind to opiate re-ceptors. Evidence for this conclusion is that following the administration of *naloxone*, a po-tent opiate antagonist, the anesthetic effects of acupuncture are blocked. In the placebo effect, pain is often relieved by indifferent medication such as saline. In these cases, the placebo effect can be shown to be blocked by naloxone.

Gastrointestinal (Gut-Brain) Peptides

These peptides were initially identified in the GI tract and were later found to be also localized within the nervous system.

Vasoactive intestinal peptide (VIP) is widely distributed in the CNS and in the intrinsic neu-rons of the gut. It is found in high concentrations in the cerebral cortex, hippocampus, amygdala, and hypothalamus. Its role in the CNS is not understood. It appears to function as an inhibi-tory modulator to smooth muscle and as an exci-tatory modulator to glandular epithelial cells.

Substance P is an excitatory modulator lo-cated in the CNS and GI tract. Its effects are of long duration. Its role in the GI tract is to influence the constriction of smooth muscles. Substance P is released in the dorsal horn of the spinal cord by A-delta and C pain fibers of the dorsal root ganglia sensory neurons (Chap. 9). Specific populations of neurons of the stria-tum contain neurons in which substance P and GABA coexist. These neurons project to the me-dial segment of the globus pallidus and to the substantia nigra (Chap. 24). Substance P is found in the neurons of the raphe nuclei of the brainstem and hypothalamus.

Neurotensin is a gut-brain peptide present in the enteric neurons and in the median eminence (hypothalamus), substantia nigra, periaqueduc-tal gray, LC, and raphe nuclei of the brain. It may have a role in the control of body tempera-ture and in the regulation of the pituitary gland (Chap. 21).

Hypothalamic-Releasing Peptides (Hormones)

Opioid hypothalamic-releasing hormones in-clude *somatostatin*, a peptide that inhibits the release of growth hormone, and *thyrotropin-re-leasing hormone* that stimulates the release of thyrotropin from the pituitary gland (Chap. 21).

Neurohypophyseal (Pituitary) Peptide (Hormone)

Vasopressin (antidiuretic hormone) is the neuro-hypophyseal peptide hormone involved with the reabsorption of water by the kidney and in the constriction of blood vessels.

Oxytocin is the peptide involved in stimulat-ing (1) the smooth muscles of the uterus to con-tract and (2) milk release in lactating women by the contraction of the myoepithelial cells of the mammary gland.

Both vasopressin and oxytocin are synthe-sized within the cell bodies of the hypothalamic neurons of the magnocellular neurosecretory system and stored in the posterior lobe of the pituitary gland (Chap. 21).

NITRIC OXIDE, CARBON MONOXIDE, AND ADENOSINE

Nitric oxide (NO) acts as a neuronal messenger in both the central and peripheral nervous sys-tems. It is an unconventional nitrergic transmit-ter that is not found in vesicles. Rather, it read-ily diffuses from its site of origin in the cell through the cell and its membranes. The possi-bility is that NO can be released from both pre-synaptic and postsynaptic neurons. Note that NO is not the nitrous oxide used as an anes-thetic.

In neurons, NO can be produced in response to the excitatory synaptic transmitter glutamate acting through an NMDA receptor that opens Ca^{++} ion channels. The resulting influx of Ca^{++} ions passing through the channels bind to the intracellular protein calmodulin that acti-vates the enzyme nitric acid synthetase. This enzyme converts the amino acid arginine into NO. This sequence is rapid, taking only milli-seconds. NO is an unstable gas which is extremely membrane permeant. It diffuses through membranes bypassing interactions with synaptic membrane receptors. It acts as a modulator in which a postsynaptic neuron can influence a presynaptic neuron. It is extremely labile and lasts for about 5 to 10 seconds. The mechanisms underlying the actions of NO remains to be elucidated.

Nitric oxide's (NO) role in dilating blood vessels (nitrovasodilator) is indicative of one mode of its activity. The parasympathetic neurotransmitter ACh binds to the endothelial cells lining blood vessels to activate the release of NO which diffuses across membranes to the smooth muscles of the blood vessel (Chap. 20). The NO causes the dilation of the blood vessel as a consequence of the relaxation of the smooth muscle cells. Thus, ACh acts through NO and not directly on the smooth muscles which lack ACh receptors. The NO relaxes the muscles through the activation of the second messenger system involving cGMP (cyclic guanosine monophosphate), which is related to cAMP (Chap. 3). The dilation is counterbalanced by the sympathetic transmitter norepinephrine which acts directly with receptor sites on the smooth muscle. The smooth muscles contract resulting in the constriction of the blood vessel. The NO formed following the absorption of nitroglycerine into the blood stream relieves the pain symptoms of angina caused by the constricted blood vessels of the heart. The NO stimulates the cardiac blood vessels to dilate and therefore restores an adequate blood flow to the heart muscle. NO is released by neurons of the myenteric plexus of the gut as a nonadrenergic-noncholinergic (NANC) agent involved in smooth muscular relaxation during peristalsis (Chap. 20).

The NO released at glutamatergic synapses is thought to have a role in developmental and synaptic plasticity exhibited by neurons (Chap. 3). This may be of significance in the synaptic plasticity underlying learning and memory associated with, for example, the hippocampus (Chap. 22). In addition, NO may participate in the acquisition of learned behavior.

Carbon monoxide (CO) is another membrane-permeant gas formed in the brain that may also have roles in molecular neurobiology.

Adenosine (a purine) is a mysterious *purinergic modulator* that is a degradation product of adenosine triphosphate (ATP). This purine acts as a chemical messenger, but more specifically as a modulator. Adenosine may exert its influences presynaptically by inhibiting the release of transmitters and postsynaptically by its action on some receptors associated with the second messenger systems. It is released by sympathetic neurons innervating, for examples, the smooth muscles of the vas deferens and the GI tract (see Neural Control of the Gut, Chap. 20) and the cardiac muscle of the heart.

SUGGESTED READINGS

Bloom F. Neurohumoral transmission and the central nervous system. In: Gilman A, Rall T, Nies A, Taylor P, eds. *Goodman and Gilman's The Pharmacological Basis of Therapeutics*. 8th ed. Elmsford, NY: Pergamon Press; 1990:244–268.

Bradford H. *Chemical Neurobiology: An Introduction to Neurochemistry*. New York, NY: WH Freeman Co; 1985.

Cooper J, Bloom F, Roth R. *The Biochemical Basis of Neuropharmacology*. 6th Ed. New York, NY: Oxford University Press; 1991.

Cooper J, Meyer F. Possible mechanisms involved in the release and modulation of release of neuroactive agents. *Neurochem Int*. 1984;6:419–433.

Cuello A, Sofroniew M. The anatomy of CNS cholinergic neurons. *Trends Neurosci*. 1984;7:74–78.

Emsom P, ed. *Chemical Neuroanatomy*. New York, NY: Raven Press; 1983.

Hökfelt T, Johansson O, Goldstein M. Chemical anatomy of the brain. *Science*. 1984;225:1326–1334.

Jones E, ed. *Molecular Biology of the Human Brain*. Vol. 72. New York, NY: Wiley; 1988.

Kandel E, Schwartz J, Jessell T, eds. Essentials of Neural Science and Behavior. Norwalk, Conn: Appleton & Lange; 1995.

Krieger D. Brain peptides, what, where, and why? *Science*. 1983;222:975–985.

Lefkowitz R, Hoffman B, Taylor P. Neurohumoral transmission: the autonomic and somatic motor nervous systems. In: Gilman A, Rall T, Nies A, Taylor P, eds. *Goodman and Gilman's The Pharmacological Basis of Therapeutics*. 8th ed. Elmsford, NY: Pergamon Press; 1990:84–121.

Reichlin S. Somatostatin. *N Engl J Med*. 1983;309:1495–1501, 1556–1563.

Rosenberg R, Harding A. *The Molecular Biology of Neurological Disease*. London: Butterworths; 1988.

Schmitt F. Molecular regulators of brain function: a new view. *Neuroscience.* 1984;13:991–1001.

Schuman E, Madison D. Nitric oxide and synaptic function. *Annu Rev Neurosci.* 1994;17:153–183.

Siegel G, Agranoff B, Albers R, Molinoff P, eds. *Basic Neurochemistry: Molecular, Cellular, and Medical Aspects.* 5th ed. New York, NY: Raven Press; 1994.

Snyder S, Bredt D. Biological roles of nitric oxide. *Sci Am.* 1992;266:68–77.

Takaki H, Oomura Y, Ito M, Otsuka M, eds. *Biowarning System in the Brain.* Tokyo: University of Tokyo; 1989.

Ungerstedt U. Stereotatic mapping of the monoamine pathways in the rat brain. *Acta Physiol Scand.* 1971;367(suppl):1–48.

Auditory and Vestibular Systems 16

The auditory system is an exteroceptive system concerned with the perception of sound. The vestibular system is proprioceptive and concerned with the maintenance of equilibrium and the orientation of the body in space. The receptors—actually mechanoreceptors—are hair cells within specialized neuroepithelial structures. They are responsible for converting mechanical energy in the form of fluid displacement from sound waves (for hearing) and head movements (for balance) into electrochemical energy to be transmitted to the auditory (cochlear) or vestibular nerves, respectively. The hair cells are located within the membranous labyrinth of the inner ear, which is a closed tubular system filled with endolymph. The auditory hair cells are in the spiral organ of Corti in the cochlea. The vestibular hair cells are located in the macula of the utricle, the macula of the saccule, and the cristae ampullares of the three semicircular canals. The cochlear and vestibular nerves merge and comprise the vestibulocochlear nerve or eighth cranial nerve (n. VIII), which enters the brainstem at the *cerebellopontine angle* (junction between the cerebellum, pons, and medulla, **Fig. 13.3**).

THE LABYRINTHS

There are two labyrinths in the auditory and vestibular systems, the osseous (or bony) labyrinth and the membranous (or otic) labyrinth. The *osseous labyrinth*, a network of canals and vesicles located within the temporal bone, forms the bony framework for the cochlea, vestibule (utricle and saccule), and the three semicircular canals (**Fig. 16.1**). The *membranous labyrinth* is enclosed within the osseous labyrinth to form a structure analogous to a tube within a tube; the outer tube is the osseous labyrinth and the inner tube is the membranous labyrinth (**Fig. 16.2**). The hair cells are located within the membranous labyrinth. The space within the osseous labyrinth (perilymphatic space) and surrounding the membranous labyrinth is filled with *perilymph*; the space within the membranous labyrinth (endolymphatic space) is filled with *endolymph*. The hair cells are located within the endolymphatic space. The endolymphatic and perilymphatic spaces are separate compartments. Their respective fluids have different chemical compositions similar to the differences between extracellular fluid (perilymph) and intracellular fluid (endolymph). Thus, they have different resting potentials allowing for the passage of charge and the stimulation of the hair cells.

The Membranous Labyrinth

The vestibular portion of the membranous labyrinth on each side consists of (1) three semicircular ducts: lateral (or horizontal), superior (or anterior), and posterior (or inferior), named for their orientation within the temporal bone; (2) the utricle; and (3) the saccule. The three semicircular ducts are in open communication via five openings with the utricle. Each semicircular duct has one bulbous portion, the ampulla. The nonampullated ends of the superior and posterior canals are joined to form the common crus. The portion of the membranous labyrinth

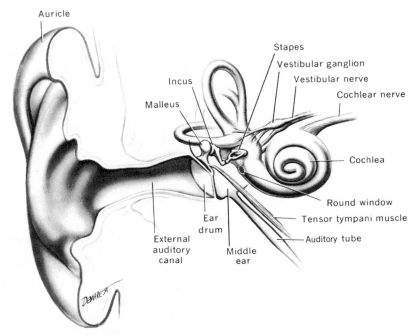

Figure 16.1: External ear, middle ear, and inner ear. (Right ear viewed from the front.)

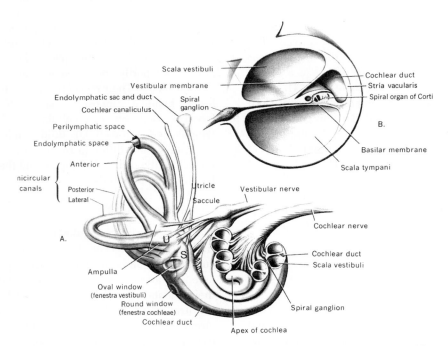

Figure 16.2: The labyrinth. **A.** Right labyrinth, from the front. The perilymphatic space is located between the bony labyrinth and the membranous labyrinth: it extends as the cochlear canaliculus. The endolymphatic space is located within the membranous labyrinth, which includes the three semicircular ducts, utricle, saccule, cochlear duct, and endolymphatic duct and sac. **B.** Cross section through the cochlea. The scala vestibuli and scala tympani are connected through a passage called the helicotrema, located at the apex of the cochlea.

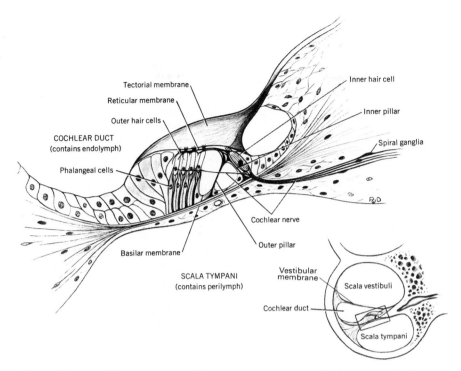

Figure 16.3: The middle turn of the spiral organ of Corti, showing four rows of outer hair cells. There are three rows of outer hair cells in the basal turn and five in the apical half turn, reflecting the fact that the basilar membrane is wider at the apex.

associated with the auditory system is the *cochlear duct (scala media)* (**Fig. 16.3**). The cochlear duct is connected to the saccule via the *ductus reuniens*. The utricular duct (from the utricle) and the saccular duct (from the saccule) merge to form the *endolymphatic duct* (within the bony vestibular aqueduct) which drains endolymph into the *endolymphatic sac* (**Fig. 16.2**). The endolymphatic sac is located between layers of a well-vascularized region of the dura mater on the posterior face of the petrous bone (**Fig. 16.2**). The entire membranous labyrinth (cochlear duct, saccule, utricle, semicircular ducts, and endolymphatic duct and sac) is filled with endolymph. Endolymph is actively formed in both the cochlear and vestibular portions of the labyrinth.

The Osseous Labyrinth

The osseous labyrinth consists of the vestibule, semicircular canals, and cochlea within the temporal bone. It develops from the primitive otic capsule. The utricle and saccule are within the vestibule. Openings into the vestibule include the vestibular aqueduct, foramina for the passage of vestibular nerve bundles, and the oval window. The three semicircular canals surround the semicircular ducts. The bony cochlea is a spiral structure that winds two and a half turns around a bony core, the *modiolus*, that contains the cell bodies (spiral ganglion) of the afferent auditory nerve fibers, as well as the efferent fibers from the brainstem passing to the auditory hair cells. The cochlea is partially divided by the *spiral osseous lamina*, a thin ridge of bone extending out laterally from the modiolus, that partially separates the perilymphatic space into the *scala vestibuli* and *scala tympani*. The separation is completed by the cochlear duct (or scala media). The scala vestibuli and scala tympani communicate at the apex of the cochlea by a small opening called the *helicotrema*. The scala vestibuli is in continuity with the perilymphatic space of the vestibule and, thus, with the oval window. At the basal end of the scala tympani, is the round window. It should be noted that the perilymphatic space is connected through the narrow cochlear aqueduct at the basal end of the scala tympani to the subarachnoid space. Perilymph is therefore in continuity with cerebrospinal fluid.

Sensory Receptor Areas

There are six specialized areas within the membranous labyrinth that contain the sensory epithelial receptors (hair cells) in contact with the terminal endings of the eighth cranial nerve. These are the three cristae ampullares (one in the ampulla of each semicircular duct), one macula utriculi, and one macula sacculi, all innervated by the vestibular neurons; and the spiral organ of Corti in the cochlea, innervated by auditory (cochlear) neurons.

The organ of Corti is located within the cochlear duct (scala media) of the membranous labyrinth.

Scala Media

The *vestibular (Reissner's) membrane* forms the roof of the scala media and separates it from the scala vestibuli. This membrane is a single layer of cells that runs obliquely from the upper limit of the spiral ligament (attached to the lateral wall of the cochlea) to the limbus on the osseous spiral lamina. The *basilar membrane*, bordering the scala tympani, forms the floor of the scala media. Resting on the basilar membrane is the spiral *organ of Corti*, the organ of hearing. The basilar membrane is suspended medially by the osseous spiral lamina and laterally by the lower extent of the spiral ligament. The lateral wall of the scala media is formed by the stria vascularis on the spiral ligament. It contains the specialized cells for active transport of ions to maintain the +80 millivolt endolymphatic potential, and thus, the current necessary for hair cell depolarization.

AUDITORY SYSTEM

Ear Anatomy and Physiology

The "ear" consists of the external ear, middle ear, and the inner ear (Fig. 16.1).

The external ear (auricle and external auditory meatus) is separated from the middle ear by the *tympanic membrane* (ear drum). The external auditory meatus works as a sound resonator, increasing the sound pressure level (usually measured in decibels) at the tympanic membrane. The auricle and head have a baffle effect and shadow effect on sound waves that aid in sound localization.

The middle ear is an air filled space bounded laterally by the tympanic membrane and medially by the inner ear. Traversing this space is a chain of three ear ossicles: the *malleus* which is attached to the tympanic membrane; the *incus* in an intermediate position; and the *stapes* whose footplate is inserted into the *oval window*. There are two small skeletal muscles in the middle ear: the *tensor tympani muscle*, which is inserted into the malleus, and the *stapedius muscle*, which is attached to the stapes. The latter is responsible for the stapedial reflex (see later). The middle ear functions as a mismatch transformer increasing the sound pressure level at the oval window as compared to that at the tympanic membrane. This is necessary because of the increased impedance of the cochlear fluids (perilymph) as compared to air in the external auditory canal. A greater amount of pressure is necessary to vibrate the higher impedance fluid. If the tympanic membrane and ossicular chain were not present, sound waves would hit the oval and round windows simultaneously, canceling out their vibrations. Also, there would be insufficient energy to stimulate the inner ear adequately. This is important clinically in patients with chronic middle ear disease.

The inner ear is the cochlea (spiral shell). Traveling waves within the perilymph, generated by movement of the oval window, displace the basilar membrane on which the organ of Corti sits. The organ of Corti contains hair cells that are the specialized auditory receptors.

Sound Reception

Vibrations may be perceived as sounds. Sound travels in the form of waves with a characteristic frequency, measured in hertz (cycles per second), and amplitude, measured in sound pressure level (decibels, dB). Frequency is a measure of pitch and amplitude is a measure of loudness. It is important to remember that the decibel scale is logarithmic, so a ten decibel increase has 100 times more energy. Zero decibels is the average threshold for human hearing and 140 dB is the threshold for pain. Normal conversational speech is 40 dB to 60 dB. Frequencies between 50 and 20,000 hertz can be detected as sound. The frequencies perceived with optimum acuity by most subjects fall between 2000 and 5000 hertz. Airborne vibrations (sound waves) pass through the external auditory meatus and set the tympanic membrane vibrating (air conduction). Some vibrations may bypass the ear ossicles and reach the perilymph directly through bone (bone conduction). The oscillations of the stapes footplate in the oval window produce pressure waves within the perilymph of the cochlea that travel variable distances, depending on frequency, up the $2\frac{1}{2}$ turns of the scala vestibuli (**Figs. 16.1 to 16.3**). High frequency waves press down on the organ of Corti and its basilar membrane near the base of the cochlea, whereas lower frequency waves impinge progressively toward the apex. Thus, each section of the basilar membrane has a characteristic tuning curve for which it is most sensitive (this is found in all levels of the auditory system). The waves cause downward, followed by upward, deflections of the basilar membrane. To allow propagation of the pressure (traveling) waves in the inner ear, the membrane of the round window bulges outward and inward in synchrony (equal and opposite) with movement of the stapes. This is necessary because perilymphatic fluid is incompressible within the bony cochlea; traveling waves would not be generated if there wasn't compensatory movement at the round window.

The Organ of Corti and Auditory Hair Cells

The spiral organ of Corti has two types of hair cells, the flask shaped inner and rectangular shaped outer (**Figs. 16.3 and 16.4**). There is one row of *inner hair cells*, and between three (at the base) and five (at the apex) rows of *outer hair cells* for a total of about 15,500. Both have efferent, as well as afferent, nerve endings; however, efferent innervation is mainly to the outer hair cells, which contain myosin. It is thought that the outer hair cells are contractile and fine

tune the basilar membrane. The inner hair cells are responsible for the perception of sound. There are several rows of *stereocilia* (actually microvilli) at the apical end of each hair cell. The *basal body*, a rudimentary kinocilium, is located adjacent to the tallest row of stereocilia.

The distal tips of the stereocilia are embedded in the rigid keratin-like tectorial membrane (**Fig. 16.3**). There are 140 or so stereocilia for each of the 3500 inner hair cells and 12,000 outer hair cells in the human organ of Corti (**Fig. 16.3**). With the vibration of the basilar membrane (**Fig. 16.3**), a shearing force is produced with an accompanying displacement of the stereocilia; this results because the tectorial membrane does not move to the same degree as the hair cells. The hair cells are polarized, with stimulation occurring when the stereocilia are bent along the axis of sensitivity, i.e., toward the basal body (**Fig. 16.4**). The hair cells act both as transducers (converting mechanical energy into electrochemical energy) and biologic amplifiers. The organ of Corti is a frequency analyzer with the highest pitches monitored at the base of the coil, the lowest at the apex, and the intermediate pitches in an organized topographic pattern between the highest and the lowest (*tonotopic organization*). In addition to physical differences in the waveforms produced by individual frequencies, hair cells along the length of the basilar membrane vary slightly in morphologic and physiologic properties to correspond with the specific frequencies that they mediate (i.e., have frequency-specific tuning curves).

Perception of loudness is related to the amplitude of the vibrations of the organ of Corti. Hair cells at rest have a basal rate of electrical activity or steady state potential. This is thought to be due to calcium gated channels at the tips of the stereocilia that are opened or closed by tip links that connect adjoining stereocilia. At rest, the channels are equally open and closed. With displacement of the stereocilia toward the basal body, the gates are preferentially opened, allowing depolarization of the cell membrane and transduction of electric signals (the generator potential) to the base of the hair cell where synaptic contact with nerve endings is made. The generator potential stimulates neurotransmitter release. Thus, each hair cell is a mecha-

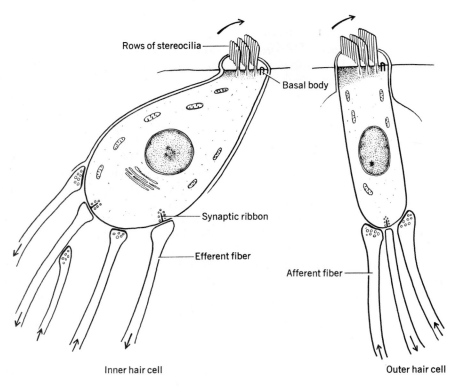

Rows of stereocilia

Basal body

Synaptic ribbon

Efferent fiber

Afferent fiber

Inner hair cell

Outer hair cell

Figure 16.4: The hair cells of the spiral organ of Corti. The axis of sensitivity of a cochlear hair cell is in the direction of the basal body.

noreceptor that transduces mechanical energy of the sound waves into graded potentials. In turn, these generator potentials stimulate the nerve endings of the bipolar cells of the spiral ganglion of the cochlear nerve.

Ascending Pathways (Fig. 16.5)

Each of the approximately 30,000 fibers of the cochlear nerve has (1) distal branches terminating as synaptic connections with, from a few to many, hair cells of the spiral organ of Corti, and (2) proximal branches synapsing with many neurons in the cochlear nuclear complex (dorsal, posteroventral and anteroventral cochlear nuclei) located on the posterolateral surface of the upper medulla (**Fig. 13.11**). Each of these nuclei is tonotopically organized (has a frequency specific tuning curve) and gives rise to at least partially separate second-order ascending fiber systems. Most fibers decussate in the caudal pons and many ascend in the contralateral lateral lemniscus. The great majority arise

from each anteroventral cochlear nucleus and cross to the opposite side as the rather conspicuous trapezoid body in the anterior pontine tegmentum; a large number terminate in the superior olivary complex. Fibers from the posteroventral and dorsal cochlear nuclei decussate more posteriorly in the pontine tegmentum as the intermediate and dorsal acoustic striae, respectively. Some fibers from the cochlear nuclei ascend as uncrossed fibers in the ipsilateral lateral lemniscus.

Intercalated within the ascending auditory pathways to the auditory cortex are several nuclei; these include the superior olivary complex, nuclei of the lateral lemniscus, inferior colliculus, and medial geniculate body. Commissural fibers interconnect the bilateral nuclei of the lateral lemniscus and inferior colliculi. The portion of the lateral lemniscus between the inferior colliculus and the medial geniculate body is called the brachium of the inferior colliculus. The fibers (auditory radiation) from the neurons

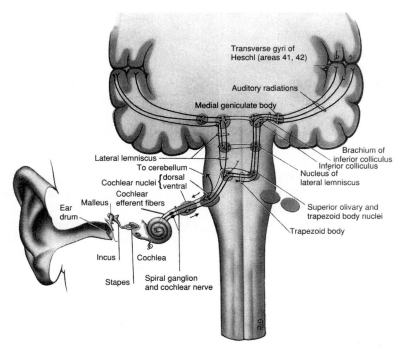

Figure 16.5: Diagram of the auditory pathways.

of the medial geniculate body ascend through the posterior limb of the internal capsule (sublenticular portion) and terminate in the transverse gyri of Heschl (areas 41, 42) of the temporal lobe (**Fig. 25.5**). The two hemispheres are interconnected via the corpus callosum.

The complexity of the auditory cortex is revealed in studies which indicate that it consists of a tonotopically organized primary cortex (area 41) in the temporal lobe and at least five other tonotopically organized auditory cortical areas in the immediate vicinity of the primary auditory cortex.

Two functionally significant features of the ascending pathways deserve mention: (1) the processing centers at each level have a multiple tonotopic organization, and (2) the output from each ear is conveyed bilaterally, i.e., via auditory pathways of both sides, with more being projected along the contralateral pathway than the ipsilateral pathway.

Descending Pathways

Projecting from the auditory cortex and the other nuclei of the auditory pathway are descending fibers, which accompany the ascend-

ing fibers (**Fig. 16.5**). These fibers have a role in processing ascending influences (they enhance signals and suppress "noise"). The nerve fibers from the superior olivary nuclei are integrated into a feedback system that courses as crossed and uncrossed projections—called the olivocochlear or cochlear efferent bundle—via the vestibulocochlear nerve, before terminating at the base of the hair cells of the spiral organ of Corti (**Fig. 16.5**). The inhibitory influences conveyed by these efferent fibers act to suppress the activity of the afferent fibers of the cochlear nerve, and fine tune the basilar membrane through the outer hair cells.

Functional and Clinical Considerations

Deafness restricted to one ear is usually associated with damage to the cochlear nerve or the cochlea itself (sensorineural hearing loss [SNHL]), or the conducting apparatus within the middle ear (conductive hearing loss) on the side of the deafness. Unilateral lesions of the ascending auditory pathways above the level of the cochlear nuclei produce only minor impairments because of the strong bilaterality of the pathway. Bilateral lesions of the central auditory pathway are rare because the tracts and nuclei are far apart, near the lateral margin of the brainstem; the auditory cortex similarly occupies a region at the lateral margin of the cerebrum. Evidence from animal studies indicates that the auditory cortex is not essential for discrimination of intensities or frequencies, but is necessary for differentiation of more complex functions such as patterns or rhythms.

An irritative lesion of the organ of Corti or the cochlear nerve may result in tinnitus—the subjective hearing of hissing, roaring, buzzing, and humming sounds. This may occur in acoustic neuromas of n. VIII in the cerebellopontine angle. Tinnitus may be followed by nerve deafness as the irritative lesion expands and all cochlear nerve fibers are interrupted. Nerve deafness is also associated with occlusion of the internal auditory artery, aging and Meniere's disease (see later for Meniere's disease).

Several commonly used drugs are ototoxic. The most common drugs to cause irreversible SNHL are the aminoglycosides, such as gentamicin. Early cessation of treatment will allow reversal of the damage. This class of antibiotic causes direct hair cell toxicity to both the auditory and vestibular hair cells. This is usually an unwanted side effect of aminoglycoside use, but in patients with severe vertigo, it is used to alleviate symptoms. Other common agents that cause ototoxicity include the loop diuretics, which cause both permanent and reversible losses, and salicylates including aspirin, which cause a reversible hearing loss. Cisplatin, a common antineoplastic agent, causes a permanent hearing loss. An early symptom of ototoxicity from all of these agents is often tinnitus.

Damage to the eardrum and the ossicles of the middle ear is usually followed by a partial deafness. This middle-ear deafness (conduction deafness in otosclerosis) is accompanied by a partial loss in the perception of low-pitched sounds and a mild loss in the entire auditory range.

Presbycusis is the gradual impairment of ability to perceive or to discriminate sounds in old age. This increasing difficulty in hearing high-pitched sound is associated with the degeneration of the hair cells near the base of the cochlear coil.

Conduction deafness may occur as a conse-

quence of middle-ear disease such as otitis media. A tuning fork test, the Rinne test, can be used to distinguish bone conduction deafness from air conduction deafness. The base of a vibrating tuning fork is applied to the mastoid process of the skull and sound is heard by bone conduction; at the moment the sound ceases the vibrating fork is placed near the external auditory meatus. A subject with normal hearing will hear the vibrations by air conduction after the bone conduction hearing ceases. In middle-ear deafness, the vibrating fork cannot be heard by air conduction. In partial nerve deafness, air conduction hearing is better than bone conduction hearing, although both are diminished.

Brainstem auditory evoked potentials are employed for diagnostic purposes. They are recorded from electrodes applied to the scalp using a computer to average multiple responses. Potentials from the various portions of the auditory pathway have different latencies and characteristics of wave form. Abnormalities in the potentials can be an aid in determining the presence of injury to the auditory pathways and its localization, as in multiple sclerosis, strokes, tumors, etc.

The auditory pathways are reflexly integrated with the cranial nerves innervating the stapedius (n. VII) and tensor tympani (n. V) muscles. Immediately after stimulation of sounds of high intensity, these two muscles contract reflexly and exert tension on the ear ossicles; this action protects the spiral organ of Corti from damage by excessive stimulation. Paralysis of these muscles results in *hyperacusis*—the increased acuity of hearing and hypersensitivity to low tones.

The *stapedial reflex* is the response to loud sounds. The cochlear nerve acts as the sensory limb of the reflex arc. The motor limb of the arc arises from neurons in the region of the superior olivary complex that project to both stapedius muscles. Contraction of the stapedius dampens the oscillations of the ear ossicles and reduces the perceived loudness of the sound. The role of the tensor tympani in this reflex remains controversial.

Other auditory reflexes involve the various brainstem nuclei and their projections to the spinal cord, especially to the motor centers innervating the neck musculature, which rotates the head in the direction of the source of the sound.

VESTIBULAR SYSTEM

The purpose of the vestibular system is to signal changes in the motion of the head (kinetic) and in the position of the head with respect to gravity (static). The information from the periphery required by the nervous system to perform these roles is obtained from three afferent sources: the eyes, the general proprioceptive receptors throughout the body, and the vestibular receptors in the inner ear. These three afferent sources are integrated into three systems—visual, proprioceptive, and vestibular systems—known as the equilibrial triad.

The vestibular system is actually the special proprioceptive system that functions to maintain equilibrium, to direct the gaze of the eyes, and

to preserve a constant plane of vision (head position), primarily by modifying muscle tone.

The receptor end organs in each inner ear of the vestibular system include the three cristae ampullares (one crista located in the ampulla of each semicircular duct) and the maculae of the utricle and saccule (**Fig. 16.6**). The three semicircular ducts, oriented at right angles to each other, represent the three dimensions of space. The membranous labyrinths of the semicircular canals, utricle and saccule, are filled with endolymph (continuous with the cochlear duct) and surrounded by perilymph in the osseous labyrinth (continuous with the scala vestibuli and scala tympani of the cochlea).

The 75 to 100 stereocilia and one kinocilium of each hair cell of the many in each crista are embedded in a gelatinous matrix (*cupula*) that abuts against the roof of the ampulla; the *kinocilium* of each hair cell is located on one side of all stereocilia (**Figs. 16.6 and 16.7**). The

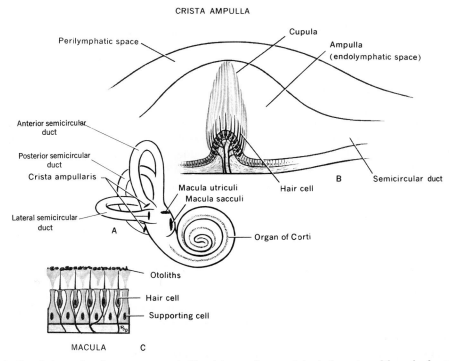

Figure 16.6: Vestibular and auditory receptors. **A.** The right membranous labyrinth as viewed from the front. Neuroepithelial areas (in black) include a crista ampullaris in the ampulla of each semicircular duct, the macula of the utricle, the macula of the saccule, and the spiral organ of Corti of the cochlear duct. **B.** The crista ampullaris of an ampulla. Note that the free border of the crista is in contact with the wall of the ampulla. **C.** The macula. Note that the tips of the hair cells are in contact with the otoliths embedded in the gelatinous mass.

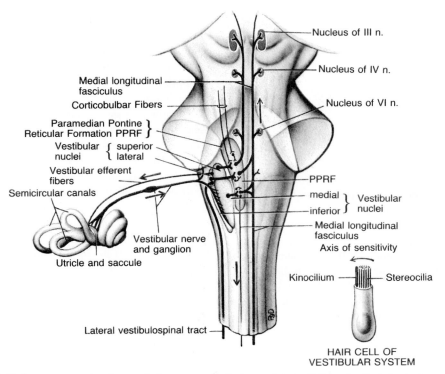

Labels in figure:
- Nucleus of III n.
- Nucleus of IV n.
- Nucleus of VI n.
- Medial longitudinal fasciculus
- Corticobulbar Fibers
- Paramedian Pontine } Reticular Formation PPRF }
- Vestibular { superior nuclei { lateral
- Vestibular efferent fibers
- Semicircular canals
- Vestibular nerve and ganglion
- Utricle and saccule
- PPRF
- medial } Vestibular inferior } nuclei
- Medial longitudinal fasciculus
- Axis of sensitivity
- Kinocilium
- Stereocilia
- Lateral vestibulospinal tract
- HAIR CELL OF VESTIBULAR SYSTEM

Figure 16.7: Pathways composing the vestibular nerve, vestibular nuclei, medial longitudinal fasciculus, and lateral vestibulospinal tract. The connections of the vestibular system with the vestibulocerebellum are illustrated in Fig. 18.4. The axis of sensitivity of a vestibular hair cell is in the direction of the kinocilium.

kinocilium is a true cilium and the stereocilia, as in the organ of Corti, are microvilli. Each vestibular hair cell is depolarized when the stereocilia bend in the direction of the kinocilium and hyperpolarized when deflected in the opposite direction. All hair cells in a crista are polarized in the same direction. The cristae ampullares respond to angular movements and only to acceleration and deceleration, not constant movement of the head. Thus, these receptors act as angular accelerometers that respond to the twists and turns of the head.

The movement of the endolymphatic fluid within the semicircular ducts as the head turns and rotates results in the bending of the gelatinous matrix and the cilia. Semicircular ducts of the two sides operate in pairs: the two horizontal ducts are yoked, as are the anterior duct of one side with the posterior duct of the opposite side. The kinocilia of the horizontal ducts, in contrast to those of the other ducts, face the utricle. Thus, rotation to the left causes: (1) deflection

of the stereocilia in the left horizontal duct toward the kinocilium and in the right duct away from the kinocilium, (2) depolarization of hair cells in the crista ampullaris of the left horizontal duct and hyperpolarization in the right crista, and (3) increased frequency of impulses in the left vestibular nerve leading from the horizontal duct and decreased frequency in the right nerve. The vestibular nerve has a spontaneous rate of firing of about 100 impulses per second.

The macula of the saccule is oriented with its long axis essentially in a vertical plane, and the macula of the utricle in a horizontal plane. The stereocilia and kinocilium of each hair cell, similar to those in the crista ampullares, are embedded in a gelatinous matrix (**Fig. 16.6**). However, in the maculae there is a layer of calcareous crystals (*otoliths*) that amplify the force caused by the deflection of the stereocilia. Additionally, the stereocilia are polarized in relation to a curved band, the *striola*, which passes through the central portion of the maculae. In the utricle all kinocilia face the striola, whereas in the saccule they face in the opposite direction (away from the striola).

The two maculae, also called otolith organs, are really linear accelerometers. The saccular macula responds to vertically directed acceleratory and deceleratory linear displacements and gravity (e.g., movements up and down in an elevator). The utricular macula responds to horizontally directed forces and gravity. Some investigators say the saccule is a sensor for the reception of vibratory stimuli.

The role of the vestibular receptors in the orientation of the head and body in space is expressed through muscular activities in the coordination of eye reflexes, head position, and body movements. These specialized proprioceptors tend to (1) reinforce the tonic activity of muscles while the subject is in a stationary position (e.g., maintain balance while he is standing in a moving vehicle), and (2) trigger muscular reflexes in response to changes in the position of the head, body, and extremities (e.g., sustain balance while walking a tightrope).

Input to the Vestibular Nuclei

The sensory neurons of the vestibular nerve (cell bodies in the vestibular ganglion) (Figs. 16.7 and 18.4) are bipolar neurons. They terminate distally by synapsing with the hair cells of the vestibular receptors (maculae and cristae ampullares). Most of their centrally directed axons terminate ipsilaterally within the brainstem in precise synaptic patterns within each of the four vestibular nuclei (superior, lateral, medial, and inferior). In general, the fibers originating from the cristae ampullares end in the medial and superior nuclei; the fibers originating in the maculae of the utricle and saccule terminate primarily in the lateral, inferior, and medial nuclei. Other fibers of the vestibular nerve course through the juxtarestiform body (part of the inferior cerebellar peduncle; Fig. 18.4) and end directly in the ipsilateral cerebellar cortex, chiefly in the flocculonodular lobe, which is sometimes called the vestibulocerebellum. In addition, this lobe and the fastigial nuclei of the cerebellum send crossed and uncrossed fibers to the vestibular nuclei. In summary, the vestibular nuclei receive their main input from both the vestibular receptors and the cerebellum. In addition, the vestibular nuclei have reciprocal connections with the flocculonodular lobe and nuclei fastigii of the cerebellum.

Output from the Vestibular Nuclei

The influences from the vestibular nuclei are projected (1) to the spinal cord via the (lateral) vestibulospinal tract and medial vestibulospinal tract (within medial longitudinal fasciculus, MLF) (Fig. 16.7); (2) to the cerebellum via fibers in the juxtarestiform body (Fig. 18.4); (3) to the brainstem primarily via the MLF (vestibulomesencephalic fibers); and (4) to the postcentral gyrus between areas 2 and 5 (see Chap. 23) via a relay in the ventral posterior inferior thalamic nucleus.

Postural Pathways

The *vestibulospinal tract*, originating from the lateral vestibular nucleus, is an uncrossed, somatotopically organized bundle of fibers terminating in laminae VII and VIII at all levels of the spinal cord (Figs. 7.5 and 11.4). It conveys excitatory influences for extensor muscle tone and extensor spinal reflexes. The *medial vestibulospinal tract*, originating from the medial vestibular nucleus, is primarily an uncrossed bundle of fibers descending in the MLF before terminating mainly in lamina VIII in the cervical and upper thoracic levels. It conveys inhibitory influences for extensor muscle tone. These descending vestibular tracts act mainly through spinal interneurons on both the alpha and gamma motoneurons. Their influence in concert with local myotatic reflexes is to maintain the tonus of the extensor muscles of the trunk (back musculature) and the limbs. These neural activities are critical for the support of the body against gravity, i.e., for the maintenance of upright posture. Fibers in the MLF participate in coordinating position of the head with eye movements.

Vestibuloocular Pathways

One of the most important tasks of the vestibular system is its role in influencing the conjugate (i.e., coupled) movements of the eyes. These

conjugate movements are controlled by inputs
from many sources, e.g., from areas 8, 18, and
19 of the cerebral cortex, and by means of inputs
to the vestibular system. The paramedian pontine reticular formation (PPRF, *pontine gaze
center*), located medially in the reticular formation, and its rostral continuation in the midbrain, is a critical staging region in the central
control of eye movements. It acts as a nuclear
processing complex and contains a variety of

cell types whose activity determines the form of
many eye movements. Input to neuronal pools
within the PPRF is derived from the cerebral
cortex, superior colliculus, cerebellum, auditory and vestibular systems, and the spinal cord.
Output from the PPRF is conveyed by circuits
utilizing the MLF and the reticular formation
and terminating in the motor nuclei of cranial
nerves III, IV, and VI, which innervate the extraocular muscles. The vestibulomesencephalic

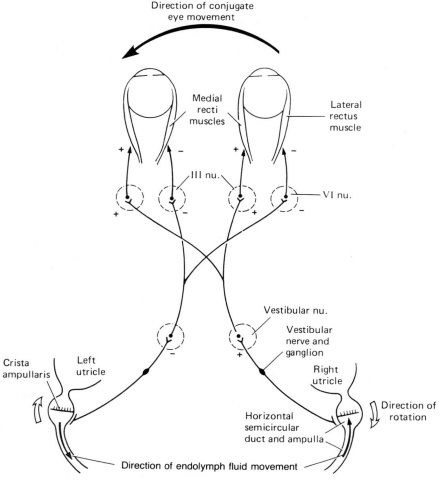

Figure 16.8: Conjugate eye movement associated with the horizontal semicircular ducts and ampullae. Rotational
acceleration of the head in a clockwise direction to the right (outlined arrows outside the ampullares) results in the
relative movement of endolymph in the paired semicircular ducts to the left (solid arrows in the ducts). Movement
of the endolymph toward the utricle results in excitatory activity (+) in the hair cells of the right ampulla and away
from the utricle results in inhibitory activity (−) in the hair cells in the left ampulla. These activities result in
excitation (+) and inhibition (−) in the medial and superior vestibular nuclei and fibers of the medial longitudinal
fasciculi; this produces excitatory and inhibitory influences in appropriate motoneurons in the abducent (lateral
rectus muscles) and oculomotor (medial rectus muscles) nuclei to stimulate conjugate eye movement to the left (solid
arrow).

circuit for conjugate eye movements comprises the vestibular nuclei to the PPRF to the nucleus of n. VI (in lower pons) and via the MLF to the nuclei of n. III and IV (in midbrain). The abducens and oculomotor nuclei also are reciprocally interconnected directly via fibers that travel in the MLF, and by way of linkages through the MLF with the PPRF (**Fig. 16.8**). Through these, the PPRF is associated with lateral gaze movements and horizontal saccades.

Vestibular influences are conveyed cephalically via relays in the ventral posterior inferior thalamic nucleus, and then to the postcentral gyrus, as noted previously. This pathway is thought to be involved in the appreciation of subjective sensations (e.g., dizziness) associated with the vestibular system.

Vestibular Tests and Disorders

Nystagmus

Nystagmus refers to involuntary rhythmic movements of the eyes with a rapid movement in one direction (called a saccade) followed by a slow movement in the opposite direction. It is related to an imbalance of synchronized impulses from vestibular sources. Nystagmus can be elicited and used in tests of vestibular function; when it occurs spontaneously it may be a symptom of a lesion.

Nystagmus in the normal individual has the following basis. As the head and body pivot and circle, the eyes attempt to fix on an object in space (slow component); as the head and body continue to circle, the eyes snap quickly in the direction in which the head is circling (fast or quick component). The action is similar to what happens when one is watching telegraph poles from a moving train—the fast component is in the direction in which the train is moving. These eye movements repeat throughout the duration of the circling. By convention, nystagmus is named by the direction of the fast saccade component. Horizontal nystagmus is the most common form. Vertical and rotatory nystagmus occur less frequently.

Nystagmus may occur following irritative or destructive lesions of a vestibular end organ, vestibular nerve, vestibular pathways, brainstem, or cerebellum. Certain toxic substances can also cause nystagmus.

Sudden recurrent attacks of vertigo and nystagmus occur in Meniere's disease. This is usually accompanied with tinnitus, unilateral deafness, and varying degrees of nausea and vomiting. The condition is thought to be a consequence of increased pressure and dilatation of the membranous labyrinth due to edema.

Rotation Test

The paired horizontal semicircular canals can be tested by placing the subject in a rotating (Bárány) chair and tilting the head forward by 30 degrees to bring the horizontal canals parallel to the ground. The chair is quickly rotated 10 to 12 turns before being abruptly stopped. The endolymph continues to "flow" in the same direction, deflecting the crista ampullaris of each horizontal canal. A whirling sensation follows. The impulses from the vestibular source stimulate the eye movements, and the visual impulses from the eyes, in turn, create the conscious spinning sensation (*vertigo*). During the spin of the chair to the right, the fast component (saccade) in the normal individual is to the right. Immediately after the spin is stopped, each saccade (postrotatory nystagmus) is reversed and is now directed to the left (called nystagmus to the left). By placing the head in appropriate planes, the other pairs of semicircular canals can be tested. The right anterior and the left posterior semicircular canals are paired, as are the right posterior and the left anterior semicircular canals.

Caloric or Thermal Test

The semicircular canals can be tested calorically by irrigating the external auditory meatus with warm (or cold) water. This sets up convection currents in the endolymph, deflecting the crista ampullaris. Each side of the vestibular apparatus can be tested separately. For example, each horizontal semicircular canal is examined by having the patient sit with the head tilted backward about 60 degrees, bringing the horizontal semicircular canal to the vertical plane. Normally, the nystagmus is to the tested side after warm water is used (and to the opposite side after cold water is used).

Motion Sickness

Dizziness, feeling of lightheadedness, headache, nausea, and vomiting are symptoms associated with motion sickness (seasickness and airsickness). Motion sickness, whether on the sea, in the air, or on the ground (highway) is apparently the response to an excess of accelerations and decelerations as monitored by the vestibular receptors and projected to the brain.

Deaf mutes, who lack receptors in the membranous labyrinths, do not experience motion sickness. Drugs such as Dramamine raise the threshold of vestibular stimulation and, thereby, ameliorate the symptoms of motion sickness. Four out of every 10 astronauts experience motion sickness during space missions. This affliction is thought to be related to a discordance of signals monitored by the eyes, proprioceptors in the body, and the vestibular receptors in the head and projected to the brain during the novel conditions of weightlessness.

Central influences are conveyed via vestibular efferent fibers which pass through the vestibular nerve and terminate on the hair cells of the vestibular end organs. These vestibular efferent fibers probably exert inhibitory effects which ameliorate influences that might result in motion sickness and nystagmus.

In a general way, the vestibular system helps us appreciate a sense of motion and assists us in keeping our balance. Perhaps its finest expression is in such maneuvers as gymnastics, but even when one runs up a spiral staircase the vestibular system is fully engaged in its remarkable coordination of the movements of the eyes, head, trunk, and extremities.

SUGGESTED READINGS

Cohen B, ed. Vestibular and oculomotor physiology: international meeting of the Bárány Society. *Ann N Y Acad Sci.*, 1981;374:1–892.

Corwin J, Warchol M. Auditory hair cells: structure, function, development, and regeneration. *Annu Rev Neurosci.* 1991;14:301–333.

Edelman G, Gall W, Cowan W, eds. Auditory Function: Neurological Basis of Hearing. New York, NY: Wiley; 1988.

Flock Å. The ear. In: Weiss L, ed. *Cell and Tissue Biology: A Textbook of Histology.* 6th ed. Baltimore, Md: Urban & Schwartzenberg; 1988: 1107–1124.

Hudspeth A. The cellular basis of hearing: the biophysics of hair cells. *Science.* 1985;230: 745–752.

Kelly J. Hearing. In: Kandel E, Schwartz J, Jessell T, eds. *Principles of Neural Science.* 3rd ed. New York, NY: Elsevier; 1991:481–499.

Kelly J. The sense of balance. In: Kandel E, Schwartz J, Jessell T, eds. *Principles of Neural Science.* 3rd ed. New York, NY: Elsevier; 1991: 500–511.

Khanna S, Ulfendahl M, Flock Å. Changes in cellular tuning along the length of the cochlea. *Acta Otolaryngol.* 1989;467(suppl):157–162.

Netter F. *Atlas of Human Anatomy.* West Caldwell, NJ: Ciba-Geigy; 1989:plates 87–93.

Roberts W, Howard J, Hudspeth A. Hair cells: transduction, tuning, and transmission in the inner ear. *Annu Rev Cell Biol.* 1988;4:63–92.

Schuknecht H. *Pathology of the Ear.* 2nd ed. Philadelphia, Pa: Lea & Febiger; 1993.

Spoendlin H. Anatomy of cochlear innervation. *Am J Otolaryngol.* 1985;6:453–467.

Strominger NL. The anatomical organization of the primate auditory pathways. In: Noback C, ed. *Sensory Systems of Primates.* New York, NY: Plenum; 1978:53–91.

von Békésy G. *Experiments in Hearing.* New York, NY: McGraw-Hill; 1960.

Webster D, Popper A, Fay R, eds. The Mammalian Auditory Pathway: Neuroanatomy. New York, NY: Springer-Verlag; 1992.

Wilson V, Melvill-Jones G. *Mammalian Vestibular Physiology.* New York, NY: Plenum; 1979.

Lesions of the Brainstem

The effect of any lesion will depend upon the anatomic and physiologic features of the nerve tracts and nuclei interrupted, as well as the total innervation of the affected regions. In general, tracts passing through and commencing within the brainstem are oriented in a plane parallel to the long axis of the brainstem. Examples are the spinal trigeminal tract, medial lemniscus, and pyramidal tract. Cranial nerves, however, course in a plane perpendicular to the long axis. For this reason they are helpful in localizing the level of the lesion. These orientations should be kept in mind in the following account.

GENERAL STATEMENT

The long ascending (sensory) and descending (motor) pathways are generally involved with sensory and motor expressions of the contralateral (opposite) side of the body. The latter occurs when the pathway is above where it decussates. Ten pairs of cranial nerves emerge from the brainstem: from the midbrain, III and IV; from the pons, V; from the pons-medulla junc-

tion, VI, VII, and VIII; from the medulla, IX, X, XI, and XII; and from the cervical spinal cord, spinal XI. They express their roles on the same side of the body. Thus, depending on its location, a unilateral lesion may result in signs on the opposite side (lesion of a pathway above its decussation) and the ipsilateral (same) side (lesion of one or more cranial nerves) of the body.

Depending on the level, a *unilateral lesion in the medial brainstem* may result in (1) contralateral loss of position and vibratory sense (medial lemniscus in medulla or pons), (2) contralateral hemiplegia (corticospinal tract in medulla, pons, and midbrain), and (3) ipsilateral lower motoneuron (LMN) paralysis of cranial nerves XII (medulla), VI (pons-medulla junction), and III (midbrain). The combination of an LMN paralysis on the ipsilateral side of the head and an upper motoneuron (UMN) paralysis on the contralateral side of the body is known as an *alternating hemiplegia*.

A *unilateral lesion in the lateral medulla* may result in (1) contralateral loss of pain and temperature on the body (lateral spinothalamic tract), (2) ipsilateral loss of pain and temperature on the face (uncrossed spinal tract and nucleus of n. V), (3) ipsilateral Horner's syndrome (see later, descending sympathetic fibers), (4) nystagmus (vestibular nuclei; Chap. 16), and (5) unsteady ipsilateral extremities (input to cerebellum; Chap. 18). The combination of the loss of pain and temperature on the ipsilateral side of the head and the contralateral side of the body is called *alternating hemianesthesia.*

Lesions of the above noted pathways within the brainstem result in signs on the contralateral side of the body and occiput because these are *crossed tracts*: spinothalamic (decussates in spinal cord), medial lemniscus (decussates in lower medulla), and corticospinal (decussates in lower medulla). In their courses through the brainstem, (1) the spinothalamic tract is located in the lateral tegmentum, (2) the medial lemniscus shifts as it ascends from its location in the anteromedial tegmentum in the medulla to the lateral tegmentum in the midbrain before terminating in the ventral posterior lateral thalamic nucleus, and (3) the corticospinal tract descends through the ventromedial portion of the brainstem.

A unilateral lesion of the auditory pathway (lateral lemniscus and brachium of the inferior colliculus) results in only subtle changes in auditory perceptual capacity because of the strongly bilateral nature of the auditory pathway. The thresholds for sound intensity are unaffected. Unilateral lesions destroying the cochlear nuclei would produce deafness on the ipsilateral side because it would interrupt the auditory fibers prior to their decussation.

A unilateral lesion of the anterior trigeminothalamic tract in the pons and midbrain is accompanied by loss of pain and temperature on the forehead, face, nasal cavity, and oral cavity on the contralateral side. This occurs because the lesion is *above* the level where the fibers of this tract decussate in the medulla.

Cranial nerves III (midbrain), VI (pons-medulla junction), and VII (medulla) emerge on the anterior aspect of the brainstem in close proximity to the descending corticospinal tract. Injury to one of these nerves and the corticospinal tract results in an *alternating hemiplegia*—the lesion to each nerve produces an LMN paralysis on the *same side* of the head, and the lesion to the corticospinal tract produces an

UMN paralysis on the *contralateral side* of the body (because the lesion is rostral to the level of the tract's decussation). The syndrome or partial paralysis of voluntary muscles innervated by LMNs is known as a *palsy*, and that by the motoneurons of the bulb (medulla) as a *bulbar palsy*. When the corticobulbar fibers (UMNs to cranial nerves) are bilaterally interrupted, the resulting paralysis is known as *pseudobulbar palsy*. Usually, unless damage to corticobulbar fibers is bilateral, unilateral lesions lead to little, if any, motor disturbances, with the exception of the lower facial muscles. A unilateral lesion of the corticobulbar fibers causes an UMN paralysis on the contralateral side of the muscles of facial expression below the level of the eye (see Chap. 11 for explanation). Signs associated with pseudobulbar palsies include dysphagia (difficulty in swallowing), dysarthria (difficulty in articulating speech), and hyperreflexia of the jaw jerk reflex (evoked by tapping the chin gently with the jaw slightly opened).

The branchiomeric nerves (V, VII, IX, X, and XI) pass close to the spinothalamic tract before emerging on the lateral side of the brainstem. Injury to one of these nerves and the spinothalamic tract results in (1) sensory loss of the region, and an LMN paralysis of the muscles innervated by that nerve and (2) loss of pain and temperature on the contralateral side of the body and back of the head due to the interruption of the decussated fibers of the spinothalamic tract.

BLOOD SUPPLY OF THE BRAINSTEM

The sequence of vertebral arteries, basilar artery, and posterior cerebral arteries forms the main trunk system supplying arterial blood to the medulla, pons, midbrain, cerebellum, and posterior medial cerebrum (**Figs. 4.1 and 4.2**). The paired vertebral arteries ascend along the anterolateral aspect of the medulla and join at the pons-medulla junction to form the single midline basilar artery, which ascends and then divides in the midbrain region into the paired posterior cerebral arteries. Branches of these arteries supply the brainstem in patterns which may be conceptually summarized as follows: in a general way, the paramedian

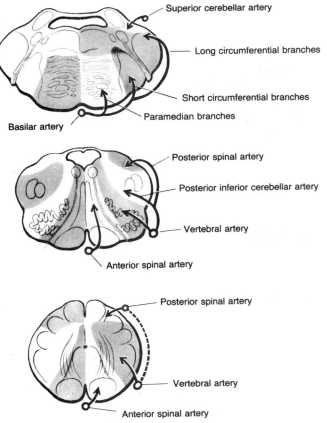

Figure 17.1: The patterns of arterial supply of the branches of the basilar artery within the pons (upper), midmedulla (middle), and caudal medulla (lower). (Refer to Fig. 4.1.)

branches are distributed to a medial zone on either side of the midsagittal plane, the short circumferential branches to an anterolateral zone, and the long circumferential branches to a posterolateral zone and to the cerebellum (**Fig. 17.1**).

MEDIAL ZONE OF THE MEDULLA

The occlusion of an anterior spinal artery and its paramedian branches to the medial zone of the medulla (**Fig. 17.2A**) may be the cause of a lesion which involves the hypoglossal nerve (n. XII), corticospinal tract of the pyramid, and medial lemniscus. The resulting *alternating hemiplegia* combines an LMN paralysis of the tongue on the ipsilateral side (n. XII) with an UMN paralysis and a loss of discriminatory gen-

eral senses (medial lemniscus) on the contralateral side of the body and both limbs. Recall that the corticospinal tract decussates at the junction of the medulla and cervical spinal cord, and that the posterior column-medial lemniscus pathway decussates in the lower medulla. During the first few weeks after the lesion, the ipsilateral half of the tongue will fibrillate (denervation sensitivity); later, the muscles atrophy and that side of the tongue appears wrinkled.

When protruded, the tongue deviates to the paralyzed side; this is due primarily to the unopposed action of the contralateral genioglossus muscle. The contralateral side of the body exhibits the signs of an UMN paralysis (corticospinal tract) and loss of position, muscle and joint sense, impaired tactile discrimination, and loss of vibratory sense (medial lemniscus), because the lesion interrupts these tracts above the level of their decussation.

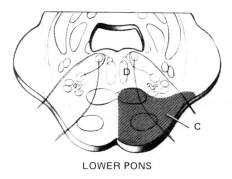

LOWER PONS

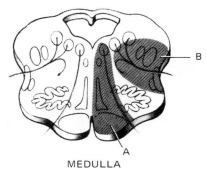

MEDULLA

Figure 17.2: Sites of lesions in the lower brainstem as described in the text. In the medulla, the lesions are located in the medial zone (A) and in the posterolateral medulla (B). In the lower pons, the lesions are located in the medial and basal portion (C) and in the medial longitudinal fasciculus (D).

Immediately after the vascular occlusion, the upper and lower limbs on the contralateral side exhibit a hypotonus with weakness, decreased stretch reflexes (deep tendon reflexes), diminished resistance to passive manipulation, loss of superficial reflexes, and loss of response to plantar stimulation. After a month or so following the onset of the lesion, the two limbs develop a spastic paralysis, hypertonia with weakness, clasp-knife resistance to passive movement (Chap. 8), hyperreflexia, loss of superficial reflexes, and the Babinski (extensor plantar) reflex.

POSTEROLATERAL MEDULLA

The failure of the posterior inferior cerebellar artery (a long circumferential artery) may be the cause of a lesion resulting in the *lateral* *medullary syndrome (Wallenberg's syndrome)* **(Fig. 17.2B).** Damage to the following structures will produce the symptoms: spinothalamic tract; spinal trigeminal tract and nucleus; fibers, and possibly nuclei, associated with the glossopharyngeal nerve, vagus nerve, bulbar portion of the accessory nerve (including the nucleus ambiguus, dorsal vagal nucleus, and tractus and nucleus solitarius) and part of the reticular formation; portions of the vestibular nuclei; and some portion of the inferior cerebellar peduncle. The symptoms include:

1. Loss of pain (*analgesia*) and temperature sensation (*thermoanesthesia*) on the contralateral side of the body, including the back of the head (crossed spinothalamic tract).
2. Loss of pain and temperature on the same side of the face and nasal and oral cavities in all three trigeminal divisions (uncrossed spinal trigeminal tract and nucleus). This combination of (1) and (2) is an *alternating hemianesthesia.*
3. Difficulty in swallowing and a voice that is hoarse and weak. This is caused by damage to the nucleus ambiguus. A lesion of the nucleus ambiguus on one side results in an ipsilateral paralysis of the palatal, pharyngeal, and laryngeal muscles, all innervated by cranial nerves IX and X. Difficulty in the initial stage of swallowing is due to paralysis of some muscles of palatal and adjacent regions. Difficulty in the later stages of swallowing (dysphagia) is due to paralysis of the pharyngeal muscles. When vocalizing, the palate and uvula deviate to the nonparalyzed side. The hoarseness occurs because of the paralysis of the musculature controlling the ipsilateral vocal cord.
4. Loss of gag reflex on the ipsilateral side and absence of sensation on the ipsilateral side of the fauces (glossopharyngeal nerve).

A bulbar palsy results following degeneration of motoneurons of the medulla. A transient tachycardia (increase in heartbeat) may result from sudden withdrawal of some parasympathetic innervation; compensatory mechanisms including influences from the contralateral vagus nerve restore normal heartbeat. The absence of visceral afferent stimulation from some visceral receptors (e.g., carotid body and carotid sinus) to the solitary nucleus is compensated for by the input from similar receptors to the normal contralateral side. The interruption of spinocerebellar and other fibers passing through the inferior cerebellar peduncle results in some signs of cerebellar malfunction on the ipsilateral side of the body—including hypotonia, asynergia, ataxia, and poorly coordinated voluntary movements (Chap. 18). Irritation of the vestibular nuclei may be expressed by nystagmus or a deviation of eyes to the ipsilateral side. Horner's syndrome (including pupillary dilatation, ptosis of eyelid, and absence of sweating from half of the face) on the same side may occur if many descending fibers of the autonomic nervous system to the thoracic sympathetic outflow are damaged. The tactile and discriminative general senses from the face are normal because the principal sensory nucleus of n. V and its ascending pathways are above the level of the lesion.

REGION OF THE CEREBELLOPONTINE ANGLE (CPA SYNDROME)

Acoustic neuromas are slow-growing tumors that originate from neurolemmal (Schwann) cells of the vestibular nerve. Those in the vicinity of the internal auditory foramen may extend into the *cerebellopontine angle (CPA)*, the junction of the cerebellum, pons and medulla near the emergence of cranial nerves VII and VIII (Fig. 13.3). In the early stages, symptoms are referable to the VIIIth cranial nerve; they include (1) tinnitus (ringing in the ears) followed by progressive deafness on the lesion side, and (2) abnormal labyrinthine (vestibular) responses, such as tilting and rotation of the head with the chin pointing to the lesion side and, at times, horizontal nystagmus. As the tumor enlarges it exerts pressure upon the brainstem and damages the fibers of the inferior and middle cerebellar peduncles, spinothalamic tract, spinal trigeminal tract, and facial nerve. The cerebellar signs that result from the involvement of the cerebellar peduncles include coarse intention tremor, dysmetria, moderate ataxic gait, dysdiadochokinesis, hypotonia, and others on the lesion side (Chap. 18). The loss of pain and temperature sensation on the ipsilateral

side of the face, oral and nasal cavities, and on the contralateral side of the body, are a consequence of damage to the spinal trigeminal tract and spinothalamic tract, respectively; this combination of ipsilateral and contralateral sensory loss is called *alternating hemianesthesia*. Injury to the facial nerve may result in an LMN paralysis of the muscles of facial expression (Bell's palsy), loss of corneal reflex, hyperacusis, and loss of taste on the anterior two thirds of the tongue ipsilaterally (Chap. 14).

MEDIAL AND BASAL PORTION OF THE CAUDAL PONS

The occlusion of paramedian and short circumferential branches of the basilar artery (Fig. 17.2C) may result in damage to the following structures within the confines of the lesion: abducent nerve (n. VI), facial nerve (n. VII), pyramidal tract, medial lemniscus, and medial longitudinal fasciculus.

The interruption of the fibers of n. VI (LMNs) and the pyramidal tract (UMNs) results in an *alternating abducent hemiplegia*. The transection of n. VI on one side produces a medial deviation of the affected eye from the unopposed pull of the medial rectus muscle (eye is cocked in). There is also horizontal diplopia (double vision) because the image of an object falls upon noncorresponding portions of the two retinas and is seen as two objects. Diplopia is maximal when the patient attempts to gaze to the lesion side. It is minimal (or absent) when gaze is directed to the side opposite the lesion because the unaffected eye and the affected eye are viewing the same visual fields. The signs occurring from damage to the corticospinal fibers, n. VII and the medial lemniscus are discussed above, and those from damage to the medial longitudinal fasciculus are discussed below.

MEDIAL LONGITUDINAL FASCICULUS

Unilateral lesions of the medial longitudinal fasciculus (Fig. 17.2D) between the abducent and oculomotor nuclei result in *internuclear ophthalmoplegia*, a disturbance of conjugate horizontal eye movements. Such a disorder is found at times in patients who have multiple sclerosis. This condition may damage fibers (by demyelination) that synchronize the contractions of the lateral rectus of one eye (abductor innervated by n. VI) and the medial rectus muscle of the opposite eye (adductor innervated by n. III). Such a unilateral lesion in the MLF results in (1) weakness of adduction of the eye on the same side as the lesion when attempting lateral gaze to the opposite side, (2) a horizontal nystagmus of the other eye (which is abducted), and (3) no impairment with convergence of the two eyes. This convergence indicates that the integration of the medial recti of both eyes by the corticobulbar fibers is preserved. The observation that the eye fails to adduct to one side upon attempted lateral gaze, but does adduct during convergence, indicates that the loss of adduction is related to a supranuclear (UMN) problem.

LATERAL HALF OF THE MIDPONS

The structures within the region of the lesion (Fig. 17.3A) include the trigeminal nerve,

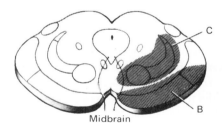

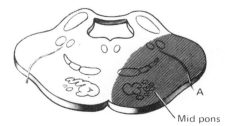

Figure 17.3: Sites of lesions in the pons and midbrain as described in the text. In the midpons, the lesion is located laterally (A). In the superior collicular level of the midbrain, the lesions are located in the basal region (B) and in the midbrain tegmentum (C).

spinothalamic tract, lateral lemniscus, and the middle cerebellar peduncle. Damage to the trigeminal nerve (n. V) results in (1) the absence of all general senses (anesthesia) on the ipsilateral side of the face, forehead, nasal, and oral cavities—including absence of corneal sensation and the corneal reflex and (2) an LMN paralysis of the muscles of mastication, with the chin deviating to the lesion side when the mouth is opened. The lesion of the medial lemniscus results in a contralateral loss of position, muscle and joint sense, impaired vibratory sense, and tactile discrimination. If the lesion is extensive enough to include the corticospinal tract, the combination of the pyramidal tract and n. V produces an *alternating trigeminal hemiplegia*. Interruption of pontocerebellar fibers may be expressed by some cerebellar signs on the same side (Chap. 18), including hypotonia, coarse intention tremor, and a tendency to fall to the side of the lesion.

Coma and the "Locked-In" Syndrome

The brain stem reticular formation contains the anatomic substrates for the reticular activating system projecting to the diencephalon and cerebral cortex (Chap. 22). The reticular system has a role in arousal, the regulation of the sleep-wake cycle, and the state of alertness (Chap. 22).

Extensive bilateral lesions involving the upper pons and midbrain reticular formation are associated with coma, which is the state of sustained unconsciousness and unresponsiveness. It differs from sleep in being less easily reversed.

Bilateral lesions of the ventral pons, usually due to an occlusion of the basilar artery, may completely interrupt the corticobulbar and corticospinal tracts on both sides. Such lesions can spare much of the reticular formation and some corticobulbar fibers to the oculomotor nuclei. These patients may be completely immobile or "locked-in" but not in a coma. They are quadriplegics who are unable to speak or have facial or tongue movements. However, such patients are fully conscious and can communicate by responding with eye movements when asked to do so because their reticular formation and corticobulbar fibers to the oculomotor nuclei are functional.

BASAL REGION OF THE MIDBRAIN (WEBER'S SYNDROME)

The occlusion of paramedian branches and short circumferential branches of the basilar and posterior cerebral arteries may produce *Weber's syndrome* (Fig. 17.3B), which is a consequence of damage to the oculomotor nerve (n. III), the corticospinal tract, and a variable number of corticobulbar and corticoreticular fibers. The interruption of all the fibers in the oculomotor nerve results in signs restricted to the ipsilateral eye, including drooping of the eyelid (*ptosis*, or inability to raise eyelid because of paralysis of levator palpebral muscle); diplopia; external *strabismus* (squint) due to unopposed contraction of the lateral rectus muscle (the eye remains maximally adducted); inability to elevate, depress, or adduct the eye; and a fully dilated pupil (the normally acting sympathetic influences are unopposed due to the absence of parasympathetic influences conveyed by the damaged parasympathetic fibers of n. III). The consensual light reflex of the contralateral eye is normal (Chap. 19). An *alternating hemiplegia* results as a consequence of the LMN paralysis of the extraocular muscles and the UMN paralysis of the contralateral side of the body from the damage to the corticospinal tract.

The unilateral interruption of the corticobulbar and corticoreticular (indirect corticobulbar) fibers results in only minimal effects upon the muscles innervated by the cranial nerves.

In general, the motor nuclei of the cranial nerves (except for the neurons of the facial nucleus innervating the lower face) receive UMN influences from both halves of the cerebrum (Fig. 11.3). Hence, unilateral lesions interrupting the UMNs to these motor nuclei usually do not produce UMN paralysis of the muscles innervated by these nerves, except for weakness of the contralateral muscles of facial expression of the lower face. In some individuals, the interruption of the UMNs to the nucleus ambiguus and hypoglossal nucleus may result in weakness of the muscles of the jaw, soft palate, and

tongue. Lesion of the UMN fibers to the motor nucleus of n. V (masticatory nucleus) may result in an exaggerated jaw jerk reflex (stretch reflex).

The explanation for these occasional observations is that the UMN innervation to the LMNs innervating these muscles is similar to the UMN innervation of the LMNs innervating the muscles of facial expression of the lower face (Fig. 11.2). The result is weakness of the muscles of the lower half of the face; the soft palate and uvula will be drawn to the same side as the lesion and the tongue will deviate to the opposite side when protruded.

The bilateral, diffuse involvement of the corticobulbar and corticoreticular fibers results in a *pseudobulbar palsy*. In this syndrome there is a bilateral paralysis or weakness without atrophy of many muscles innervated by cranial nerves. The muscle groups affected control chewing, swallowing, speaking, and breathing. Unrestrained crying and laughing occur in many subjects with pseudobulbar palsy. These emotional outbursts may be related to release from influences from the cerebral cortex and subcortical centers.

UPPER MIDBRAIN TEGMENTUM

A unilateral lesion in the midbrain tegmentum (Fig. 17.3C) limited to the region including the fibers of the oculomotor nerve, red nucleus, superior cerebellar peduncle, medial lemniscus, and spinothalamic tract results in *Benedikt's syndrome*. The damage to the red nucleus and the fibers of the superior cerebellar peduncle results in such signs of cerebellar damage as coarse intention tremor, dysdiadochokinesis, cerebellar ataxia, and hypotonia on the contralateral side of the body (Chap. 18). The injury to the third cranial nerve results in an LMN paralysis of the ipsilateral extraocular muscles and in a dilated pupil (mydriasis) from absence of parasympathetic influences (see "Basal Region of the Midbrain" above). The eye cannot be elevated, lowered, or adducted beyond the midline.

The interruption of the crossed spinothalamic tract, trigeminothalamic tract, and medial lemniscus results in loss of the sense of pain, temperature, light touch, vibratory sense, pressure touch, and other discriminatory senses on the opposite side of the body and head. Touch and other discriminatory senses on the contralateral side of the head may be retained if the uncrossed posterior trigeminothalamic tract is intact.

LESIONS OF BOTH SUPERIOR COLLICULI (PARINAUD'S SYNDROME)

Tumors of the pineal gland may compress both the superior colliculi and pretectum. The resulting lesion produces a paralysis of upward gaze (gaze in a vertical plane).

The pupils may be dilated with loss of the light reflex, but they are capable of accommodation.

SUGGESTED READINGS

Adams R, Victor M. *Principles of Neurology.* 5th ed. New York, NY: McGraw-Hill; 1993.

Bogousslavsky J, Meienberg O. Eye-movement disorders in the brain-stem and cerebellar stroke. *Arch Neurol.* 1987;44:141–148.

Gilman S, Newman S. *Manter and Gatz's Essentials of Clinical Neuroanatomy and Neurophysiology.* 8th ed. Philadelphia, Pa: FA Davis Co; 1992.

Rowland L, ed. *Merritt's Textbook of Neurology.* 9th ed. Philadelphia, Pa: Williams & Wilkins; 1994.

Rowland L. Clinical syndromes of the spinal cord and brain stem. In: Kandel E, Schwartz J, Jessell T, eds. *Principles of Neural Science.* 3rd ed. New York, NY: Elsevier; 1991:711–731.

Cerebellum

18

Gross anatomy
Subdivisions of the cerebellum
Salient features of function
General cerebellar circuitry
Functional considerations
Cerebellar dysfunction

The cerebellum is the great coordinator of muscle action and has a major function in the learning of motor tasks. It synchronizes the contractions of muscles within and among groups of muscles, smoothing out their responses by delicately regulating and grading muscle tensions. Thus, it also plays an important role in equilibrium and muscle tone. Located in the posterior cranial fossa, beneath the tentorium cerebelli and behind the pons and medulla, the cerebellum processes sensory input related to ongoing motor activity, all of it on the unconscious level. Additionally, an increasing body of evidence suggests that the cerebellum plays a role in cognitive functions.

The sensory input to the cerebellum is derived from the vestibular system, stretch receptors (neuromuscular spindles and Golgi tendon organs), and from other general sensors in the head and body. Some information is derived from the auditory and optic systems. This input is functionally integrated into the motor pathway systems and into the cerebellar feedback circuits from and to the cerebral cortex, vestibular system, and brainstem reticular formation.

GROSS ANATOMY

The cerebellum consists of (1) an outer gray mantle, the *cortex*, (2) a *medullary core* of white matter composed of nerve fibers projecting to

and from the cerebellum, and (3) four pairs of *deep cerebellar nuclei (fastigial n., globose n., emboliform n.,* and *dentate n.)*. The globose and emboliform nuclei together are often called the *interposed nucleus.*

The cerebellar surface is corrugated into parallel long narrow "gyri" called *folia*; about 15% of the cortex is exposed to the outer surface, whereas 85% faces the sulcal surfaces between the folia. The cerebellum is connected to the brainstem by three cerebellar peduncles: (1) the *inferior cerebellar peduncle* is the bridge between the medulla and the cerebellum and is composed of fibers projecting both to and from the cerebellum, (2) the *middle cerebellar peduncle* is the bridge between the basilar portion of the pons and the cerebellum and is composed of fibers projecting to the cerebellum, and (3) the *superior cerebellar peduncle* is the bridge between the midbrain and the cerebellum and is composed mainly of fibers projecting from the cerebellum to the brainstem and the thalamus; it also contains some fibers of the anterior spinocerebellar tract projecting to the cerebellum.

SUBDIVISIONS OF THE CEREBELLUM

Hemispheres, Lobes, and Zones

The cerebellum has been subdivided in three different ways on the basis of several criteria (Fig. 18.1).

251

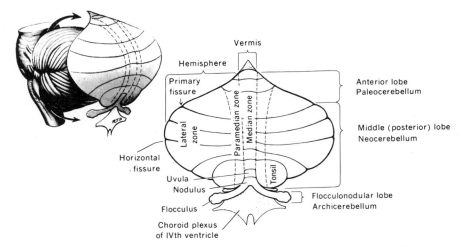

Figure 18.1: Major subdivisions and some landmarks as viewed on the surface of the cerebellum (after surface is unfolded and flattened). Serial *Roman numerals* refer to designated lobules of the vermis (some numerals are not on the vermis). Lobules of the hemispheres on either side of horizontal fissure are named crus I and crus II.

1. In a longitudinal organization, the cerebellum consists of two large bilateral *hemispheres* separated by a narrow *vermis*.
2. In a transverse organization, the cerebellum comprises three divisions: (a) flocculonodular lobe, (b) anterior lobe, and (c) middle or posterior lobe.
   a. The flocculonodular lobe consists of paired appendages called *flocculi* located posteriorly and inferiorly and joined medially by the *nodulus* (part of the vermis). It is also called the *archicerebellum* because it is phylogenetically the oldest cerebellar structure, and the *vestibulocerebellum* because this lobe is integrated with the vestibular system. The flocculonodular lobe plays a significant role in the regulation of muscle tone, maintenance of equilibrium, and posture through influences on the trunk (axial) musculature.
   b. The *anterior lobe* is located rostral to the primary fissure. It is also called the *paleocerebellum* because it is phylogenetically the next oldest cerebellar structure. This lobe, especially the vermal portion, receives proprioceptive and exteroceptive inputs from the body and limbs via the spinocerebellar pathways and from the head via fibers from the brainstem

(Fig. 10.4). It plays a role in the regulation of muscle tone.
   c. The large *posterior lobe* is located between the primary fissure and the posterolateral fissure. This phylogenetically new lobe (*neocerebellum*) receives input from cerebral cortex via a relay in the basilar pons. It performs a significant role in planning and programming of movements important for muscular coordination during phasic activities.
3. In another longitudinal organization, the cerebellum is divided into mediolaterally oriented zones. They are the (1) medial or vermal zone, (2) paramedian or paravermal zone, and (3) lateral or hemispheric zone. Each consists of a zone of cortex, underlying white matter, and a deep cerebellar nucleus to which it projects topographically. The *vermal zone* includes the *vermal cortex* and the *fastigial nuclei*. The *paravermal zone* includes the *paravermal cortex* and the *interposed nuclei*. The *hemispheric zone* includes the cortex of the cerebellar hemisphere and the *dentate nucleus*.

Cerebellar Cortex

There are three cortical layers: the outer *molecular layer*, the middle or *Purkinje cell layer*, and the *granular layer* (**Fig. 18.2**). The Purkinje

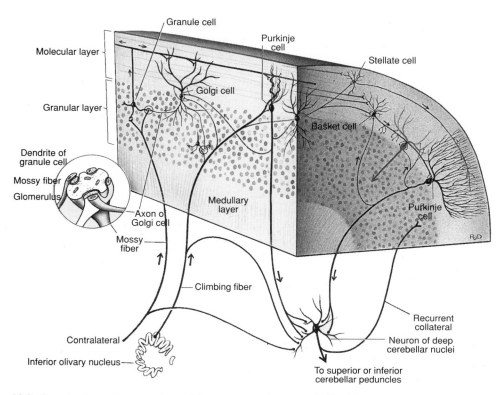

Figure 18.2: Organization and connections of the neurons within a cerebellar folium. A sagittal section through the cerebellum is represented on the right and a transverse section on the left. The long axis of a folium is in the transverse plane. The thin Purkinje cell layer, between the molecular and granular layers, is not labeled. The cerebellar glomerulus, represented in the insert, is encapsulated by a glial sheath.

layer is a thin layer characterized by the cell bodies of the Purkinje cells. All folia have the same neuronal organization. The billions of cerebellar neurons, most of which are granule cells, are arranged and oriented as follows:

A *granule cell* has a cell body and 4 to 6 short dendrites located within the granular layer; its axon projects to the molecular layer, where it bifurcates as a T into two branches (called *parallel fibers*) that course in opposite directions parallel to the long axis of the folium. The parallel fibers form excitatory synapses with the dendrites of Purkinje cells, stellate cells, Golgi cells, and basket cells. One parallel fiber synapses with the dendrites of thousands of Purkinje cells and, in turn, each Purkinje cell receives synapses from thousands of parallel fibers. Quantitatively, the granule cells in the cerebellum are estimated to at least equal the number of neurons in the cerebral cortex.

The *stellate cells* and *basket cells* are found wholly within the molecular layer. Each of these neurons has its axon oriented at right angles to the long axis of a folium. A single stellate cell axon has inhibitory synaptic connections with the dendrites of several Purkinje cells. Each basket cell axon has inhibitory synaptic connections with cell bodies of several Purkinje cells. Note that these inhibitory synapses are near the initial segment of the axon where the action potential is initiated (Chap. 3).

Each *Golgi cell* has its dendritic tree within the molecular layer; its axon terminates within glomeruli of the granular layer by forming inhibitory synapses with dendrites of granule cells. A *glomerulus* (**Fig. 18.2**) is a synaptic processing unit, encapsulated by a glial lamella, consisting of: (1) an excitatory axon terminal of a mossy fiber, (2) dendritic endings of one or more granule cells, and (3) an inhibitory axon terminal of a Golgi cell synapsing with a dendrite of the granule cell.

Each *Purkinje cell* has its cell body in the middle layer of the cortex. In fact, Purkinje cell bodies define this layer. Its dendritic tree arborizes in the molecular layer in the sagittal plane, perpendicular to the long axis of the folium, and its axon passes into the white matter to form inhibitory synaptic connections with neurons of the deep cerebellar nuclei, releasing gamma aminobutyric acid (GABA) as the neurotransmitter. This corticonuclear projection has a precise topographic organization; each cerebellar nucleus contains a complete representation of the body surface. Some Purkinje cells from the archicerebellum, as well as from the vermis of the anterior and posterior lobes, emit axons that project out of the cerebellum and form inhibitory synapses with neurons of the lateral vestibular nucleus. Recurrent axon collaterals of each Purkinje cell have inhibitory connections with other Purkinje cells, basket cells, and Golgi cells. Through these inhibitory influences, the Purkinje cells modulate the output of the deep cerebellar nuclei and of the lateral vestibular nucleus. The latter conveys excitatory influences on extensor reflex activity (Chap. 16).

SALIENT FEATURES OF FUNCTION

Climbing and *mossy fibers* convey excitatory input directly from the spinal cord and brainstem, through the cerebellar peduncles, to the deep cerebellar nuclei and cerebellar cortex. The climbing fibers in each cerebellar hemisphere originate exclusively from the contralateral inferior olivary nucleus and enter the cerebellum via the inferior cerebellar peduncle (Fig. 18.2). They exert powerful excitatory influences not only on the cells of the deep cerebellar nuclei, but also on Purkinje cells. Every climbing fiber divides within the granular layer into up to ten branches (also called climbing fibers) each of which enters the molecular layer and makes up to several hundred synaptic contacts on dendrites of a single Purkinje cell. Whereas collateral branches may contact several adjacent Purkinje cells, an individual Purkinje cell receives input from only one climbing fiber.

The mossy fibers originate from nuclei in the spinal cord, receptors of the vestibular nerve, and vestibular, trigeminal, pontine, and reticular nuclei of the brainstem. These fibers, which branch profusely, exert excitatory influences on numerous granule cells within the glomeruli of the granular layer. Collaterals of mossy fibers, as well as of climbing fibers also may, depending on the source, form excitatory synapses with the deep nuclei of the cerebellum. Through their parallel fibers, the packed granule cells make excitatory synaptic connections with the dendrites of the Purkinje cells and, in addition, with the dendrites of the stellate cells, basket cells, and Golgi cells of the molecular layer. After excitation, the stellate cells and basket cells exert inhibitory influences on Purkinje cells. Similarly, the Golgi cells inhibit the granule cells within the glomeruli.

The following is an account of how the output from the cerebellar cortex is orchestrated. The Purkinje cells, through their axons, are the only outlet for processed information from the cerebellar cortex. Their output, directed to the deep cerebellar nuclei and the lateral vestibular nucleus, is solely inhibitory. Insofar as mossy and climbing fibers supply only excitatory inputs, it is the Purkinje fibers that modulate, through inhibition, the output from the deep cerebellar nuclei to targets outside the cerebellum (and output from the lateral vestibular nucleus). As mentioned, Purkinje cells are excited, as well as inhibited, by stimuli from other cells. The climbing fibers and granule cells contribute excitatory influences; the stellate and basket cells convey inhibitory stimuli.

A final element of this mosaic concerns the granule cells. Granule cell output is modulated by inhibitory influences from Golgi cells. The latter in turn depend on granule cells for their own activation. This negative feedback circuit consists of the sequence (1) granule cell, (2) Golgi cell, and (3) Golgi cell axons that extend back to form inhibitory synapses on granule cells within glomeruli.

In summary, the wholly excitatory input to the cerebellum is via mossy and climbing fibers. Of the neurons whose cell bodies are located within the cerebellar cortex, the granule cells are the only excitatory ones. The Golgi, Purkinje, stellate, and basket cells are inhibitory neurons, whose neurotransmitter is GABA. They act as modulators. The cerebellar nuclei also convey excitatory input to the granular layer of cerebellar cortex via nucleocortical connections, some of which are collaterals of fibers that project out of the cerebellum.

In addition, aminergic cell groups such as the locus ceruleus and raphe nuclei of the brainstem provide another input to the cerebellum. Their projections terminate in the deep cerebellar nuclei and the cerebellar cortex, including from the locus ceruleus directly on Purkinje cell somata. The projections from the locus ceruleus are noradrenergic and those from the raphe nuclei are serotoninergic. Input from these sources is thought to have generalized effects on the tone of cerebellar activity.

GENERAL CEREBELLAR CIRCUITRY

Input to the Cerebellum

There are approximately 3 times as many cerebellar afferent fibers as cerebellar efferent fibers.

The *inferior cerebellar peduncle (restiform body)* is composed of fibers of the posterior spinocerebellar tract, cuneocerebellar tract, rostral spinocerebellar tract, reticulocerebellar fibers, olivocerebellar fibers, and trigeminocerebellar fibers. The *juxtarestiform body* (bundle of fibers on medial aspect of the inferior cerebellar peduncle) contains vestibulocerebellar fibers (Chap. 16). The posterior spinocerebellar, cuneocerebellar, and rostral cerebellar tracts convey information from the stretch and exteroceptive receptors of the body via the spinal cord to the anterior lobe of the cerebellum (Chap. 10). The reticulocerebellar fibers project from the lateral reticular nucleus of the medulla (input to this nucleus is from the spinal cord, red nucleus, and fastigial nucleus) and paramedian nuclei of the medulla, largely as uncrossed components, to the anterior lobe and vermis. The olivocerebellar fibers originate in the contralateral inferior olivary nucleus of the medulla and terminate in all cortical areas of the cerebellum. The accessory olivary nuclei project to the vermis, and the principal olivary nucleus projects to the opposite cerebellar hem-

isphere. Input to the inferior olivary nuclei is derived from the cerebral cortex, brainstem reticular nuclei, dorsal column nuclei, and red nucleus, as well as from the cerebellum. The *inferior olivary nucleus* is the only source of climbing fibers to the cerebellum. The trigeminocerebellar fibers convey influences from stretch and exteroceptive receptors of the head. Primary fibers from the vestibular nerve and secondary fibers from vestibular nuclei pass, as vestibulocerebellar fibers, through the juxtarestiform body before terminating in the flocculonodular lobe and adjacent cortex (referred to as the *vestibulocerebellum*). Secondary vestibular fibers emit collaterals to the fastigial nuclei as well.

The *middle cerebellar peduncle (brachium pontis)* is composed of crossed pontocerebellar fibers projecting from the pontine nuclei in the basilar pons to the neocerebellum and paleocerebellum. This tract conveys influences from the cerebral cortex transmitted via the corticopontine tract (see below under "Feedback Loops").

The *superior cerebellar peduncle (brachium conjunctivum)* contains fibers of the anterior spinocerebellar tract, which terminate in the anterior lobe. (See p. 197 and **Fig. 13.13**; see also Chap. 10.)

Output from the Cerebellum

The cerebellum influences motor coordination almost entirely through indirect pathways (**Figs. 18.3 and 18.4**). There is some evidence supporting the presence of a small projection directly to the spinal cord.

The outflow through the juxtarestiform body includes (1) crossed and uncrossed fastigiobulbar fibers from the fastigial nuclei to the vestibular nuclei and reticular nuclei of the pons and medulla, (2) a few fibers that synapse monosynaptically on lower motoneurons in the contralateral upper cervical spinal cord, and (3) some direct fibers from the cortex of the vestibulocerebellum (flocculonodular lobe) to the vestibular nuclei. Some fibers from the fastigial nuclei pass around the rostral aspect of the superior cerebellar peduncle as the *uncinate (hooked) fasciculus* before passing through the juxtarestiform body (**Figs. 13.12 and 18.4**).

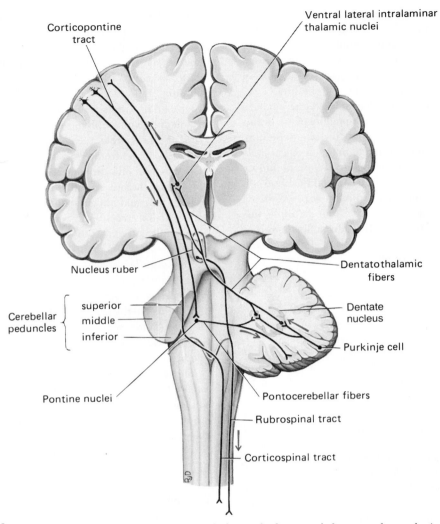

Figure 18.3: Cerebellar (neocerebellar) connections with the cerebral cortex, thalamus, and some brainstem nuclei.

Each fastigial nucleus receives input from the vestibular nuclei and archicerebellum.

The *superior cerebellar peduncle* consists primarily of efferent fibers from the dentate, emboliform, and globose nuclei. Those arising from the large dentate nucleus are called the dentatorubral, dentatothalamic, and dentatoreticular tracts. The entire outflow crosses over in the lower midbrain as the decussation of the superior cerebellar peduncle. Most fibers from the dentate nucleus project rostrally to the ventral lateral (VL) and intralaminar thalamic nuclei, with some fibers terminating in the rostral (parvocellular) third of the red nucleus that

gives rise to the rubroolivary tract; other fibers turn caudally as the *descending branch of the superior cerebellar peduncle* to terminate in the brainstem reticular nuclei (reticulotegmental nucleus) as well as the principal inferior olive. The globose and emboliform nuclei project to the caudal (magnocellular) part of the red nucleus that is the source of the rubrospinal tract, and also emit fibers to the brainstem reticular nuclei; some fibers go to the dorsal and medial accessory olives and a few to the upper cervical the spinal cord where they terminate upon interneurons in the intermediate grey.

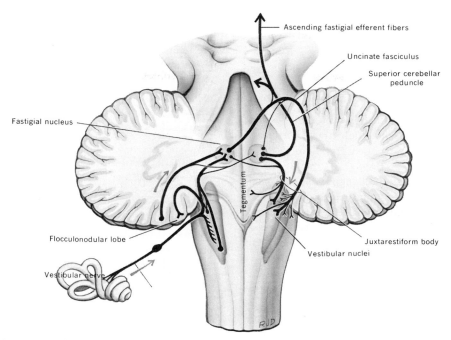

Figure 18.4: The vestibulocerebellar pathways. Left, input to the cerebellum; right, output from the cerebellum.

FUNCTIONAL CONSIDERATIONS

The cerebellum may be divided into four anatomic zones: (1) median zone or vermis, (2) paramedian zone or intermediate hemisphere, (3) lateral zone or lateral hemisphere, and (4) floccular-nodular lobe or vestibulocerebellum (**Fig. 18.1**). Three recognized functional divisions include the (1) *spinocerebellum*, that comprises the median zone and paramedian zone, (2) *cerebrocerebellum*, that comprises the lateral zone, and (3) *vestibulocerebellum* or flocculonodular lobe.

The spinocerebellum is involved in the control of movements of the body axis (posture) and primarily proximal limbs. It receives somatosensory input from the spinal cord, telling about the progress of ongoing movements, and generates information to correct errors. The cerebrocerebellum receives strong input from the cerebral cortex and is involved in the planning of movement and learning of sequences in complex movements such as playing a piano. The vestibulocerebellum receives input from the vestibular receptors and is involved in the maintenance of balance and regulation of head and eye movements. It is important to realize that these circuits are indicative of the complex anatomic circuitry by which the cerebellum is integrated into the control of motor activity of the muscles of the body (see subsequent section concerning circuitry).

These functional divisions of the cerebellar cortex have similar patterns in the organization of their intrinsic circuitry, as described previously in this chapter. Each division differs, however, from the others with respect to the specific sources of afferent input and the specific neural centers to which it projects.

Each of the circuits outlined subsequently is organized to become involved in specific aspects of the functional control of certain muscle groups. In brief, the vermis is associated with the control of axial muscles, the intermediate hemisphere with the control of limb muscles, the cerebrocerebellum with the planning of movement, and the vestibulocerebellum with the maintenance of balance and control of eye movements. Recall that the deep cerebellar nuclei receive excitatory input from the climbing fibers, with all these projections derived from the inferior olivary nucleus. Note that these circuits are organized to relay their influences selectively to both the medial and lateral descending systems (Chap. 11).

Circuitry Associated with the Vermis (Vermal Zone)

Somatic sensory information from the body and limbs is conveyed somatotopically via the dorsal spinocerebellar and cuneocerebellar tracts to the cortex of the vermis (Fig. 10.7; Chap. 10). In addition, afferent input from the head is derived from the spinal trigeminal nucleus and vestibular, auditory, and visual systems. The vermal cortex projects to the fastigial nucleus, which, in turn, projects to two different regions via fibers passing through the inferior cerebellar peduncle. (1) Most of the fibers descend in the juxtarestiform body and central tegmental tract of the brainstem to the pontine and medullary reticular nuclei. (2) A few fibers ascend and terminate mainly in the contralateral VL nucleus of the thalamus. Projections from this part of VL ascend and terminate in the regions of the primary motor cortex which give rise to the anterior corticospinal tract. The pontine and medullary reticular nuclei give rise respectively to the medial and lateral reticulospinal tracts. All three of these tracts belong to the *medial descending systems* (Chap. 11), which terminate in the medial column of spinal gray matter, from which originate the lower motoneurons innervating axial musculature. *Thus, the linkage between the vermis (vermal zone) and the control of the axial and girdle musculature.*

Circuitry Associated with Intermediate Lobe (Paravermal Zone)

Somatic sensory information is conveyed via the dorsal spinocerebellar and cuneocerebellar tracts to the cortex of the intermediate lobe (Chap. 10). This cortex projects to the interposed nuclei. Fibers from these nuclei pass through the superior cerebellar peduncle and cross in the decussation of the superior cerebellar peduncle. Some fibers terminate in the magnocellular portion of the nucleus ruber. Others ascend and terminate in the VL. The latter projects to the primary motor cortex (area 4) and the supplementary motor cortex (area 6). The *lateral descending systems* originate from

these sources: the rubrospinal tract from the magnocellular portion of the nucleus ruber, and the lateral corticospinal tract from the primary motor and supplementary cortices. These tracts control the activity of the musculature of the extremities. *Note the linkage between the intermediate lobe (paravermal zone) and the control of musculature of the extremities.*

Circuitry Associated with the Cerebrocerebellum (Lateral Hemisphere or Zone)

The cerebellar hemisphere is reciprocally interconnected with the cerebral cortex. The output originates from many areas of the cerebral cortex, but largely from the motor cortices (areas 4 and 6) and the somatic sensory cortices (areas 1, 2, 3, and 5). These projections comprise the corticopontine fibers that pass successively through the posterior limb of the internal capsule, the crus cerebri of the midbrain, and terminate in the ipsilateral pontine nuclei. From these nuclei, pontocerebellar fibers decussate and form the middle cerebellar peduncle; they terminate in the contralateral cerebellar cortex of the lateral hemisphere. Axons of Purkinje cells arising from this cortex, project to the dentate nucleus. This nucleus gives rise to fibers that course through the superior cerebellar peduncle to terminate in two different structures. (1) Some fibers contribute to the following circuit: They cross in the decussation of the superior cerebellar peduncle and terminate in the contralateral parvocellular division of the red nucleus which gives rise to the rubroolivary fibers that terminate in the inferior olivary complex. A few postdecussational fibers in the peduncle turn caudally and go directly to the inferior olivary complex. This complex is the source of the olivocerebellar fibers that decussate and enter the inferior cerebellar peduncle to terminate as climbing fibers. The inferior olive is the only source of climbing fibers; they terminate and synapse with the neurons in both the deep cerebellar (fastigial, interpositus, and dentate) nuclei and axodendritically on the Purkinje cells of the cerebellar cortex. (2) The largest number of fibers cross over in the decussation of the superior cerebellar peduncle and ascend to terminate in the VL. This nucleus projects to primary motor cortex and premotor cortex. The primary motor cortex gives rise to the lateral corticospinal tract of the *lateral descending systems* and anterior corticospinal tract of the *medial descending system*. The premotor cortex gives rise to corticoreticular fibers to the pontine and medullary reticular nuclei, which give rise to the medial and lateral reticulospinal tracts of the *medial descending system. Note the linkage between the lateral hemispheric zone and the cerebrum for the planning of movement.*

Circuitry Associated with the Vestibulocerebellum (Flocculonodular Lobe)

The input to the vestibulocerebellar cortex is derived from the vestibular nuclei and, in addition, directly from the vestibular labyrinth via some fibers of the vestibular nerve. Purkinje cell axons from this cortex project ipsilaterally to the fastigial nucleus and to the medial, inferior, and superior vestibular nuclei. Cortex of the uvula, which may in terms of connectivity be considered as part of the vestibulocerebellum, sends fibers to the lateral vestibular nucleus. The projections to the vestibular nuclei (the only projections from the cerebellar cortex to a noncerebellar site) indicate that these nuclei are similar to deep cerebellar nuclei. The medial vestibular nucleus gives rise to the medial vestibulospinal tract of the *medial descending system*. A few fibers from the fastigial nucleus ascend and pass through the superior cerebellar peduncle and terminate in the contralateral VL nucleus. These VL neurons project to those sites of primary motor cortex that give rise to the anterior corticospinal tract of the *medial descending system. Note the linkage between the flocculonodular lobe and the axial musculature* (see discussion of the vestibular system in Chap. 16).

Thalamic Projections of the Cerebellar Nuclei

As noted, the dentate, interposed, and fastigial nuclei all project to the ventrolateral nucleus of the thalamus. Fibers originating in these nuclei terminate in a relatively acellular zone sandwiched between, and separate from, the projection fields of the somatosensory pathways (more posteriorly) and of the basal ganglia (more anteriorly). The entirely crossed terminations from the dentate and interposed nuclei are separate but interdigitating. The small number of fibers from the fastigial nucleus are distributed bilaterally to a more limited region. This indicates that the functional differences of the cerebellar zones are retained at thalamic levels.

Internal Feedback Connections to the Cerebellum

The anterior spinocerebellar and the rostrocerebellar tracts that terminate in the vermis (Chap. 10) probably do not relay sensory information derived from the periphery to the cerebellum. Rather these tracts are thought to be in an *internal feedback circuit* to the cerebellum. *These nuclei may be monitoring neural activity of the descending motor pathways and then informing the cerebellum.*

Postulated Role of Cerebellum in Cognitive and Language Function

The presence of reciprocal connections between the phylogenetically new cerebellar structures (ventrolateral parts of the dentate nucleus, referred to as the neodentate, and some of the lateral lobe cortex) and the frontal association areas of the cerebral cortex suggest that the cerebellum has a role in cognitive function. Evidence from imaging studies (MRI and PET) support the view that the "computational power of the cerebellum" is used for some non-motor activities such as solving a puzzle and language processing. Deficits in the latter and in error-detection have been reported in a PET documented case with unilateral cerebellar damage.

CEREBELLAR DYSFUNCTION

The key to cerebellar function is thought to be the inhibitory control by the cerebellar cortex through the Purkinje cells upon the level of excitability of the deep cerebellar nuclei and their output. The delicate and subtle interactions of the cerebellar cortex with these deep nuclei are basic to the precision, speed, and coordination essential for motor activities. These are expressions of *synergy*, which is the cooperative activity of all the muscles utilized in each motor act.

Lesions of the cerebellum, that is, of its input

fibers, output fibers or cortex, result in symptoms which are actually the result of the activity of noncerebellar centers, e.g., the VL nucleus of the thalamus. These centers, released from cerebellar influences, produce so-called *release phenomena* that are the expression of the loss of negative feedback. For instance, in moving the upper extremity to touch an object with the tip of a finger there is an *intention tremor*—the extremity, especially the hand and finger, oscillates back and forth as the tip of the finger approaches the object. This resembles an airplane's automatic-pilot control system, in which each correction is followed by a small overshoot. In the normal cerebellum, negative feedback activity reduces each overshoot to insignificance. Thus, the cerebellum acts as servomechanism in a negative feedback system, functioning to prevent oscillations (tremor) during motion and thereby maintaining stability in a movement.

Unilateral cerebellar lesions have *homolateral* effects. The symptoms are expressed on the same side of the body because the pathways from the cerebellum decussate and integrate with pathway systems that, in turn, cross over to the side of the original cerebellar output to exert their effects. For example, one side of the cerebellum projects via the crossed dentatothalamocortical pathway to the contralateral red nucleus and cerebral cortex. In turn, the rubrospinal and corticospinal tracts are crossed descending pathways. In effect, the cerebellum exerts its influences through a double crossing of (1) the ascending fibers of the decussating superior cerebellar peduncle and (2) the decussating descending rubrospinal and corticospinal tracts.

Lesions of the cerebellum result in disturbances expressed as a *constellation* of symptoms and neurologic signs (noted below). Small lesions may produce no symptoms or only transient symptoms, whereas large lesions produce severe symptoms. The cerebellar cortex possesses a good margin of physiologic safety; with sufficient time the neurologic symptoms attenuate, and the resulting compensation, presumably by other mechanisms in the brain, markedly reduces the severity of the deficits.

Lesions of the lateral cerebellum result in

asynergia of the limbs on the same side. Lesions in the vermis result in titubation (see later).

Neocerebellar Lesions

With neocerebellar lesions, the tendon reflexes are diminished (*hypotonia*); this effect is expressed as a pendular knee jerk that swings freely back and forth. Muscles tire easily (*asthenia*). An arm extended horizontally gradually drifts downward when the eyes are closed because proprioceptive sense is used improperly. *Asynergia*, or loss of muscular coordination, is expressed by jerky, puppetlike movements including the decomposition of movement, dysmetria, past pointing, and dysdiadochokinesis.

The *decomposition of movement* is the breaking up of a movement into its component parts; instead of a smooth, coordinated flow of movement in bringing the tip of the finger of the extended upper extremity to the nose, each joint of the shoulder, elbow, wrist, and finger may flex independently (puppetlike) in an almost mechanical fashion. *Dysmetria*, or the inability to gauge or measure distances accurately, results in the overshooting of an intended goal by consistent pointing toward the lesion side of the object (*past pointing*). *Dysdiadochokinesis* is the impairment of the ability to execute alternating and repetitive movements, such as supination and pronation of the forearm, in rapid succession with equal excursions. *Intention tremor* is expressed during the execution of a voluntary movement. It is absent or diminished during rest. These tremors are particularly noted at the end of the movement. Such *terminal tremor* is exhibited when the patient is asked to touch the tip of his nose with the tip of the index finger. As the limb approaches the nose, the hand and finger will exhibit terminal tremor. The larger the cerebellar lesion, the more pronounced the tremor.

The *ataxic gait*, or the asynergic activity elicited during walking, is a staggering movement resembling that of drunkenness. The ataxia is due to incoordination of the trunk and proximal girdle muscles. A tendency to veer or to fall to the side of the lesion is apparent. To counteract the unsteadiness, the patient will stand or walk with legs far apart (broad-based stance). Clinicians usually equate asynergy with ataxia.

Lack of check (rebound phenomenon) is demonstrable in neocerebellar lesions. Lack of check is the inability of a rapidly moving limb to stop quickly and sharply; in the attempt to stop the limb there is an overshoot and then a rebound (overshoot in the opposite direction). For example, the forearm is flexed at the elbow against a strong resistance exerted by the examiner; when the examiner suddenly removes the resistance, the forearm jerks forward and the subject is unable to check the motion before the hand strikes the chest.

A *scanning speech*, or *dysarthria*, is the result of the incoordination of the muscles used in speaking. The speech is hesitating, slurred and explosive in quality, with a telegram-staccato pace (pauses in the wrong places). Although the mechanism of speech is impaired, there is no aphasia (Chap. 25).

Lesion of the Vermal and Paravermal Zones

These zones comprise the vermis, flocculonodular lobe, and fastigial nuclei. Stance and gait are affected. The patient stands and walks with a broad base and feet several inches apart. A truncal tremor may occur. The subject has difficulty in placing the heel of one foot in front of the other foot in a sequential order (impairment in *walking in tandem*). The head may be rotated or tilted to one side or the other. The choice of side is not an accurate clue to the location of the lesion site. *Titubation* is expressed. Titubation is a truncal tremor occurring when the patient is sitting or standing; this rapid rhythmic tremor of the head or body occurs several times per second. Nystagmus often results.

Cortical degeneration affecting both the vermis and the anterior lobe, seen in some alcoholic patients, is described in the next section.

Lesion of Paleocerebellum (Anterior Lobe)

A lesion involving the anterior lobe occurs in a form of cerebellar cortical degeneration affecting certain alcoholic subjects. It involves the lower limbs and gait. The gait is ataxic and wide-based. The asynergia of the lower limbs can be demonstrated by the *heel-shin test* in which the heel of one foot is made to slide down the shin of the opposite leg.

Archicerebellar Lesions

Lesions of the flocculonodular lobe may result in ataxia of the trunk muscles without any signs of tremor or hypotonia. Children with nodular lobe tumors have a tendency to fall backward, sway from side to side, and walk with a wide base and an ataxic gait. They may be unable to maintain an upright balance.

SUGGESTED READINGS

Arshavsky Y, Gelfand I, Orlovsky G. The cerebellum and control of rhythmical movements. *Trends Neurosci.* 1983;6:417–422.

Asanuma C, Thach W, Jones E. Brainstem and spinal projections of the deep cerebellar nuclei in the monkey, with observations on the brainstem projections of the dorsal column nuclei. *Brain Res Rev.* 1983;5:299–322.

Dietrichs E, Walberg F. Cerebellar nuclear afferent—where do they originate? A re-evaluation of the projections from some lower brain stem nuclei. *Anat Embryol (Berl).* 1987;177:165–172.

Eccles J, Ito M, Szentagothai J. *The Cerebellum as a Neuronal Machine.* New York, NY: Springer Verlag; 1967.

Fiez J, Petersen S, Cheney M, Raichle M. Impaired non-motor learning and error detection associated with cerebellar damage. A single case study. *Brain.* 1992;115:155–178.

Gilman S, Bloedel J, Lechtenberg R. *Disorders of the Cerebellum.* Philadelphia, Pa: FA Davis Co; 1981.

Ghez C. The cerebellum. In: Kandel E, Schwartz J, Jessell T, eds. *Principles of Neural Science.* 3rd ed. New York, NY: Elsevier; 1991:626–646.

Gould B. The organization of afferents to the cerebellar cortex in the cat. Projections from the deep cerebellar nuclei. *J Comp Neurol.* 1979;184:27–42.

Ito M. *The Cerebellum and Neural Control.* New York, NY: Raven Press; 1984.

Kim S, Ugurbil K, Strick P. Activation of a cerebellar output nucleus during cognitive processing. *Science.* 1994;265:949–951.

King J, ed. New Concepts in Cerebellar Neurobiology. New York, NY: Liss; 1987.

Leiner H, Leiner A, Dow R. Cognitive and LAnguage functions of the human cerebellum. Trends Neurosci. 1993;16:444–447.

Llinás R, Sotelo C, eds. *The Cerebellum Revisited.* New York, NY: Springer Verlag; 1992.

Middleton F, Strick P. Anatomical evidence for cerebellar and basal ganglia involvement in higher cognitive function. *Science.* 1994;266:458–461.

Oscarsson O. Functional units of the cerebellum-sagittal zones and microzones. *Trends Neurosci.* 1979;2:143–145.

Stein J. Role of the cerebellum in the visual guidance of movement. *Nature.* 1986;323:217–221.

Thach W, Goodkin H, Keating J. The cerebellum and the adaptive coordination of movement. *Annu Rev Neurosci.* 1992;15:403–442.

Zagon I, McLaughlin P, Smith S. Neural populations in the human cerebellum: estimations from isolated cell neuclei. *Brain Res.* 1977;127:279–282.

Visual System 19

Eye
Pathways of the visual system
Visual cortex
Reflex pathways
Control of eye movements
Lesions within the visual pathways

Sight is our dominant sense—we live largely in a visual world. Yet our eyes detect only a small part of the broad spectrum of electromagnetic radiation engulfing us. They are sensitive only in the wavelengths ranging from 400 to 700 nm, i.e., from blue to red. This is the visual spectrum. The visual system conveys its influences from the eyes via several pathways or channels associated with different functional aspects of vision.

EYE

The eye is a globe that is composed of three coats (Fig. 19.1). The outer coat, moving from posterior to anterior, consists of the sclera and the cornea; the middle layer consists of the choroid, ciliary body, and iris diaphragm; and the inner layer consists of the retina, which is the neural portion of the eye. The lens is suspended behind the iris diaphragm by fine "guy ropes" called *zonula fibers* that are anchored in the folds of the ciliary body.

The cornea is the nonadjustable lens of the eye, whereas the lens proper is adjustable. The ciliary body contains involuntary muscles that vary the tension exerted on the lens by the zonula fibers. Such adjustment alters the shape of the lens and is called *accommodation*.

The iris diaphragm surrounds the pupil. Action by the muscles of the iris causes the pupil

to be enlarged or reduced, thereby regulating the amount of light passing into the depths of the eye. Contraction of the radial muscles of the iris causes dilation of the pupil. Contraction of the circular (sphincter) muscles causes constriction of the pupil.

Retina

The retina is the mobile portion of the central nervous system (CNS) (i.e., the eyes move). It functions as a relatively simplified and miniaturized brain. Its five neuronal cell types include the receptor (rods and cones), bipolar, horizontal, amacrine, and ganglion cells (Fig. 19.2). The axons of the ganglion cells are the fibers that transmit action potentials via the optic nerves and tracts to the brain. The other cells communicate, not via action potentials, but only via local potentials.

The environment viewed by the eyes is called the *visual field*. Light waves from the visual field enter the eyes and stimulate the photopigments in the disks of the outer segments of the *rods* and *cones*, which are the photoreceptor neurons of the visual system (Fig. 19.3). The photopigments are the light absorbing molecules concerned with visual transduction. The rods are light sensitive because they contain the visual pigment *rhodopsin*, which absorbs photons. Each rhodopsin molecule is composed of two components—*retinal* (a prosthetic group) and *opsin* (protein moiety). Retinal, a form of vita-

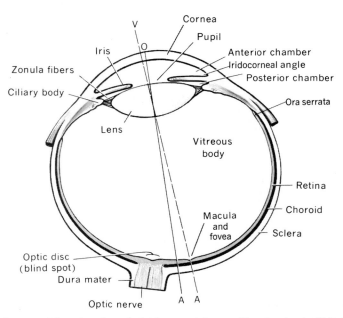

Figure 19.1: Horizontal equatorial section through the human right eye. The visual axis (VA) is the line joining the fixation or "nodal point" (center of object in focus) within the lens with the fovea. The optical axis (OA) is the line passing through the optical centers of the principal refracting surfaces of the cornea and lens.

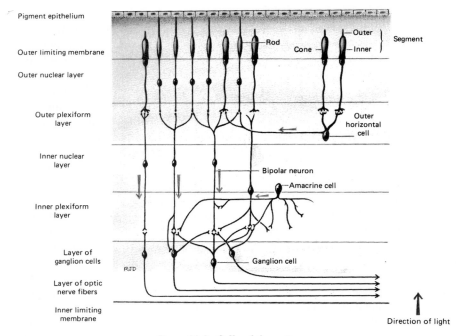

Figure 19.2: Cells of the retina.

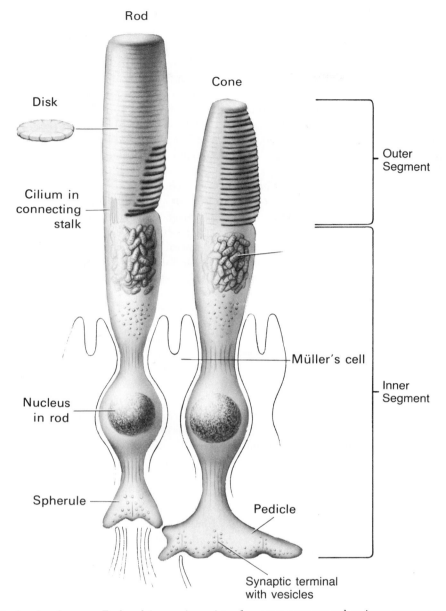

Figure 19.3: A rod and a cone. Each rod (or cone) consists of an outer segment and an inner segment connected by a cilium. The outer segment of the rod is rod-shaped and that of a cone is cone-shaped. In both, the receptor disks are specialized structures of the plasma membrane that contain the photopigments (integral proteins). The new disks of a rod are continuously formed by repeated infolding of the plasma membrane at the base of the outer segment. The disks of the cones are not continuously replaced. The inner segment contains the biosynthetic organelles and the synaptic terminals.

min A, is the light absorbing chromatophore molecule. It is attached to opsin, an integral protein of the plasma and disk membranes. Rhodopsin mediates vision in dim light absorbed maximally at 495 nm. The critical event regarding vision is the trapping of photons of light by the photopigment. The photon converts retinal from the II-cis form to the all-trans form. This triggers changes in the opsin which, in turn, activates *second messengers* that are involved in the neural signal of the rod. This exposure to light results in the *hyperpolarization* of the plasma membrane and *is the only light-dependent phase of visual excitation*. Light has performed its role. Amazingly, photoreceptors are normally excited in the dark. Darkness excites (depolarizes through an increase in sodium conductance) the rods and cones so that they spontaneously release an inhibitory transmitter. Following the action of light, the hyperpolarization decreases the amount of inhibitory transmitter released at the synapses with the bipolar cells. This results in the depolarization of the bipolar cells followed by excitation of the ganglion cells (Fig. 19.2). The horizontal cells and amacrine cells are the interneurons that affect the neural processing by modulating the activity of the bipolar and ganglion cells.

The *cones* are the mediators of color vision. Like rhodopsin, the visual pigments of the cones are composed of opsin and retinal. Unlike the rods, there are three types of cones in the human retina. Each cone type contains a different cone opsin, which absorbs a different part of the visual spectrum. The three cone pigments involved with color vision have their absorption spectra maxima at approximately 420 nm (blue-sensitive pigment), 530 nm (green-sensitive pigment), and 560 nm (red-sensitive pigment).

The light receptors in each eye include more than 100 million rods and 7 million cones (Fig. 19.2). Within the retina there is considerable convergence from the receptor rods and cones to the million ganglion neurons whose axons terminate in the brain. The exception is the direct private line connections of a cone to bipolar neurons to ganglion neurons within the *fovea centralis*. The fovea is an area within the macula where visual acuity is sharpest and color vision is optimal (Fig. 19.1); it contains cones, but no rods. In summary, the rod system (rods and

their projections) is a convergent pathway with high sensitivity and low visual acuity. The cone system is color coded, with low sensitivity and high visual acuity. In the fovea, where the cones also are smaller than further peripherally, it is a point-to-point private line pathway.

Each of the 1 million ganglion cells in each retina receives stimulation from a spot in the environment. The cell's view of the environment is called its *center-surround receptor field* and consists of a small circle composed of either an *on* excitatory center (like a hole in a doughnut) and an *off* inhibitory surround (the doughnut), or an *off* center and an *on* surround (Fig. 19.4). Each cell relays signals concerning the contrast between the intensity of illumination in the center and that in the surround. The neurons of the optic system respond to contrasts. The opponent or antagonistic organization between the center and the surround is called center-surround opponency. The retina is like a mosaic of ganglion cells sending a stream of center-surround signals. Those directed to the lateral geniculate body (LGB) of the thalamus are received by cells of similar orientation that relay the signals to the primary visual cortex (area 17, V1).

In primates, there are two main functional classes of retinal ganglion neurons, called P and M cells, and a third minor class without designation. The *P cells*, which are the most common type, have small cell bodies whose axons project to the parvocellular layers of the LGB. These neurons are color coded and also mediate fine detail at high contrasts. The *M cells* have larger cell bodies and wider dendritic fields, whose axons project mainly to the magnocellular layers of the LGB, although some also send collaterals to the tectum of the midbrain (superior colliculi). These neurons provide information concerning patterns and are very sensitive to smaller contrasts in illumination. They also detect moving stimuli. The *third class* of ganglion cells, less than 10% of the total, has variably sized cell bodies with axons of varied conducting rates that project to both the LGB and the tectum. Their functional role is enigmatic. The functional significance of the P and M cell concept is that two classes of ganglion cells are projecting information from the retina via separate channels. Thus, the visual pathways are organized to express the *principle of parallel*

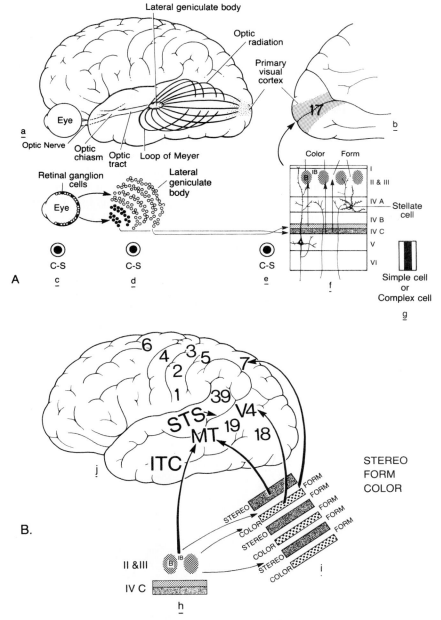

Figure 19.4: Diagram of the functional segregation of the visual system. **A.** (a) Lateral view of visual pathway. The fibers projecting from the lateral geniculate body (LGB) to the primary visual cortex (area 17, visual area 1, V1) comprise the optic radiation (geniculocalcarine pathway). (b) Medial view of occipital lobe illustrating the primary visual cortex. (c) Ganglion cells of retina with center-surround (C-S) receptive field. (d) LGB: the magnocellular neurons (laminae I and II) are functionally color blind, have fast response, high-contrast sensitivity, and low resolution; parvocellular neurons (laminae III through VI) are functionally color selective, have slow response, low-contrast sensitivity, and high resolution. All neurons have center-surround receptive fields. (e) Cell of lamina IV (area 17) with center-surround receptive field. (f) Section through primary visual cortex and its laminae (see text for explanation). (g) Simple cell and complex cell, each with a receptive field comprised of the on-slit flanked by off-slits. **B.** (h) Lateral view of a cerebral hemisphere with some of Brodmann's areas and extrastriatal areas indicated. (i) Representation of portion of area 17 (refer to f above). (j) Surface view of functional segregation of area 18 (visual area 2). B = blob, C-S = center surround receptive field (on-center off-surround illustrated), IB = interblob, ITC = inferotemporal cortex, LGB = lateral geniculate body and its layers 1 through 6 (layers 1 and 2, solid circles; layers 3–6, open circles), MT = middle temporal area (movement and stereopsis), STS = superior temporal sulcus, V 4 = visual area 4 (color). (Adapted from Livingstone M, Hubel D. Segregation of form, color, movement, and depth: anatomy, physiology, and perception. *Science.* 1988;240:740–749.)

processing. It should be mentioned that ganglion cells in primates are functionally different from those in cats; the latter have only two types of cone receptors, and appear to perceive color poorly.

The retina of each eye is divided into a temporal (lateral) half or *hemiretina* and a nasal (medial) half by a vertical line passing through the macula, near the posterior pole of the eye. Hemiretinae are subdivided into upper and lower quadrants by a horizontal line through the macula. The retina is further subdivided by three concentric circles: a small macular area, a pericentral (paramacular) area, and a peripheral (monocular) area.

Images from the environment are inverted (upside down) and reversed (temporal/nasal) by the lens before reaching the retina. In this sense, the eye resembles a camera, with the retina being the film. Hence, the temporal visual field is projected to the nasal hemiretina, the nasal visual field to the temporal hemiretina, the upper visual field to the lower hemiretina, and so on **(Fig. 19.5)**. Most of the visual field

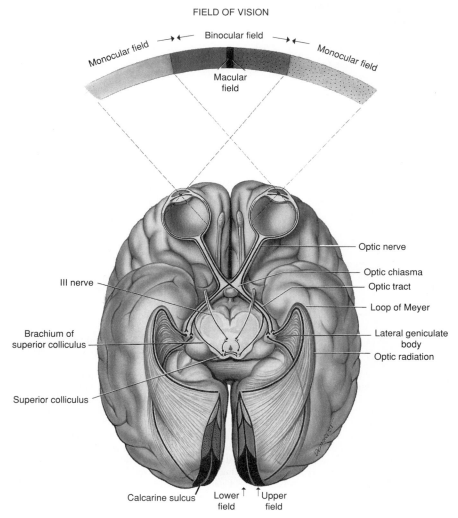

Figure 19.5: The visual pathways from the retina to the lateral geniculate bodies and to the primary visual cortex. The macular field projects to the posterior aspect of the primary visual cortex (solid black). The area just rostral to this receives the rest of the binocular field, and still more rostral is the area for the monocular visual field. The upper half of the visual field projects to the cortex below the calcarine sulcus, i.e., the lingual gyrus. The lower half of the visual field projects to the cortex above the sulcus, known as the cuneus.

is shared by the two eyes (binocular field), but the monocular area (monocular crescent) in the extreme temporal field is seen by each eye alone when the eyes are at rest.

PATHWAYS OF THE VISUAL SYSTEM

Pathways from the retina can be divided into three systems.

1. The *retinogeniculostriate pathway*, the principal one for vision, includes the LGB and the *primary visual cortex (visual area 1, V1, area 17 or striate cortex)*—striate cortex because of a stripe (stria) of myelinated fibers in layer IV, visible on gross inspection (**Fig. 19.4**). *Cortical area 18 (visual areas 2 and 3; V2, V3), cortical area 19 (visual areas 4 and 5; V4, V5, middle temporal area [MT]),* and others (e.g., *inferotemporal cortex [ITC]*) are involved in the higher processing of visual input (**Fig. 19.4**). The visual cortex, aside from the striate cortex, is called the *extrastriate cortex* or *visual association area*. This pathway system appears to mediate fine grain pattern analysis leading to the perception of the visual image.

   The cortical visual areas are hierarchically organized with ascending and descending anatomic connections encompassing both serial and parallel processing. Several functional streams exist so that each area is subdivided into subareas, each involved with processing different types of visual information (e.g., color, stereopsis). In general, the striate cortex distributes much of its output in an orderly fashion to V2 and V3 in area 18. In turn, area 18 projects to several small areas including V4 and V5 within area 19, and ITC (**Fig. 19.4**). Thus, each area has connections with successively higher areas and, in turn, each higher area projects back to the area or areas from which it receives input. In addition, these areas have connections with structures deep in the brain. For example, there are projections to the superior colliculus involved with accommodation (focusing) and reciprocal connections with certain nuclei of the thalamus (e.g., pulvinar) somehow involved with additional processing.

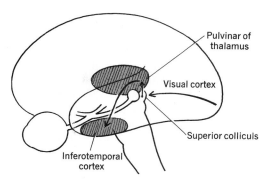

Figure 19.6: The tectal system.

2. The *tectal pathway* is primarily a reflex pathway projecting from the retina to the superior colliculus in the midbrain tectum, as well as to the pretectum. Further processing is carried out by connections from the superior colliculus to the pulvinar and lateral posterior nucleus of the thalamus, and from there, to the ITC (**Fig. 19.6**). The tectal pathway is involved with visual attention and detection of movement, as well as with the light and accommodation reflexes.

3. The *retinohypothalamic tract* links the retina with the hypothalamus (suprachiasmatic nucleus). Functionally, it is involved with circadian rhythms (e.g., sleep-wake, day-night), the reproductive cycle, and other periodic events (Chap. 21).

Retinogeniculostriate Pathway

This pathway includes (1) ganglion cell axons of the retina, which, upon emerging from the eye, become (2) fibers of the optic nerve (cranial nerve II), pass through the optic chiasma (from which point they are part of the optic tracts), and terminate in the LGB of the thalamus; (3) fibers from the LGB to the primary visual cortex on the upper and lower "banks" of the calcarine sulcus (area 17, striate cortex); and (4) fibers from area 17 to visual association areas of the cortex (areas 18, 19, and others). The processing sites in this pathway are the retina, LGB, and visual cortical areas (**Figs. 19.5, 25.5, and 25.6**).

Lateral Geniculate Body

Fibers from the ganglion cells in the *temporal hemiretina* of each eye terminate in the ipsilateral LGB. They do not decussate in the optic chiasma (**Fig. 19.5**). The fibers from the *nasal hemiretina* decussate in the optic chiasma and project to the contralateral LGB. In effect, the temporal hemiretina of one eye and the nasal hemiretina of the other eye (hemiretinae that view the same visual hemifield) project to the same LGB. The projections from the hemiretinae are separate (no overlap), with the fibers from each temporal hemiretina terminating on neurons of layers 2, 3, and 5 of the ipsilateral LGB and those from each nasal hemiretina, contralaterally in layers 1, 4, and 6. Each LGB consists of 6 layers with the ventral layers 1 and 2 called the magnocellular (large-cell layers) and the dorsal 3 to 6 layers called the parvocellular (small-cell) layers (**Fig. 19.4**). In effect, the influences from the right visual fields project to the left LGB and those from the left visual fields project to the right LGB (**Fig. 19.5**). Furthermore, the axons of retinal ganglion cells terminate in a precise point-to-point (*retinotopic*) configuration in the six layers of the LGB. In addition, the receptive field of the neurons of the LGB show center-surround opponency responses (**Fig. 19.4**).

This structural distinction of magnocellular and parvocellular layers is also expressed physiologically in four major ways—*color, acuity, speed*, and *contrast sensitivity*. The cells of the magnocellular layers are color-blind (have black and white responses), are involved with higher contrast sensitivity (have larger receptive field centers), respond faster (have a role in detecting movement), and express low resolution (are less sensitive to detail and perception of form). Conversely, the cells of the parvocellular layers are color sensitive (cells are spectrally sensitive, red-, green-, and blue-selective), are involved with lower contrast sensitivity (smaller receptive field centers), respond slower, and express higher resolution (more sensitive to detail and perception of form). These distinctions are the initial indication of the designation of a (1) *magnocellular system (pathway)* and (2) a *parvocellular system (pathway)*.

The precise function of the LGB is incompletely understood. The LGB does not simply relay center-surround field information from the retina to area 17. Rather, transmission within this nucleus is altered or gated by the feed back

circuits from the cortex and other higher centers. Thus gate control may serve to modulate visual input to the ordinary visual cortex associated with, for example, visual attention.

The fibers from the LGB pass in a retinotopic organization through the *retrolenticular portion of the internal capsule* and continue posteriorly as the *optic radiation* along the lateral aspect of the lateral ventricle before terminating in lamina IV of the primary visual cortex (Chap. 25). Fibers in the upper half of the optic radiation convey information from the upper hemiretinae, and those in the lower half of the optic radiation, from the lower hemiretinae. Fibers receiving input from the lower peripheral retinae arch ventrally and rostrally through the temporal lobe, as the *loop of Archambault (Meyer)*, before coursing posteriorly (**Figs. 19.4 and 19.5**). In a sense, a visuotopic map of the retina is present in some form throughout the retinogeniculostriate pathway. The primary visual cortex is organized so that the projections from each upper hemiretina terminate within area 17 of the cuneate gyrus (above the calcarine sulcus), and those from each lower hemiretina terminate within area 17 of the lingual gyrus (below the calcarine sulcus). As a consequence, area 17 of the cuneus "looks down to see" the lower half of the visual field, and area 17 of the lingual gyrus "looks up to see" the upper half of the visual field.

VISUAL CORTEX

The visual cortex has been divided into the primary visual cortex (area 17, striate cortex, visual area V1) and extrastriate cortex (**Figs. 19.4 and 19.5**). The striate cortex consists of six layers, with layer IV consisting of several sublayers (**Fig. 19.4**). The axon of each lateral geniculate neuron terminates in a small locale in lamina IV of the striate cortex. This input is processed in local cortical loops within the other laminae. Neurons in laminae II and III project to other cortical areas, those in lamina V to the superior colliculus, and those from lamina VI back to the LGB. Neurons of lamina I project to other parts of the striate cortex.

Cortical neurons that are receptive to visual stimuli have been classified on the basis of their receptive fields as "center-surround," "simple," "complex," or "hypercomplex" cells. The *center-surround cells* are located only in lamina IV of area 17; they receive direct input from cells in the LGB. *Simple cells* respond to either a dark bar on a light background or a light bar on a dark background and, in addition, the bar must be oriented at a specific angle. A simple cell is presumed to express this feature because its input comes from the convergence of thalamic neurons whose center-surround fields fall along a straight line (**Fig. 19.4**). *Complex* and *hypercomplex cells* respond optimally to edges, bars, and corners, and have special movement and orientation properties (**Fig. 19.4**). These properties are explained, at least in part, by the convergence of input from simple cells. The simple and complex cells are detectors of receptive fields of straight lines, while hypercomplex cells are detectors of angles and curved lines. Area 17 has simple and complex cells; areas 18 and 19 contain complex and hypercomplex cells.

Primary Visual (Area 17, Striate) Cortex

Axons of the geniculate neurons (center-surround cells) convey influences through a point-to-point retinotopic projection to the center-surround cells in lamina IV of area 17. More specifically, the LGB cells project to area 17 via two channels: (1) the magnocellular layers more superficially to lamina IVCa, and (2) the parvocellular layers slightly deeper to lamina IVCb (**Fig. 19.4**). Following processing, several channels project from the neurons of lamina IV to laminae II, III, and IVB (**Fig. 19.4**). The projections to laminae II and III of visual area 1 terminate in clusters of cells called *blobs* (contain cells that stain intensely for the mitochondrial enzyme cytochrome oxidase) or in bands of cells between the blobs called *interblobs* (**Fig. 19.4**). In the portions of visual area 2 adjacent to V1, the mitochondrial stain reveals alternating stripes and interstripes; each is several millimeters wide and oriented perpendicular to the border between V1 and V2.

There are three major parallel channels (pathways) from the retina to the neocortex, each of which conveys primarily one feature of visual information and is named by its connections in the LGB and V1.

(1) The *magnocellular system* (channel, pathway) is involved with the location and movement of the visual image—*where the object is* (see later). This channel projects from the magnocellular laminae of the LGB to laminae IVCa to IVB and to interblobs of laminae II and III of V1, and then to V2 and V3, and to V4 and MT (V5) of area 19 (**Fig. 19.4**). These are areas involved in visual aspects of depth and motion. The cells in lamina IVB are orientation selective (respond to lines of a particular orientation) and show selectivity to direction of movement. The MT (motion) area and an area within the superior temporal sulcus (STS) are specialized for the analysis of movement (visual motion), stereoscopic depth, and associated subjective perceptions of motion during a visual task. Lesions in this system are associated with deficits in eye movements directed toward objects in motion.

(2) The *parvocellular system* is involved more with color and form of vision—*what the object is* (see later). These are (A) the *parvocellular-blob channel* from the parvocellular layers of LGB to IVCb to blobs in layers II and III. It is involved with color vision and (B) the *parvocellular-interblob channel* from the parvocellular layers to IVCb to interblobs. It is involved in the perception of form and depth. The cells of the blobs are color and brightness selective, and are not concerned with orientation. The cells of the interblobs are orientation selective and may be responsible for high resolution form perception. The main output of the parvocellular channels is from V1 and V2, forming the pattern of stripes and interstripes. Visual area 2 projects to V4 (and other visual areas including the middle temporal area). Lamina IVCa also projects to the MT area (**Fig. 19.4**). Visual area 4, in the fusiform gyrus of the temporal lobe, is specialized for color perception, and V5 for motion. The parvocellular blob and interblob pathways eventually reach the inferotemporal cortex—a cortical area concerned with color, form, and depth perception. The parvocellular-interblob channel is sensitive to the outline and orientation of images that are essential to the perception of form. The property of high resolution is requisite for seeing detail in stationary objects. Lesions in the inferotemporal cortex result in

deficits associated with the recognition of complex objects such as faces.

Ocular Dominance and Orientation Columns of the Striate Cortex

The primary visual cortex, like the rest of the neocortex, is organized into six laminae oriented parallel to the cortical surface (Fig. 19.7). Because the axons and dendrites of the cortical cells are primarily perpendicular to the laminae, their processes extend from one lamina into other laminae. Most of the input from the LGB terminates on the stellate cells of lamina IV and is conveyed by other cells to the lamina above

and below lamina IV. This is the structural basis of the "functional columns" (e.g., ocular dominance and orientation columns noted below) oriented perpendicular to the cortical surface (Fig. 19.7).

Within each column of the striate cortex are center-surround, simple and complex cells. Each point in the visual field is represented only once. If the point is in the binocular field, the stimulus travels from the retinae as two center-surround receptive fields that terminate in one locale within the striate cortex. Processing fuses these two inputs. It is this fusion which permits us to see one visual image viewed by two eyes.

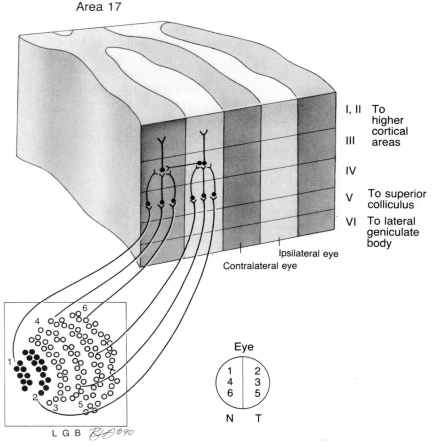

Figure 19.7: Schema of the relation of ocular dominance columns (slabs) in area 17. Orientation columns (not illustrated) are also present in area 17. The nasal half of the retina projects to laminae 1, 4, and 6 and the temporal half of the retina to laminae 2, 3, and 5 of the lateral geniculate body. The magnocellular laminae 1 and 2 are represented by solid circles and the parvocellular 3, 4, 5, and 6 by open circles. N = nasal half of retina, T = temporal half of retina. (Adapted from Hubel D, Wiesel T. Functional architecture of the macaque monkey visual cortex. *Proc R Soc Lond B Biol Sci.* 1977;198:1–59.)

The inputs and processing within the striate cortex produce two types of independent and overlapping functional columns, ranging from 30 to 100 μm wide, namely (1) ocular dominance (preference) columns and (2) orientation preference columns. The cells in each lamina of the column respond to some degree to the preference exhibited by that column. Each ocular dominance column receives input from both eyes, but a given column will receive more from one (preferred eye) than the other eye. Thus, each column is binocularly driven, but more by one eye than by the other. Each of the orientation columns responds to specifically oriented lines or edges (linear stimuli) in the visual field, with each column being responsive to the line at a slightly different angle of orientation. An individual striate cortical neuron may be integrated in both an ocular dominance column and an orientation preference column. In summary, the striate cortex has two principal roles: (1) to perform the act of fusion of the inputs from both eyes into one image, and (2) to analyze the visual world with respect to the orientation of the stimuli in the visual fields. In addition, these functionally characterized columns are indicative of a modular (selectively responsive modules) organization.

The macular, pericentral, and monocular retinal areas are represented in the posterior (occipital pole), intermediate, and anterior portions of area 17, respectively **(Fig. 19.5)**. The large representation of macular vision is associated with the sharp visual acuity monitored by the macula where the cone receptors are smaller and more densely packed than in the pericentral retina. The pericentral area, which registers less visual acuity, is represented by a smaller cortical area. Each monocular area, with the least cortical representation, receives retinal input derived from the peripheral field of vision of only the opposite eye.

Channels and Pathways of the Visual System

The retinogeniculostriate pathway may be conceived as being functionally structured (1) to relay visually derived influences to hierarchically organized centers with each successively higher level furthering the processing, and (2) to convey various features abstracted by the eyes from the visual spectrum by several independent parallel pathways (channels). (1) The former is an expression of serial (sequential) processing where successive higher levels "see more" and have an increased capacity for abstraction. It is illustrated by the sequence of center-surround fields at the retinal, geniculate, and striate levels followed by successive groups of cells known as simple, complex, and hypercomplex cells. At each higher level, the cells "see more" and abstract more. (2) The latter is an expression of the parallel processing of different features of the visual world. Some degree of cross-talk between parallel channels presumably exists. It is illustrated by separate pathways previously noted for color selectivity, speed, acuity, and contrast sensitivity.

The previously held notion of a hierarchically organized single serial processing pathway of the visual system has yielded to the current concept of many hierarchically organized parallel processing multichannels (multipathways) in the visual system. According to the latter theory, each channel (pathway), acting as a single pathway, is concerned with a specific visual feature that is conveyed from the retina to a representation in the visual cortex. As many as 32 representations of the retina are estimated to be located in the extrastriate cortex. As yet, there is no known area in the brain that integrates and synthesizes all the information to produce the final image. Semir Zeki addresses the enigma as follows: *"There is no single cortical area to which all other cortical areas report exclusively, either in the visual or in any other system. In sum, the cortex must be using a different strategy for generating the integrated visual image."*

The case for parallel processing along separate channels can explain *prosopagnosia*, a rare syndrome in which an individual may lose the ability to recognize faces, including the faces of parents, children, spouses, and even the patient's own face in a mirror. Some patients with brain damage can recognize expressions, but not familiar faces. This condition is thought to occur following a stroke or head injury to a small area of the brain. Such is the condition described by Sacks in his book, *The Man Who Mistook His Wife for a Hat*. This individual was essentially normal except for an unusual visual flaw such as that noted in the title of the book.

This is explicable by the occurrence of small bilateral cerebral lesions involving the inner aspect of the temporal lobes caudally and extending into the inferior part of the occipital lobes; probably one of a number of hierarchically organized channels may be causative. "The fact that an object's shape, color, position, and motion appear unified, even though each compartment is analyzed separately, can be compared in the experience of listening to someone speak. You hear the person's voice and see the mouth move without being aware that the two are processed independently."

Some groups of channels remain segregated as functionally distinct regions of the visual association areas. The *occipitoparietal pathway system* is the *"where" system* involved with the assessment of visual relationships such as the position of objects. The *occipitotemporal pathway system* or *"what" system* is essential for learning to identify objects by their appearance (object vision and pattern discrimination) (Chap. 25). This distinction is called the "what" and "where" of vision.

On the basis of physiologic evidence, two other major functional streams are indicated within the many visual areas of the cortex. One stream is involved in the analysis of visual motion (tracking the trajectories and speed of moving objects in space). The other stream is associated with the analysis of form and color (form and object perception, spatial localization).

Tectal Pathway

The tectal pathway (Fig. 19.6) comprises the sequence from retina (M ganglion neurons) to the superior colliculus of the tectum to the lateral posterior nucleus and pulvinar of the thalamus (called the "tectal recipient zone") to the ITC (areas 20 and 21). The tectal system is thought to be involved with visual attention and movement detection in the visual fields. This extrageniculate system interacts with the retinogeniculostriate system in two ways: (1) the superior colliculus receives input from the visual association areas of the cerebral cortex, the so-called extrastriate visual areas. Following processing, the colliculus projects output through the "tectal recipient zone" to the ITC. (2) The

ITC interacts through cortical circuitry with other extrastriate visual association areas.

Superior Colliculus

The laminated superior colliculus and the rostrally located pretectum (Fig. 13.16) are complex reflex centers. The pretectum is involved in the direct light response and the consensual light reflex (see below). The superficial layers of the superior colliculus receive direct input from the retina and indirect input from the visual cortex. The deep layers receive input from the auditory and somatosensory systems; they also are the source of tectospinal and tectopontine fibers (for relay to the cerebellum) as well as of fibers that go to the accessory oculomotor nucleus of Edinger-Westphal (see later, Accommodation Reflex) and to the paramedian pontine and midbrain reticular formation. The superior colliculus has roles in orienting the head and eyes toward a visual stimulus, particularly through its outputs to the cervical spinal cord via the tectospinal tract for turning the head, and to the paramedian pontine reticular formation (PPRF) "gaze center" for control of saccadic eye movements (see later; Chap. 16). The superior colliculus is topographically organized; neurons in a vertical column are activated by auditory or visual stimuli from a given location, and stimulation of deep layers of that column causes a saccade to the same location.

REFLEX PATHWAYS

Light Reflexes (Fig. 19.8)

When a bright light is directed into an eye, the pupils of both eyes constrict following the contraction of the constrictor muscles of the iris. The response in the stimulated eye is called the *direct light response*, and that in the unstimulated eye is called the *consensual light response*. The sequence and course of neurons in this arc are as follows:

1. Axons of the ganglion cells of each eye pass through the optic nerve, chiasma, tract, and brachium of the superior colliculus before terminating in both sides of the pretectum of the midbrain (some fibers cross and some

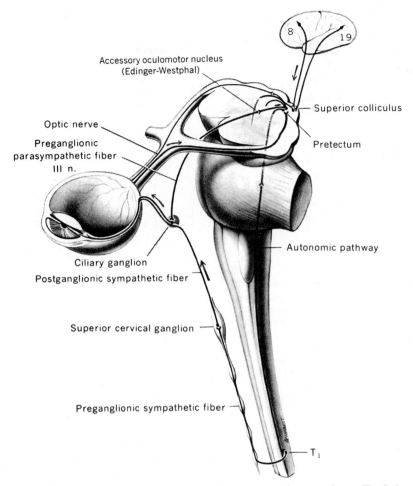

Figure 19.8: The light reflex pathway (pupillary reflex) and the accommodation pathway. The light reflex pathways relay (1) through the midbrain pretectum and the parasympathetic outflow of the oculomotor nerve (for pupillary constriction), and (2) through the sympathetic pathways of the brainstem, upper thoracic level, and ascending cervical paravertebral sympathetic trunk (for pupillary dilation). Accommodation is mediated via a pathway that includes corticocollicular fibers from occipital lobe (area 19) and frontal lobe (area 8), superior colliculus and parasympathetic outflow through the oculomotor nerve.

do not cross as they pass through the optic chiasma).

2. The two halves of the pretectum are interconnected by fibers passing through the posterior commissure.

3. Axons of pretectal neurons project to the pupillomotor cells in the *accessory oculomotor nuclei of Edinger-Westphal* of the same and opposite sides.

4. The preganglionic parasympathetic neurons emit fibers that pass through the oculomotor nerve and terminate on postganglionic neurons in the ciliary ganglion.

5. The latter innervate the constrictor smooth muscle of the iris.

The consensual light reflex involves the unstimulated eye by fibers that cross in the optic chiasma and the posterior commissure of the midbrain. These reflexes are carried out unconsciously, without any cortical involvement. This reflex is preserved even with lesions located in the lateral geniculate bodies, optic radiations, or visual cortex. Individuals afflicted with cortical blindness resulting from complete destruction of both striate cortices retain the light reflexes.

Accommodation Reflex (Fig. 19.8)

The adjustments of the lens by the action of the ciliary body to bring an object into focus are known as accommodation. Unlike the light reflexes, the accommodation reflex includes the visual cortex; an individual does exert some control in selecting the object brought into focus. Visual influences from the eye are relayed via the visual pathways to the visual cortex. Neurons in the visual areas have axons which descend through the optic radiation to the superior colliculus of the midbrain. In turn, collicular neurons project to the preganglionic parasympathetic neurons of the accessory oculomotor nucleus of Edinger-Westphal which, after passing through the oculomotor nerve, synapse with postganglionic parasympathetic neurons in the ciliary ganglion. These neurons innervate the smooth muscles in the ciliary body, which regulate the tension on the lens.

Accommodation-Convergence Reaction

Immediately after the eyes are shifted from a distant object to a near one (near-sight vision), several activities occur. The ciliary muscles cause the lens to thicken in order to bring the object into focus by accommodation. The eyes converge as the medial recti muscles contract. The pupils constrict to increase the definition of the image.

Argyll-Robertson Pupil

The Argyll-Robertson pupil may occur in syphilis of the CNS. In this syndrome, the pupil is small in dim light and does not constrict further when the eye is exposed to bright light. The same pupil will constrict further during the accommodation-convergence reaction. This syndrome is presumed to be caused by lesions in the pretectum.

Pupillary Dilatation

Descending sympathetic pathways pass through the brainstem and anterior half of the spinal cord before terminating on preganglionic neurons of the intermediolateral cell column at C8 and T1 spinal levels. The preganglionic fibers ascend through the sympathetic chain and synapse in the superior cervical ganglion. Postganglionic sympathetic axons course along branches of the internal carotid artery to reach the pupillary dilator fibers in the iris. Interruption of the preganglionic or postganglionic fibers results in an ipsilateral Horner's syndrome (Chap 17); the syndrome may occur following lesions in the brainstem. A phenomenon called the *paradoxic pupillary response* is discussed in Chapter 20.

CONTROL OF EYE MOVEMENTS

The congruent and convergent movements of the eyes are mediated through the superior colliculus and the PPRF (Chap. 16). Four basic types of eye movements are recognized; each is activated by an independent control system involving different regions of the brain.

1. *Fast saccadic eye movement, movement on command, searching movement.* This movement is the saccade (fast component in nystagmus, as an example) in which the eyes are searching for an object upon which to fix. Activation of motor area 8 of the cortex by a "command," or stimulation of the superior colliculus, evokes this quick voluntary movement of the eyes. The visual image is suppressed during a saccade. Electrical stimulation of area 8, or of the superior colliculus, will cause the eyes to deviate to the opposite side.

2. *Slow pursuit or tracking an ongoing motion.* This action occurs while following a moving object (following a bird in flight). Activation of cortical areas 18 and 19 evokes this movement.

3. *Vestibuloocular reflex (VOR) eye movements.* VOR eye movements serve to maintain the fixation of the eyes on an object while the head is in motion. It requires coordinated contractions of the neck musculature, mediated through the vestibular system, to maintain head position (Chap. 16). This "keep eyes on target" activity is expressed as the head turns in one direction and the eyes move in the opposite direction so the gaze remains fixed on the object.

4. *Vergence eye movements.* Influences from cortical areas 19 and 22 direct convergence so that both eyes remain upon an object, be it near or far away.

A duck hunter sitting in a gently rocking boat in a tidal marsh illustrates the action of these four systems. The hunter scans the sky for a duck using saccadic eye movements from point to point (a visual image is not recognizable during saccades because they are so fast). The duck, once spotted, is followed by smooth pursuit movements. If the duck flies close by, the vergence (convergence) eye movements combine with the pursuit movements as the hunter's vision shifts from far to near vision. During the entire sequence, the hunter employs the VOR movements to compensate for the movements of the head caused by the rocking of the boat.

LESIONS WITHIN THE VISUAL PATHWAYS

Impairment of a small area of the retina results in a blind spot (*scotoma*) in that eye. The *optic disk*, where the optic nerve fibers converge to leave the retina, is a natural blind spot; it contains no rods or cones. The complete interruption of the optic nerve results in permanent blindness in one eye (Fig. 19.9A). However, this blind eye can still accommodate and can exhibit the consensual light reflex because the normal eye activates the intact efferent part of the reflex arcs to the blind eye.

A *midline lesion of the optic chiasma* (following compression from a tumor of the pituitary gland or from a craniopharyngioma located immediately behind the chiasma) can interrupt the decussating fibers from both eyes (Fig. 19.9B). This results in blindness in the nasal half of the retina (the temporal half of the visual field of each eye); it is called *bitemporal heteronymous hemianopsia* (or *hemianopia*). By convention, lesions of the optic pathways are described in terms of resulting field deficits. Damage to the nondecussating fibers on one (right) side of the optic chiasma results in a *right nasal hemianopsia* (Fig. 19.9C), i.e., blindness in the temporal half of the retina (nasal half of the visual field of one eye). The complete interruption of the optic tract, LGB, optic radiations, or the entire primary visual cortex on one (right) side results in a *contralateral homonymous hemianopsia*, or blindness in

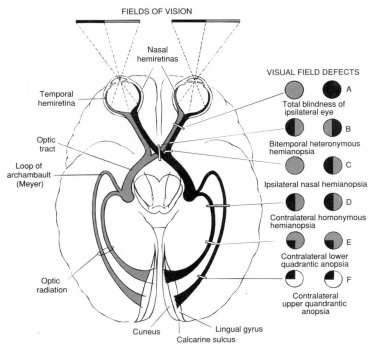

Figure 19.9: Some common lesions at various levels within the visual pathways. The corresponding visual field defects are represented on the right side of the drawing. The nerve fibers of the optic radiations terminate throughout the visual cortex of the lingual gyrus and cuneus respectively (not so represented in the illustration).

the field of vision on the opposite (left) side of the lesion (**Fig. 19.9D**). *Macular sparing* (preservation of the visual field of the maculae) sometimes occurs following strokes involving the visual cortex. This phenomenon is attributable to a dual vascular supply to this region from branches of both the middle and posterior cerebral arteries as well as to the extensive cortical representation of the central visual field. Visual defects limited to a single visual field are *homonymous*, whereas those located in both fields are *heteronymous*. Partial lesions produce partial defects in the fields of vision. A lesion of the entire cuneus (includes entire primary visual cortex above the calcarine sulcus) on one side results in *contralateral lower quadrantic anopsia* (**Fig. 19.9E**) because pathways from the upper temporal quadrant of the ipsilateral retina and upper nasal quadrant of the contralateral retina are interrupted. Conversely, a lesion of the lingual gyrus, or interruption of the optic radiations on one side as they pass through the temporal lobe (loop of Archambault [Meyer]), results in *contralateral upper quadrantic anopsia* (**Fig. 19.9F**), because pathways from the lower temporal quadrant of the ipsilateral retina and lower nasal quadrant of the contralateral retina are interrupted.

A lesion in cortical area 8 in one hemisphere results in the deviation of the eyes to the same side.

SUGGESTED READINGS

Baylor D. Photoreceptor signals and vision. Proctor Lecture. *Invest Ophthalmol Vis Sci.* 1987;28: 34–49.

DeYoe E, Van Essen D. Concurrent processing streams in monkey visual cortex. *Trends Neurosci.* 1988;11:219–226.

Dowling J. *The Retina: An Approachable Part of the Brain.* Cambridge, Mass: Harvard University Press; 1987.

Dowling J. *Neurons and Networks: An Introduction to Neuroscience.* Cambridge, Mass: Belknap; 1993.

Fawcett D, Raviola E. *Bloom and Fawcett, A Textbook of Histology.* 12th ed. New York, NY: Chapman & Hall; 1994.

Fox P, Miezin F, Allman J, Van Essen D, Raichle M. Retinotopic organization of the human visual cortex mapped with positron-emission tomography. *J Neurosci.* 1987;7:913–922.

Gouras P. Color vision. In: Kandel E, Schwartz J, Jessell T, eds. *Principles of Neural Science.* 3rd ed. New York, NY: Elsevier; 1991:467–480.

Hubel D. *Eye, Brain and Vision.* New York, NY: Freeman & Co; 1987.

Hubel D, Wiesel T. Functional architecture of the macaque monkey visual cortex. *Proc R Soc Lond B Biol Sci.* 1977;198:1–59.

Huerta M, Harting J. Connectional organization of the superior colliculus. *Trends Neurosci.* 1984;7: 286–289.

Kaneko A. Physiology of the retina. *Annu Rev Neurosci.* 1979;2:169–191.

Kuwabara T. The eye. In: Weiss L, ed. *Cell and Tissue Biology: A Textbook of Histology.* 6th ed. Baltimore, Md: Urban & Schwartzenberg; 1988: 1067–1106.

Livingstone M, Hubel D. Segregation of form, color, movement and depth: anatomy, physiology, and perception. *Science.* 1988;240:740–749.

Maunsell J, Newsome W. Visual processing in monkey extrastriate cortex. *Annu Rev Neurosci.* 1987; 10:363–401.

Mishkin M, Ungerleider L, Macko K. Object vision and spatial vision: two cortical pathways. *Trends Neurosci.* 1983;6:414–417.

Netter F. *Atlas of Human Anatomy.* West Caldwell, NJ: Ciba-Geigy Corp; 1989:plates 82–86.

Perry V, Cowey A. Retinal ganglion cells that project to the superior colliculus and pretectum in the macaque monkey. *Neuroscience.* 1984;12: 1125–1137.

Sacks O. *The Man Who Mistook His Wife for a Hat.* New York, NY: Harper & Row; 1987.

Shapley R, Perry V. Cat and monkey retinal ganglion cells and their visual functional roles. *Trends Neurosci.* 1986;9:229–235.

Sherman S, Koch C. The control of retinogeniculate transmission in the mammalian lateral geniculate nucleus. *Exp Brain Res.* 1986;63:1–20.

Ts'o D, Frostig R, Lieke E, Grinvald A. Functional organization of primate visual cortex revealed by high resolution optical imaging. *Science.* 1990; 249:417–420.

Van Essen D, Anderson G, Felleman D. Information processing in the primate visual system: an integrated systems perspective. *Science.* 1992;255: 419–423.

Van Essen D, Maunsell J. Hierarchical organization and functional streams in the visual cortex. *Trends Neurosci.* 1983;6:370–375.

Walsh C, Guillery R. Fibre order in the pathways from the eye to the brain. *Trends Neurosci.* 1984; 7:208–211.

Zeki S. The visual image in mind and brain. *Sci Am.* 1992;267:69–76.

Zeki S. *A Vision of the Brain.* London; Blackwell; 1993.

Autonomic Nervous System 20

The somatic and autonomic nervous systems

Subdivisions of the autonomic nervous system

Sympathetic (thoracolumbar) system

Parasympathetic (craniosacral) system

Enteric nervous system ("Gut brain," "Minibrain")

Descending pathways

Denervation sensitivity and sympathectomy

Activity on specific organs and structures

The functional activity of the nervous system is usually expressed by the contraction (or relaxation) of muscles and the secretion of glands. These actions are mediated through the somatic motor system and the visceral motor system (autonomic nervous system). The *somatic motor system* innervates the voluntary (skeletal, striated) muscles, whereas the *autonomic nervous system* influences the activities of involuntary (smooth) muscles, cardiac (heart) muscle, and glands. The autonomic nervous system is often called the *general visceral efferent system* or *vegetative motor system* because the effectors are associated with the visceral systems (e.g., cardiovascular, digestive, and respiratory systems) over which only minimal, if any, direct conscious control can be exerted.

THE SOMATIC AND AUTONOMIC NERVOUS SYSTEMS

The basic role of the somatic motor system is to regulate the coordinated muscular activities associated with the maintenance of posture and phasic locomotor movements; these expressions are related to adjustments to the external environment. The general role of the autonomic nervous system is to influence those visceral activi-

ties which are directed toward maintaining a relatively stable internal environment within the body. For example, the maintenance of (1) the blood pressure commensurate with the demands of the organism and (2) a constant body temperature are functional expressions of the activity of the autonomic nervous system. These two systems are not independent; they do interact. For example, the somatic nervous system responds to a drop in body temperature by generating heat through contraction of voluntary muscles, and the autonomic nervous system stimulates the constriction of cutaneous blood vessels to reduce the heat loss by radiation. In general, the somatic nervous system reacts rapidly to stimulation, whereas the autonomic nervous system responds with a greater time lag.

The two systems differ significantly with reference to the anatomic organization of the final neuronal linkage between the central nervous system and the peripherally located effectors. The somatic motor system has a *one-neuron linkage* (alpha and gamma motoneurons); the autonomic nervous system has a *two-neuron linkage* (**Fig. 20.1**). From its cell body in the brainstem or spinal cord, each somatic lower motoneuron has an axon which courses through a cranial or spinal nerve to make synaptic connections (at motor end-plates) with voluntary muscle fibers (Chap. 11). In contrast, the first

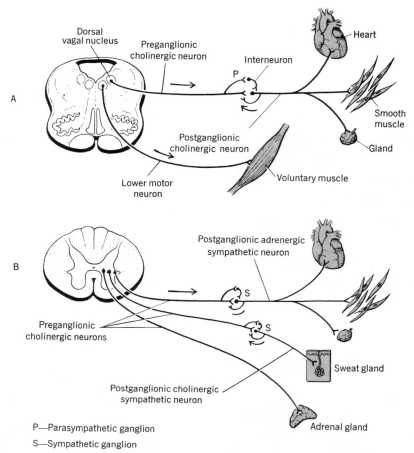

Figure 20.1: Motor innervation to the peripheral effectors. **A.** The parasympathetic outflow from the medulla innervates the heart, smooth muscle, and glands. The lower motoneuron innervates a voluntary muscle. **B.** Sympathetic outflow from the spinal cord innervates the heart, smooth muscle, and glands. See text for discussion of the various types of neurons. S = small intensely fluorescent (SIF) cells. The SIF cells of sympathetic ganglia contain catecholamine fluorescent dopamine and norepinephrine.

neuron of the autonomic nervous system, called a *preganglionic neuron*, originates in the brainstem or spinal cord and has an axon which courses through a cranial or peripheral nerve and terminates by synapsing with a second neuron (or neurons) located in an autonomic ganglion outside the central nervous system. This second neuron, called a *postganglionic neuron*, has an axon which extends peripherally to terminate in endings associated with smooth muscles, cardiac muscle, or glands. The preganglionics are myelinated B fibers and the postganglionics are unmyelinated C fibers. When denervated, smooth muscles and glands generally show significant levels of activity independent of intact innervation.

The autonomic nervous system is conventionally considered to be a motor system—the general visceral efferent motor system.

SUBDIVISIONS OF THE AUTONOMIC NERVOUS SYSTEM

The autonomic nervous system is divided into three systems: (1) sympathetic nervous system, (2) parasympathetic nervous system, and (3) enteric nervous system.

1. The *sympathetic nervous system* stimulates those activities which are mobilized by the organism during emergency and stress situa-

tions—the so-called "fight, fright, and flight" responses. These include the acceleration of the rate and force of the heartbeat, an increase in the concentration of blood sugar, and an increase in blood pressure. In contrast, the parasympathetic system stimulates those activities associated with conservation and restoration of body resources of the organism. These include a decrease in the rate of the heartbeat and the rise in gastrointestinal activities associated with increased digestion and absorption of food.

The sympathetic system is also called the *thoracolumbar* or *adrenergic system* because (1) its preganglionic fibers emerge from all thoracic and the upper two lumbar levels (T1 through L2) and (2) the neurosecretory transmitter released by the postganglionic fibers is usually norepinephrine (noradrenalin).

2. The *parasympathetic nervous system* is also called the *craniosacral* or *cholinergic system* because (1) its preganglionic fibers emerge with cranial nerves III, VII, IX, X, and at sacral spinal levels S3 and S4 (sometimes also S2 and S5) and (2) the neurosecretory transmitter released by the postganglionic fibers usually is acetylcholine.

3. The *enteric nervous system*, also called the "*gut brain*" or "*minibrain*," is the intrinsic network of neurons and their connections that extend from the esophagus to the rectum, otherwise known as the gut or gastrointestinal (GI) tract (enteron). A key feature of this system is its anatomical and physiological independence. With this system intact, the gut can function autonomously even when completely deprived of sympathetic and parasympathetic innervation.

This complex system consists of approximately 100 million neurons—roughly the equivalent of the number of neurons in the spinal cord. The 10 or so different neuronal types that have been described release as many as 20 different transmitters and modulators. The preganglionic autonomic innervation to the gut is relatively sparse, although the terminal branching of the postganglionic fibers can be profuse (Fig. 15.3). For example, of the 5000 neurons of the vagus nerve innervating the gut, about

90% are afferent neurons and 10% are preganglionic parasympathetic neurons. The diffuse and extensive branching pattern is characteristic of each postganglionic noradrenergic nerve of the sympathetic nervous system. A single neuron may have many terminal branches with lengths of over 14 cm and over several thousand varicosities containing transmitter (norepinephrine) and modulators (neuropeptides). These varicosities make numerous *en passage "synaptic junctions"* with muscle and glandular cells (Fig. 15.3). The visceral effector is a muscle bundle rather than a single cell; its individual muscle cells are linked and coupled by gap junctions which allow for electrotonic spread of activity between the muscle fibers of each muscle.

SYMPATHETIC (THORACOLUMBAR) SYSTEM

Preganglionic fibers of the sympathetic system (Fig. 20.2) originate from cell bodies located in the intermediolateral nucleus of lamina VII which extends from spinal levels T1 through L2. These fibers pass successively through the ventral roots (where they are referred to as the *thoracolumbar outflow*) of the spinal nerves, the white rami communicantes (branches of the spinal nerves), and the sympathetic trunk, after branching, they terminate by synapsing within either (1) the paravertebral ganglia of the sympathetic chain or (2) the prevertebral (collateral) ganglia. The paravertebral ganglia of the sympathetic chain (trunk), which are located along the centra of the vertebral column from the upper cervical through coccygeal levels, receive their input exclusively from the thoracolumbar sympathetic outflow. The paired sympathetic chains meet in the midline in a terminal ganglion on the coccyx, called the *ganglion impar* or coccygeal ganglion. The prevertebral ganglia are located in the abdomen adjacent to the abdominal aorta and its main branches—the celiac, aorticorenal, superior mesenteric, and inferior mesenteric ganglia (derived from T6 through L2 spinal levels). The sympathetic ganglia contain inhibitory interneurons that mainly use dopamine as the neurotransmitter.

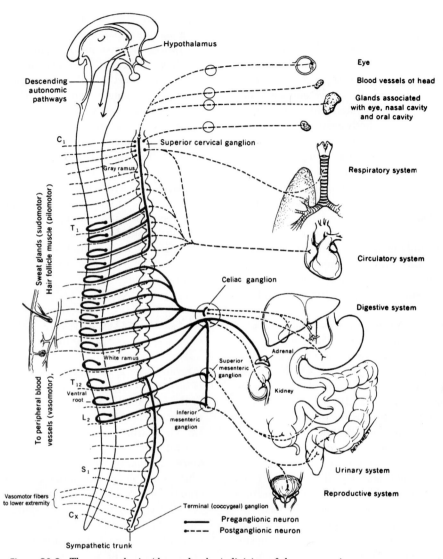

Figure 20.2: The sympathetic (thoracolumbar) division of the autonomic nervous system.

The postganglionic fibers from cells in the paravertebral ganglia pass via (1) the gray rami communicantes and the spinal nerves before terminating in the sweat glands and the smooth muscles of blood vessels and hair (erector pili muscles) of the body wall and extremities and (2) small nerves and perivascular plexuses to the visceral structures of the head, neck, and thorax (e.g., pupillary dilator muscle, heart, bronchioles). The postganglionic fibers from cells in the prevertebral ganglia form the perivascular plexuses innervating the abdominal and pelvic viscera.

In general, the sympathetic outflow is distributed as follows: T1 to T5 to the head and neck, T1 and T2 to the eye, T2 to T6 to the heart and lungs, T6 to L2 to the abdominal viscera, and L1 and L2 to the urinary, genital, and lower digestive systems.

The *neurotransmitter* released by the preganglionic nerve terminals is *acetylcholine*, which is deactivated rapidly by *acetylcholinesterase*; that released by the postganglionic nerve terminals is *norepinephrine (noradrenalin, levarterenol)*, which is deactivated slowly by *monoamine oxidase (MAO)* and *catechol-o-methyl transfer-*

ase (COMT) or taken up again by the nerve terminals. The MAO is located intracellularly, while the COMT is found extracellularly.

Adrenal Gland

The cells of the medulla of the adrenal gland are actually specialized postganglionic neurons. Preganglionic cholinergic fibers from T6 to T9 stimulate the adrenal chromaffin cells to release both epinephrine and norepinephrine into the circulatory system, which distributes these neurosecretions through the body. Within the medulla there are about eight cells that release epinephrine to one cell that releases norepinephrine. The adrenal medulla-released transmitters act in conjunction with the norepinephrine released by sympathetic postganglionic fibers.

Systemic Effects of Sympathetic Innervation

The sympathetic system is structurally and functionally organized to exert its influences over widespread body regions or even the entire body for sustained periods of time. Each preganglionic neuron has a relatively short axon which synapses with many postganglionic neurons, each of which has a long branching axon forming numerous neuroeffector junctions over a wide area. The widespread and sustained sympathetic effects are due to the slow deactivation of norepinephrine and to the systemic distribution of norepinephrine and epinephrine released by the adrenal medulla.

PARASYMPATHETIC (CRANIOSACRAL) SYSTEM

The cranial portion of the parasympathetic system (Fig. 20.3) is associated with (1) four cranial nerves (III, VII, IX, and X) that supply the parasympathetic innervation to the head, thorax and most of the abdominal viscera and (2) the sacral spinal cord that supplies the innervation to the lower abdominal and pelvic viscera. The body wall and the extremities do not have a parasympathetic innervation.

From cell bodies in the accessory oculomotor nucleus of Edinger-Westphal (in midbrain), preganglionic fibers pass via the IIIrd cranial nerve and terminate in the ciliary ganglion.

Postganglionic neurons innervate the sphincter (constrictor) muscles of the pupil and ciliary muscles involved with accommodation (focusing of lens of eye).

From cell bodies in the superior salivatory nucleus, preganglionic fibers pass via the VIIth cranial nerve and terminate in the pterygopalatine and submandibular ganglia. Postganglionic neurons innervate numerous glands in the head including lacrimal, submandibular, and sublingual glands and glands of the nasal, oral, and pharyngeal cavities.

From cell bodies in the inferior salivatory nucleus, preganglionic fibers pass via the IXth cranial nerve and terminate in the otic ganglion whose postganglionic neurons innervate the parotid gland.

From preganglionic cells in the dorsal vagal nucleus, preganglionic fibers pass via the Xth cranial nerve and synapse within terminal ganglia (located adjacent to or within visceral organs) with postganglionic neurons which innervate the viscera of the thorax and abdomen (e.g., heart, lungs, and gastrointestinal tract). The sacral portion of the parasympathetic system originates from cell bodies in the gray matter of sacral levels 3 and 4 (sometimes also S2 and S5); these preganglionic neurons pass via the pelvic splanchnic nerves to synapse in terminal ganglia with postganglionic neurons which innervate the lower abdominal and pelvic viscera (colon distal to left colic flexure, urinary, and genital viscera). The sacral parasympathetic outflow is involved with the "mechanisms of emptying"—urination and defecation—and with erection.

In general, the parasympathetic system has preganglionic fibers with long axons which synapse with a few postganglionic fibers with short axons. The neurotransmitter secretion at the terminals of both the preganglionic and postganglionic neurons is acetylcholine.

Systemic Effects of Parasympathetic Innervation

The parasympathetic system is primarily organized to respond to a specific stimulus in localized and discrete regions transiently for short durations. Each preganglionic neuron, a long axon synapsing with a few postganglionic neurons with short axons, exerts influences over a

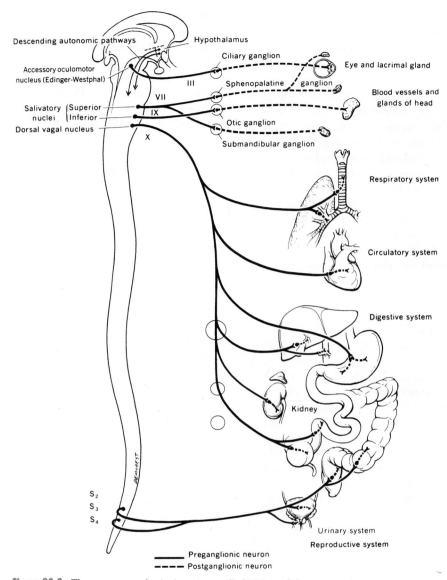

Figure 20.3: The parasympathetic (craniosacral) division of the autonomic nervous system.

small area. The rapid deactivation of acetylcholine by acetylcholinesterase restricts the time course over which a specific quantity of acetylcholine is effective.

ENTERIC NERVOUS SYSTEM ("GUT BRAIN," "MINIBRAIN")

The enteric nervous system comprises the intrinsic neural networks of sensory neurons, interneurons, and motor neurons. The motor neurons are postganglionic parasympathetic neurons which receive neural influences from (1) the intrinsic sensory neurons and interneurons within the gut and (2) the extrinsic preganglionic parasympathetic neurons and postganglionic sympathetic fibers. The *sensory neurons* with cell bodies located in the submucosa and external muscularis layer of the gut have dendritic processes that extend into the mucosal layer. These neurons respond to alterations in the tension within the gut proper and to the chemical environment within its lumen. Their axons interact with interneurons of the submucosal plexus (Meissner's plexus located in the connective tissue of the submucosa) and of myenteric plexus (Auerbach's plexus located between the circular and longitudinal layers of the external muscularis layer of the gut). The axons of the neurons of Meissner's plexus extend both orally and caudally. They are linked with motor neurons that regulate the secretory activity of a variety of cells and with the control of the muscles of the gut and blood vessels. The axons of Auerbach's plexus are oriented radially. Some neurons are integrated into feedback circuits with their axons projecting centripetally to the prevertebral ganglia (celiac, superior, and inferior ganglia), and from these ganglia back to the gut. The complex neural organization has a major role in *homeostasis* by its control of the gut blood vessel tone, motility, fluid transport, and enteroendocrine cell secretion. In essence, the neurons of the gastrointestinal system are organized into a *mini nervous system.*

The enteric nervous system has roles in the motility of the gut, the absorption of nutrients, the rate of proliferation of epithelial lining cells of the GI tract, and the release of hormones and neuropeptides by enterochromaffin cells of the *enteroendocrine system.* The substances released by the latter system include such agents as gastrin, gastrin intestinal peptide (GIP), motilin, secretin (elicits pancreatic secretion), and cholecystokinin (elicits contraction of gall bladder). Gastrin stimulates the release of hydrochloric acid by the parietal cells of the stomach and first part of the duodenum. Other cells release serotonin which influences gut motility in the stomach and small intestine. Somatostatin is released by cells in the entire gut. Cells in the intestine secrete gastrin intestinal peptide (GIP), which is a peptide antagonistic to gastrin. Motilin and substance P are neuropeptides associated with the regulation of intestinal motility. Vasoactive intestinal peptide (VIP) is involved with water and ion secretion as well as intestinal motility.

Responding to alterations in the tension in the wall of the gut and in the chemical environment, the sensory neurons can be involved in a *peristaltic reflex.* This expression of the activity

of the intrinsic neural circuitry within the gut is generally initiated by moderate distention. In the *"law of the intestine,"* stimulation of the gut causes contraction of the musculature rostral to the point of stimulation and relaxation below. Inhibition of intestinal tone and motility produced by distension of some other part of the gut is known as the *intestino-intestinal inhibitory reflex.* In addition, the myogenic smooth muscle activity is modulated by extrinsic excitatory motor (parasympathetic) and inhibitory (sympathetic) influences.

Two other features are also involved in the intrinsic reflex activity of the gut. (1) The smooth muscle cells, either individually or in groups, exhibit spontaneous waves of electrical depolarization linked to rhythmic contractions. The contractions spread from one muscle cell to another because the cells are electrically coupled by low-resistance gap junctions (Chap. 3). Because responses to the depolarization wave are facultative (optimal), each wave of depolarization may or may not be realized depending, in part, on the magnitude of the depolarization. (2) The fundus of the stomach and first part of the duodenum are two sites in the gut that have roles as pacemakers (equivalent to the pacemakers in the heart). In the human, the basic depolarization rhythm of the pacemaker (a) in the fundus governs the 3 (three) per minute waves of contraction prevalent in the stomach and (b) in the duodenum governs the 11 (eleven) per minute waves of contraction prevalent in the small intestine. The overall control and regulation of contractile activity of the gut is not focused at the pacemaker sites, but, rather, it is directed to the smooth muscle fibers throughout the gut. The control system effecting this regulation involves (1) the enteric circuitry, (2) the feedback circuits of afferent fibers from the gut to the prevertebral ganglia and efferent fibers back to the gut, and (3) influences from the sympathetic and parasympathetic systems. A major role of this system is to act as the coordinator of the "law of the intestine" by modulating, through inhibition, the spontaneous rhythmic contractile activity of the gut.

Transmitters and Modulators of the Autonomic Nervous System

The following are some of the putative transmitters and modulators identified in the peripheral nerves and ganglia of the autonomic nervous system (including adrenal medulla). The transmitter of the preganglionic autonomic neurons is predominately acetylcholine. Small intensely fluorescent (SIF) cells in the sympathetic ganglia contain the catecholamines dopamine and norepinephrine.

Sympathetic Nervous System

Norepinephrine, epinephrine, substance P, acetylcholine, enkephalins, serotonin, VIP, neuropeptide Y, cholecystokinin, and adenosine triphosphate (ATP).

Parasympathetic Nervous System.

Acetylcholine, VIP, substance P, and neuropeptide Y.

Enteric Nervous System

Gamma amino butyric acid (GABA), acetylcholine, VIP, serotonin, substance P, enkephalins, and somatotrophin.

DESCENDING PATHWAYS

The stimuli influencing the activity of the preganglionic neurons of the autonomic nervous system are derived from a variety of sources. Much input is conveyed from somatic and visceral sensory receptors via afferent fibers in the cranial and spinal nerves. Influences from the cerebrum are projected to the lower brainstem reticular formation by (1) the corticoreticular fibers from the cerebral cortex and (2) the hypothalamotegmental, mammillotegmental, and dorsal longitudinal fasciculus from the hypothalamus and the limbic lobe. Other input to the brainstem reticular formation is derived from the spinal cord via the ascending spinoreticular fibers and from the cranial nerves. In turn, the influences from the brainstem reticular formation are conveyed via some of the reticulospinal fibers located in the anterior half of the spinal cord to the preganglionic neurons. Many fibers descend in the periaqueductal gray matter to the brainstem parasympathetic nuclei and to the intermediolateral nuclei in the T1 to L2 levels (sympathetics) and to the sacral levels

(parasympathetics). These descending pathways are considered to be the upper motoneurons of the autonomic nervous system.

Interruption of the descending autonomic fibers in the brainstem or cervical spinal cord may result in Horner's syndrome (Chap. 12).

DENERVATION SENSITIVITY AND SYMPATHECTOMY

Some effectors are dependent upon their innervation for their structural and functional integrity. When denervated, they eventually become functionless and atrophy. This is the fate of denervated voluntary muscle as noted in a lower motoneuron paralysis (Chap. 12).

Other effectors are not wholly dependent upon their innervation to retain their functional status. Denervated involuntary muscles, cardiac muscles, and glands continue to function. For example, the transplanted heart may function adequately; however, when deprived of the autonomic nervous system influences, these effectors do not function absolutely normally, in that, they do not respond as effectively as they should to satisfy the changing demands of the organism.

When an effector is deprived of its innervation, it may become extremely sensitive to chemical mediators (neurotransmitters). For example, the rate of beat of the totally denervated heart will increase if the heart is exposed to but 1 part of epinephrine in 1,400 million. This *denervation hypersensitivity* is lost following the regeneration of the fibers and the reinnervation of the heart. Denervation hypersensitivity is noticeable in clinical situations following sympathectomy. In Horner's syndrome, the pupil of one eye is constricted and does not normally dilate because it is deprived of sympathetic stimulation; however, when a patient with Horner's syndrome is extremely excited, the epinephrine and norepinephrine released by the adrenal medulla can stimulate the hypersensitive denervated dilator muscle of the iris to respond so that the pupil dilates; this is known as the *paradoxic pupillary response.*

ACTIVITY ON SPECIFIC ORGANS AND STRUCTURES

The response of a specific effector to a specific neurotransmitter is not solely determined by the neurotransmitter; the nature of the receptor sites on the effector is also significant in predicting the response to a stimulation. The response of an effector is determined by the nature of the neurotransmitter-receptor linkages. For example, norepinephrine stimulates the contraction of smooth muscles of an arteriole (vessel constricts) and the relaxation of smooth muscles of the bronchial tubes (tubes dilate) in the lungs. The different responses to the same neurosecretion are explained by the differences in the nature of the receptor sites on the smooth muscles. Different neurotransmitters may stimulate different effectors to respond in a similar way. For example, the radial muscle of the iris of the eye contracts when stimulated by norepinephrine, whereas the sphincter muscles of the iris contract when stimulated by acetylcholine; both are smooth muscles. (Refer to **Table 20.1** to determine the response of various organs to sympathetic and parasympathetic stimulation.)

A dual innervation of the body by both the sympathetics and parasympathetics is general, but not universal: (1) The heart has a true reciprocal (dual) innervation, with the sympathetics acting to increase, and the parasympathetics acting to decrease, the rate of the heartbeat. (2) The salivary glands are stimulated synergistically, with sympathetic activity producing a thick, viscous secretion and parasympathetic activity producing a profuse, watery secretion. (3) The constriction and dilatation of the pupil exemplifies an activity resulting from the stimulation of different muscle groups. The pupil of the eye dilates when the radial (dilator) muscles (innervated only by sympathetic fibers) are stimulated by the sympathetics, and it constricts when the sphincter (constrictor) muscles (innervated only by parasympathetic fibers) are stimulated by the parasympathetics. (4) Some structures are innervated by only one system; hair muscles (when goose pimples are formed) and sweat glands are stimulated only by sympathetic fibers.

Non-Adrenergic, Non-Cholinergic (NANC) Transmission in the Autonomic Nervous System

Recent advances have uncovered many new significant insights into the neurobiology of the autonomic nervous system. Over 20 putative transmitters and modulators have been identified and added to the two classical transmitters, acetylcholine and norepinephrine, of this system. These new neuroactive *non-adrenergic, non-cholinergic (NANC)* agents are active in neurotransmission at synapses of sympathetic, parasympathetic, and enteric neurons. Most autonomic neurons contain two to a multiple number of agents, which include acetylcholine, amino acids, biogenic amines, neuropeptides, and others (Chap. 15). The current thesis is that many, if not all, neurons of the autonomic nervous system store and release more than one agent. For example, note the large vesicles containing a neuropeptide and small vesicles containing norepinephrine in the varicosities in **Figure 15.3**. For example, acetylcholine and VIP are cotransmitters of the parasympathetic fibers innervating the salivary glands with the former increasing salivary secretion and the latter acting as a modulator enhancing the action of the former. Within the prevertebral sympathetic ganglia (**Fig. 20.2**) are SIF cells, containing monoamines and neuropeptides. The cotransmission of specific combinations of transmitter and modulator has been suggested to be a form of "chemical coding," especially in the enteric system. The neuropeptides are presumed to act as neuromodulators (peptidergic) rather than neurotransmitters.

The purinergic transmitters responsible for most NANC inhibition are ATP or related purine compounds such as adenosine. The nitrergic transmitter responsible for some NANC inhibition is nitric oxide (NO—the free radical of nitric acid) (Chap. 15) (Hoyle, Lincoln, and Burnstock, 1994).

The autonomic nerves exhibit a functional form of plasticity—the capacity of a neuron to modify and to alter its synaptic transmitter or receptor activity—during development, and even aging (Chap. 6). For example, the postganglionic sympathetic nerves innervating the sweat glands in the human are adrenergic before birth and become cholinergic after birth.

Table 20.1: Some Comparisons Between the Sympathetic and Parasympathetic Nervous Systems

GENERAL		
	Sympathetic Nervous System	*Parasympathetic Nervous System*
Outflow from CNS	Thoracolumbar levels	Craniosacral levels
Location of ganglia	Paravertebral and prevertebral ganglia close to CNS	Terminal ganglia near effectors
Ratio of preganglionic to postganglionic neurons	Each preganglionic neuron synapses with many postganglionic neurons	Each preganglionic neuron synapses with a few postganglionic neurons
Distribution in body	Throughout the body	Limited primarily to viscera of head, thorax, abdomen, and pelvis

SPECIFIC STRUCTURES		
Structure	*Sympathetic Function*	*Parasympathetic Function*
Eye		
Radial muscle of iris	Dilates pupil (mydriasis)	
Sphincter muscle of iris		Contraction of pupil (miosis)
Ciliary muscle (accommodation)	Relaxation for far vision	Contraction for near vision
Glands of head		
Lacrimal gland		Stimulates secretion
Salivary glands	Scanty thick, viscous secretion	Profuse, watery secretion
Heart		
Rate	Increase	Decreased
Force of ventricular contraction	Increase	
Blood vessels	Generally constricts*	Slight effect
Lungs		
Bronchial tubes	Dilates lumen	Constricts lumen
Bronchial glands		Stimulates secretion
Gastrointestinal tract		
Motility and tone	Inhibits	Stimulates
Sphincters	Stimulates	Inhibits (relaxes)
Secretion	May inhibit	Stimulates
Gallbladder and ducts	Inhibits	Stimulates
Liver	Glycogenolysis increase (blood sugar)	
Adrenal medulla	Secretion of epinephrine and norepinephrine*	
Sex organs	Vasoconstriction, constriction of vas deferens, seminal vesicle, and prostatic musculature (ejaculation)	Vasodilation and erection
Skin		
Sweat glands	Stimulated*	
Blood vessels	Constricted	Slight effect
Neurotransmitter at neuroeffector junction	Usually norepinephrine*	Acetylcholine
Inactivation of transmitter	Slow and reuptake	Rapid
Reinforcement in body	Secretion of norepinephrine and epinephrine by adrenal medulla	

* Exceptions: Some postganglionic neurons of the sympathetic nervous system are cholinergic neurons. Sympathetic neuroeffector transmission mediated by acetylcholine includes (1) some blood vessels in skeletal muscles and (2) most sweat glands. The postganglionic sympathetic neurons that innervate the sweat glands are, before innervating the sweat glands, adrenergic neurons. Following the innervation of the sweat glands they become cholinergic neurons (see section concerning neural specificity and plasticity, Chap. 6). The sweat glands of the palm are innervated by adrenergic neurons. The cells of the adrenal medulla are actually postganglionic cells: they are innervated by preganglionic cholinergic sympathetic neurons.

The above are indicators that the previously held distinction between cholinergic and adrenergic (catecholaminergic) neurons underlying "the dual hypothesis of antagonism in the autonomic nervous system, is no longer tenable" (Bannister and Mathias).

Neural Control of the Pelvic Organs

The neural control of the urogenital pelvic organs is complex, and, as yet, not fully understood. The following is a general account of the patterns of control (Hoyle, Lincoln, and Burnstock, 1994). The urinary bladder is predominately under parasympathetic control; the motor limbs of the voiding reflexes (a) comprise the parasympathetic contraction of the detrusor muscle (smooth muscle of the walls of the bladder) stimulated by cholinergic and purinergic transmitters (Chap. 15) and (b) coordinate with the parasympathetic relaxation of the musculature of the proximal urethra modulated by nitrergic messengers (Chap. 15). In contrast, the primary neural control of the male accessory sex organs is via the adrenergic and purinergic sympathetic activity that stimulates motor reflex limbs involved with emission associated with the vas deferens, prostate glands, and seminal vesicles. In addition, there is adrenergic sympathetic control over the proximal urethra that results in its constriction during emission and ejaculation. This prevents retrograde ejaculation into the bladder. There appears to be parasympathetic control over the actual secretion of glandular fluid by the accessory glands into the seminal fluid. Erection of the penis appears to be under cholinergic, peptidergic, and nitrergic parasympathetic control for tumescence (swelling) and adrenergic sympathetic control for detumescence. Thus, the sympathetic and parasympathetic nervous systems act both antagonistically and synergistically to complement their functional activities. In addition, the somatosensory and motor pathways are involved in the control of storage of urine in the bladder, urination, emission, ejaculation, and probably in the maintenance of the rigidity of the penis.

Vasomotor and Sudomotor Pathways

The pathways of the autonomic nervous system involved with constriction and dilation of blood vessels (vasomotor fibers) and with secretion of the sweat glands (sudomotor fibers) descend in the ventrolateral columns of white matter. These fibers terminate and synapse with preganglionic sympathetic neurons in the intermediolateral cell column. Interruption of these descending pathways results in loss of sweating and vasodilation and an orthostatic hypotension below the level of the lesion. This occurs in paraplegia (Chap. 12). The hypotension is orthostatic (resulting when assuming the upright posture) because the central nervous system cannot produce sufficient vasoconstriction. As a consequence, the hydrostatic pressure from the pull of gravity results in the pooling of blood in the dilated blood vessels and in a reduction of the blood flow to the heart. The patient will faint because the heart does not pump enough blood to the brain.

The selective degeneration of neurons of the autonomic nervous system results in the *Shy-Drager syndrome* in which the patient faints because of orthostatic hypotension.

Congenital Megacolon (Hirschsprung's Disease)

In this serious condition in infants, a portion of the large bowel is continuously constricted, while the colon proximal to this obstructed segment is enormously dilated. The constricted segment contains the flaw responsible for the disease. Within it, intrinsic neurons of the intramural plexuses are missing, hence this aganglionic segment is unable to relax; however, this region does have an autonomic innervation consisting of both cholinergic and adrenergic axons, illustrating the significance of the intrinsic neurons of the gut in peristalsis.

SUGGESTED READINGS

Appenzeller O. *Clinical Autonomic Failure: Practical Concepts.* New York, NY: Elsevier; 1986.

Appenzeller O. *The Autonomic Nervous System: An Introduction to Basic and Clinical Concepts.* 4th ed. New York, NY: Elsevier; 1990.

Bannister R, Mathias C, eds. *Autonomic Failure: A Textbook of Clinical Disorders of the Autonomic Nervous System.* 3rd ed. New York, NY: Oxford University Press; 1992.

Burnstock G, Milner P. Structural and chemical organization of the autonomic nervous system with special reference to non-adrenergic, non-cholinergic transmission. In: Bannister R, Mathias C, eds. *Autonomic Failure: A Textbook of Clinical Disorders of the Autonomic Nervous System*. 3rd ed. New York, NY: Oxford University Press; 1992:107–125.

Cechetto D, Saper C. Evidence for a viscerotopic sensory representation in the cortex and thalamus in the rat. *J Comp Neurol*. 1987;262:27–45.

Cervero F, Morrison J, eds. Visceral sensation. *Prog Brain Res*. 1987;67.

Elfvin L-G, Lindh B, Hökfelt T. The chemical neuroanatomy of the synaptic ganglia. *Annu Rev Neurosci*. 1993;16:471–508.

Furness J, Bornstein J, Murphy R, Pompolo S. Roles of peptides in transmission in the enteric nervous system. *Trends Neurosci*. 1992;15:66–71.

Gershon M. The enteric nervous system. *Annu Rev Neurosci*. 1981;4:227–272.

Harris-Warwick R, Marder E, Silverson A, Meulens M, eds. *Dynamic Biological Networks: The Stomatogastric Nervous System*. Cambridge, Mass: Bradford Books, MIT Press; 1992.

Hoyle C, Lincoln J, Burntock G. Neural control of pelvic organs. In: Rushton D, ed. *Handbook of Neuro-Urology*. New York, NY: Marcel Dekker; 1994:1–54.

Karczmar A, Koketsu K, Nishi N, eds. *Autonomic and Enteric Ganglia*. New York, NY: Plenum; 1986.

Lefkowitz R, Hoffman B, Taylor P. Neurohumoral transmission: the autonomic and somatic nervous systems. In: Gilman A, Rall T, Nies A, Taylor P, eds. *Goodman & Gilman's The Pharmacological Basis of Therapeutics*. 8th ed. Elmsford, NY: Pergamon; 1990:84–121.

Loewy A, Spyer K, eds. *Central Regulation of Autonomic Functions*. New York, NY: Oxford University Press; 1990.

Luitin P, ter Horst G, Karst H, Steffens A. The course of paraventricular hypothalamic efferents to autonomic structures in medulla and spinal cord. *Exp Brain Res*. 1985;329:374–378.

Miller N. Biofeedback and visceral learning. *Annu Rev Psychol*. 1978;29:373–404.

Nathan P, Smith M. The location of descending fibres to sympathetic neurons supplying the eye and pseudomotor neurons supplying the head and neck. *J Neurol Neurosurg Psychiatry*. 1986;49:187–194.

Reis D, Ruggiero D, Granata A. Central nervous system control of the heart. Brainstem mechanisms governing the tonic and reflex control of the circulation. In: Stober T, et al, eds. *Central Nervous System Control of the Heart: Proceedings of IIIrd International Brain Heart Conference*. Boston, Mass: Martinus Nijhoff; 1986:19–36.

Singer M, Goebell H, eds. *Nerves and the Gastrointestinal Tract (Falk Symposium)*. Lancaster, UK: Klüver Academic Pub; 1988.

Smith O, DeVito J. Central neural integration for the control of autonomic responses associated with emotion. *Annu Rev Neurosci*. 1984;7:43–65.

Swanson L, Mogenson G. Neural mechanisms for the functional coupling of autonomic, endocrine and somatomotor responses in adaptive behavior. *Brain Res Rev*. 1981;3:1–34.

van Zweiten P. Adrenergic and cholinergic receptors. In: Bannister R, Mathias C, eds. *Autonomic Failure: A Textbook of Clinical Disorders of the Autonomic Nervous System*. 3rd ed. New York, NY: Oxford University Press; 1992:94–106.

General functional considerations

Basic circuits of the hypothalamus

Neurohumoral reflexes

Autonomic nervous system

Temperature regulation

Regulation of water balance

Food intake and energy balance

Expressions of emotion and behavior

Sleep-wake cycle, circadian rhythms, and the suprachiasmatic nucleus

Circumventricular (CV) organs

The hypothalamus functions primarily in homeostasis—the maintenance of a relatively constant internal body environment. Its effects are exerted through the autonomic nervous system, the endocrine system, and the somatic motor system. Its influence is widespread and is even involved with emotions and behavior.

The 4 gram hypothalamus is located in the basal region of the diencephalon adjacent to the third ventricle. In its rostrocaudal extent from the lamina terminalis to the midbrain, the hypothalamus is divided into nuclei and four major areas (Figs. 21.1 and 21.2): (1) a rostral or preoptic area, (2) a supraoptic area located above the optic chiasma, (3) a tuberal area (the region of tuber cinereum extends from the optic chiasma to the mammillary body), and (4) a caudal or mammillary area that grades into the midbrain central gray. The *hypophysis* (pituitary gland) extends ventrally from the tuberal area. Some important hypothalamic nuclei include the suprachiasmatic nucleus (SCN) of the preoptic area, the paraventricular nucleus and supraoptic nucleus of the supraoptic area, the lateral and ventral nuclei of the tuberal area, and the mammillary nuclei of the mammillary area. Developmentally, the preoptic area is a telencephalic structure, whereas the rest of the hypothalamus is diencephalic. The preoptic area is so closely associated with the hypothalamus, however, that it is considered to be a part of the hypothalamus.

The hypophysis (pituitary gland) comprises two major subdivisions—the *adenohypophysis* (an epithelial structure) and the *neurohypophysis* (a neural structure). The adenohypophysis develops as an outpocketing from the embryonic pharynx, while the neurohypophysis originates as an outgrowth from the region of the neural tube giving rise to the hypothalamus. The adenohypophysis consists of the pars distalis (anterior lobe), pars tuberalis, and pars intermedia (Fig. 21.1). The neurohypophysis comprises the median eminence of the tuber cinereum, infundibular stem, and infundibular process (pars nervosa, neural lobe). The median eminence, which extends from the optic chiasma to the infundibular stem, differs from the rest of the hypothalamus. The median eminence and the infundibular stem are known as the *hypophysiotropic area*, where the neurally derived hypothalamic releasing hormones are released and transferred to the hypophyseal portal system (Fig. 21.2).

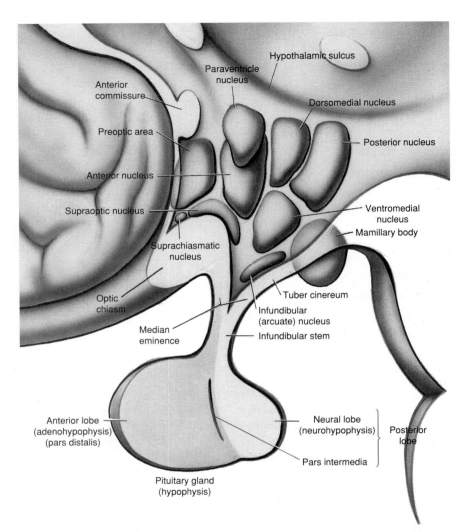

Figure 21.1: Some hypothalamic nuclei and the hypophysis. The hypothalamus is composed of four nuclear areas: (1) the rostral or preoptic area, including the suprachiasmatic nucleus; (2) the supraoptic area, including the supraoptic, anterior, and paraventricular nuclei; (3) the tuberal area, including the infundibular, ventromedial, and dorsomedial nuclei; and (4) the caudal or mammillary area, including the posterior nucleus and mammillary body.

GENERAL FUNCTIONAL CONSIDERATIONS

The hypothalamus functions primarily through the activities of regulatory centers and modulating centers. A *regulatory (integration) center* is a crucial control center that is essential to the expression of a specific function; an example is the "thermostat" monitoring and controlling body temperature, located in the hypothalamus. A *modulating center* is a nuclear pool influencing a regulation center. It is not vital to a spe-

cific function. The hypothalamus can influence the blood pressure regulatory centers in the medulla. Through these roles the hypothalamus exerts its influences on behavioral responses in both visceromotor and somatomotor spheres.

The roles of the hypothalamus are expressed primarily through (1) the endocrine system and (2) the autonomic nervous system. It regulates endocrine activity (a) directly through neurons of the supraopticohypophyseal tract that release hormones into capillaries of the general circulation within the posterior lobe (neurohypo-

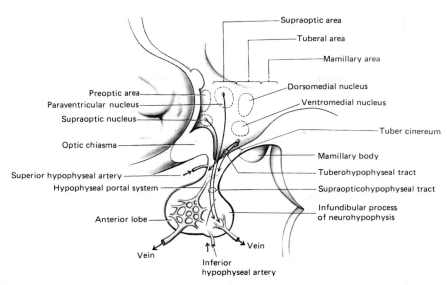

Figure 21.2: Some hypothalamic nuclei and the hypophysis. The supraopticohypophyseal tract extends from the supraoptic and paraventricular nucleus to the capillary bed of the neurohypophysis. The hypophyseal-portal system is a vascular network extending from the base of the hypothalamus and upper neurohypophysis to the anterior lobe of the hypophysis.

physis), and (b) indirectly via the blood vessels of the hypophyseal portal system from the hypophysiotropic area of the hypothalamus to the adenohypophysis (anterior pituitary gland). The hypothalamus is involved in the regulation of most functional expressions of the autonomic nervous system—called the "head ganglion of the autonomic nervous system." These include basic physiologic functions and expressions related to behavior. The former include temperature regulation, water balance, heart rate, blood pressure, and gastrointestinal activity. The latter include anger, rage, sexual behavioral patterns, and calmness.

The nervous system and the endocrine system actually form a continuum as indicated in the fields of neuroendocrinology and endocrine neurology. The nervous system is, in essence, a gland comprised of neurons that secrete neurotransmitters. The hypothalamus acts as an endocrine gland with certain neurons secreting releasing hormones that regulate the secretory activity of the hypophysis. Receptor sites for hormones are present in the plasma membranes of neurons. Hormones are involved in modulating some processing within the nervous system that, in turn, influences behavioral activities.

Intrinsic Hypothalamic Receptors

Some neurons within the hypothalamus act as intrinsic receptors involved in several vital functional activities—thermal receptors for temperature regulation and osmoreceptors for water metabolism. For example, hypothalamic receptors monitor the temperature of the blood flowing through the hypothalamic capillaries, enabling the organ to perform its role as the integrator of body temperature. The efferent limb of the reflex includes (1) descending autonomic pathways to the sweat glands and peripheral blood vessels, and (2) descending somatic pathways to the trunk musculature for panting and shivering.

Neurohumoral Reflexes

The neurohumoral reflex arc utilizes both the nervous system (neuro-) and the blood vascular system (humoral). To perform its role in water metabolism, for example, the hypothalamus utilizes an intrinsic hypothalamic receptor to monitor the osmolality of the blood flowing through the brain. The neuron receptors are stimulated to release a neurosecretion, antidiuretic hormone (ADH), that is conveyed via nerve fibers (*supraopticohypophyseal tract*) to the infundibular process of the hypophysis (Fig. 21.2), where it is stored and released into the systemic blood system and conveyed to its target structures in the kidney. Such reflexes are discussed more fully below.

Hypophyseal Portal System and Hypothalamic Releasing Hormones

The hypophysis receives its blood supply from several arteries (Fig. 21.2). A pair of inferior hypophyseal arteries from the internal carotid arteries furnish blood to the infundibular process and infundibular stem. Several superior hypophyseal arteries from the internal carotid arteries form a capillary plexus in the median eminence, pars tuberalis, and infundibular stem; this capillary plexus collects into the hypophyseal portal system of blood vessels (hypothalamic portal system and hypophyseal portal vein). This portal system is a vascular network commencing as a capillary bed in the median eminence and collecting into several main channels before arborizing into a capillary (sinusoidal) bed in the adenohypophysis.

The hypophyseal portal system is the vascular pathway through which the neural language from the hypophysiotropic area, in the form of releasing hormones (RH), is transferred and conveyed to the pars anterior to trigger the endocrine language of the hypophysis. More specifically, the hypothalamic nerve fibers liberate the releasing hormones from these nerve endings into the capillary plexuses of the median eminence and infundibular stem; these hormones are conveyed through the hypophyseal portal vessels to the adenohypophysis, where they stimulate or inhibit the release of a number of the hypophyseal hormones (see later).

BASIC CIRCUITS OF THE HYPOTHALAMUS

The hypothalamus is strategically located between the cerebrum and the brainstem. The complex neural circuits associated with the hypothalamus have reciprocal and widespread connections with these regions. The hypothalamus derives its major input from the nonspecific reticular pathways and little, if any, from the specific lemniscal pathways. The structures projecting to, and receiving from, the hypothalamus include the brainstem reticular formation, limbic lobe (including hippocampus and amygdaloid body), thalamus, and olfactory pathways. The major pathway of the hypothalamus is the medial forebrain bundle. This is an intricate complex of short, multisynaptic, multineuronal chains extending from parts of the limbic lobe through the lateral hypothalamus to the paramedian tegmentum of the midbrain.

Input

The *input to the hypothalamus* (Fig. 21.3) is conveyed via (1) ascending pathways from the brainstem tegmentum and periaqueductal gray matter (PAG), (2) descending fibers from the forebrain, and (3) the blood vascular system. The neurons of the hypothalamus respond to a variety of messengers. They contain receptor sites for (1) such neurotransmitters as acetylcholine, norepinephrine, dopamine, serotonin, and numerous neuropeptides and (2) such agents as sex steroid hormones, thyroxin, and hormones released by the adenohypophysis.

1. The *ascending pathways from the brainstem* include fibers of the mammillary peduncle from the dorsal and ventral tegmental nuclei, fibers of the dorsal longitudinal fasciculus (DLF) from the PAG, fibers of the medial forebrain bundle from the midbrain tegmentum and catecholamine pathways from some brainstem nuclei (Figs. 15.1 and 15.2), and central tegmental tract (Chap. 22).
2. The *descending fibers from the forebrain* include (Fig. 21.3):
   a. fibers of the fornix originating in the hippocampus and the septal nuclei of the limbic system. The hippocampus is a significant channel for afferent and neocortical input to the hypothalamus.
   b. fibers originating in the cortex of the uncus and amygdaloid body. These project via the stria terminalis and ventral amygdalofugal pathway to the hypothalamus. The primary olfactory cortex projects via fibers of the medial forebrain bundle. The olfactory system is the only sensory system with a direct route to the

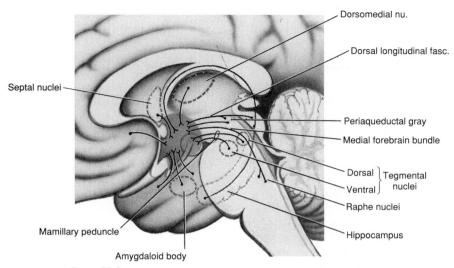

Figure 21.3: The major tracts conveying input to the hypothalamus.

hypothalamus. A few fibers from the retina terminate in the hypothalamus (suprachiasmatic nucleus).

c. the orbitofrontal cortex and septal nuclei, the source of fibers of the medial forebrain bundle.

d. the dorsomedial and midline nuclei of the thalamus that project to the hypothalamus and amygdaloid body.

3. the *blood vascular system* conveys influences to which the hypothalamus may respond. These include hormones, temperature of the blood, and osmolality of the blood plasma.

Output

The *output from the hypothalamus* (**Fig. 21.4**) is conveyed via (1) ascending fibers to the fore-

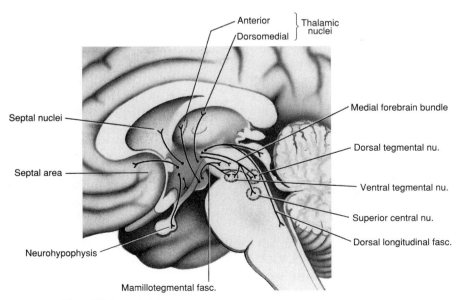

Figure 21.4: The major tracts conveying output from the hypothalamus.

brain, (2) descending fibers to the brainstem and spinal cord, and (3) fibers and blood vessels to the hypophysis (endocrine effector projections).

1. The *ascending fibers from the hypothalamus to the forebrain* include those projecting to the anterior and dorsomedial thalamic nuclei, septal nuclei, and septal (subcallosal) area.
2. The *descending fibers* to the midbrain and pons project to the dorsal and ventral tegmental nuclei, superior central nucleus (a raphe nucleus), and the PAG. The dorsal vagal nucleus and adjacent nuclei in the medulla also receive projections from the hypothalamus. The descending tracts from the hypothalamus include the DLF, medial forebrain bundle, and mammillotegmental fasciculus.
3. The influences from the *hypothalamus to the hypophysis* are conveyed via the hypophyseal portal system to the adenohypophysis and via the supraopticohypophyseal tract to the neural lobe (see below).

These projections to and from the hypothalamus are involved with the functional activities of the autonomic nervous system (Chap. 20), limbic system (Chap. 22), and endocrine system (see below).

NEUROHUMORAL REFLEXES

The hypothalamus is integrated into distinct neurohumoral reflexes in which two separate fiber pathways extend from the hypothalamus to the hypophysis. The neurons of these pathways are involved with both neurally and humorally conveyed stimuli.

Tuberohypophyseal Tract

The tuberohypophyseal tract projects from the hypothalamic nuclei located in the hypophysiotropic area found in the medial basal hypothalamus (includes the tuber cinereum) and terminates in the infundibular stem (**Fig. 21.2**). The neurons of this tract elaborate and convey hypophysiotropins (hypothalamic releasing hormones) to the capillary loops of the hypophyseal portal system, and via this vascular system, to the adenohypophysis of the pituitary gland. These hypophysiotropins are peptides that exert their influences upon the release (or nonrelease) of various hypophyseal hormones into the systemic circulation. The neurons of the tuberohypophyseal tract constitute the parvocellular neurosecretory system, so-called because its neurons have axons with small diameters. In a sense, the portal system into which the hypophysiotropins are released is actually a huge synaptic cleft; the portal system bridges the gap between the presynaptic tuberohypophyseal tract and the postsynaptic cells of the anterior lobes. In another context, the portal veins are a "final common pathway."

Releasing Hormones

1. *Gonadotropin releasing hormone* (GnRH) regulates the release of follicle stimulating hormone (FSH, follitropin) and luteinizing hormone (LH, lutropin) from the hypophysis.
2. *Thyrotropic hormone-releasing hormone* (TRH) regulates the release of thyrotropin (thyroid stimulating hormone, TSH) and prolactin from the hypophysis.
3. *Corticotropin-releasing hormone* (CRH) regulates the release of adrenocorticotropin (adrenocorticotropic hormone [ACTH]) and β-lipotropin from the hypophysis. (β-lipotropin hormone is a precursor of endorphins and ACTH.)
4. *Growth hormone-releasing hormone* (GRH or GHRH) regulates the release of growth hormone (somatotropin) from the hypophysis.
5. *Prolactin-releasing factor* (PRF) is the putative releasing hormone that regulates the release of prolactin (lactogenic hormone, mammotropic hormone) from the hypophysis.
6. *Melanocyte-stimulating hormone-releasing hormone* is the putative releasing hormone that stimulates the release of melanocyte stimulating hormone and β-endorphin from the hypophysis. In man, melanocyte-stimulating hormone (MSH) stimulates the formation of melanin pigment and its dispersion in melanocytes.

Inhibiting Hormones

1. *Growth hormone release-inhibiting hormone* (GIH, GHRIH) also called *somatostatin* (SS)

or *somatotropin release-inhibiting hormone* (SRIH) acts to inhibit the release of growth hormone and thyrotropin from the hypophysis.

2. *Prolactin release-inhibiting hormone* (PIH) or *dopamine* (DA) acts to inhibit the release of prolactin from the hypophysis.

3. *Melanocyte-stimulating hormone release-inhibiting hormone* (MIH) acts to inhibit the release of melanocyte stimulating hormone.

A complex series of feedback systems to the hypothalamus and to the hypophysis have a significant role in regulating and controlling the secretory activity of these hormones. They comprise (1) a *long feedback loop*, in which the hypothalamus monitors hormones synthesized by the peripheral target organs (e.g., thyroxine released by the thyroid gland is fed back via the bloodstream to be monitored by the hypothalamus); (2) a *short feedback loop*, in which each tropic hormone of the pituitary gland is fed back to, and monitored by, the hypothalamus; (3) an even shorter feedback loop, in which the releasing hormones feed back to and are monitored by the hypothalamus; and (4) a feedback loop in which each tropic hormone within the tissues is fed back to the hypophysis to influence and regulate the release of the same tropic hormone (e.g., growth hormone).

All of the hypophysiotropic peptides originally found in the hypothalamus are now known to be ubiquitous in the brain, though located in certain neurons. They are also found in the tissues of the gastrointestinal tract. The vasoactive intestinal peptide (VIP), which was originally identified in the gut, is also found in the central nervous system (CNS). The role of hypophysiotropic peptides in these organs has not yet been resolved. In addition, receptors for these substances have been found in many peripheral organs, but it is not clear what role these peptides play.

The peptides, once released into the synaptic space, are not recovered by a neuronal uptake mechanism similar to that for norepinephrine. Apparently, all the peptides available to presynaptic release sites are totally dependent on ribosomal synthesis in the cell body and are transported by axoplasmic flow to the synaptic terminals. The neuropeptides within neurons of the CNS coexist with the classical neurotransmitters. When released in the synaptic cleft, they act to alter the excitability of the postsynaptic membrane.

Supraopticohypophyseal Tract

The supraopticohypophyseal tract (**Fig. 21.2**), composed of about 100,000 unmyelinated fibers, extends from the supraoptic and paraventricular nuclei to the capillary bed of the neurohypophysis (posterior lobe). The fibers convey, via axoplasmic transport: (1) *antidiuretic hormone* (ADH, vasopressin), which is involved with the homeostatic role of conserving water regulating the tonicity of body fluids and (2) *oxytocin*, which has a role in stimulating the contraction of smooth muscles of the uterus and in promoting the ejecting of milk from the lactating mammary glands by stimulating contractions of its myoepithelial cells.

The neurons of this tract constitute the magnocellular neurosecretory system with its large diameter axons. They synthesize the precursors (prohormones) of the hormones that are conveyed by axoplasmic flow to the neural lobe. Oxytocin and ADH are synthesized in the cell bodies in different neurons. Both types of neurons are located in both the supraoptic nucleus and paraventricular nucleus. With the appropriate stimulus, an axon potential is conveyed to the axon terminals. This triggers the inflow of calcium followed by the release of the ADH or oxytocin at this neurovascular synapse with the fenestrated capillary wall into the systematic circulation.

AUTONOMIC NERVOUS SYSTEM

The hypothalamus is the chief *subcortical* center regulating all kinds of visceral activities and some somatic functions; it acts primarily as a modulator of autonomic centers in the brainstem and spinal cord (Chap. 20).

The *anterior hypothalamus* (preoptic and supraoptic regions) has an excitatory parasympathetic (or inhibitory to sympathetic activity) role. The stimulation of this region may produce: a decrease in the rate of the heartbeat; a decrease in blood pressure; dilatation of the cutaneous blood vessels; an increase in motility, peristalsis and secretion in the gastrointestinal tract; constriction of the pupil; and increased sweating. Activity in this region produces a parasympathetic (vagal) tone and such somatic responses as panting. Lesions in this area may result in the production of sympathetic effects.

The *posterior hypothalamus* has an excitatory sympathetic role. Activation of this region may produce: an increase in the rate of the heartbeat; an increase in blood pressure; constriction of cutaneous blood vessels; a decrease in motility, peristalsis, and secretion in the gastrointestinal tract; dilatation of the pupil; and erection of hair. Activity in this region produces a sympathetic tone and such somatic responses as shivering, running, and struggling.

The *descending projections* from the hypothalamus are involved with regulating a variety of bodily functions through its influences on the autonomic nervous system (Chap. 20). Some of its influences are involved with certain somatic functions. The latter include a role in (1) shivering produced by the activity of voluntary muscles and (2) the activities of the voluntary palatal and pharyngeal muscles associated with the ingestion of food (the latter are innervated by the nucleus ambiguus, a brainstem nucleus).

The descending fibers influencing the autonomic nervous system include the (1) DLF in the medial brainstem tegmentum and (2) fibers in the dorsolateral tegmentum. The DLF extends caudally in the medulla and innervates the superior and inferior salivatory nuclei and the dorsal motor nucleus of the vagus nerve—all are the source of parasympathetic outflow (Chap. 20). Some fibers terminate in the nucleus solitarius, a visceral sensory nucleus (Chap. 14). These fibers may constitute a *reflected feedback pathway* modulating visceral sensory input. The fibers in the dorsolateral tegmentum extend throughout the length of the spinal cord. Some of their fibers may terminate in the parasympathetic nuclei of the brainstem and they also terminate (1) in the lateral intermediate zone of T1 to L2, the location of the outflow of the sympathetic system and (2) S2 to S4, the location of the outflow of the parasympathetic system.

A lesion in the dorsolateral tegmentum of the medulla can interrupt the descending sympathetic fibers and result in Horner's syndrome (Chap. 12). This can be the consequence of an obstruction of the posterior inferior cerebellar artery (PICA) (Chap. 4). The symptoms include miosis of the pupil, ptosis of the eyelid, decreased sweating, and increased warmth and redness on the side of the face; all occur on the ipsilateral side, indicating that these fibers descend without crossing to the opposite side.

TEMPERATURE REGULATION

The hypothalamus has an essential role in body temperature; it regulates the balance between heat production and heat loss. More specifically, the hypothalamus has thermal receptor neurons which monitor the temperature of the blood. This "thermostat" regulates the heat-producing and heat-conserving control systems. In effect, the continuous fine adjustments necessary for maintaining a constant normal body temperature depend upon the hypothalamus.

The anterior hypothalamus acts to prevent a rise in body temperature. It activates those processes which favor heat loss including vasodilatation of cutaneous blood vessels, sweating (evaporation of water for cooling), and panting. Destruction of this "heat-dissipating region" may produce a highly elevated body temperature (hyperthermia).

The posterior hypothalamus contains a region which triggers those activities concerned with heat production and heat conservation. These include the metabolic heat-producing systems (oxidation of glucose), vasoconstriction (especially of cutaneous blood vessels), erection of hair (goose pimples), and shivering. The malfunctioning of this region may produce a cold-blooded mammal that cannot sustain a uniform body temperature.

Pyrogenic substances, produced in some diseases, affect the hypothalamus. A fever known as *neurogenic hyperthermia* results.

REGULATION OF WATER BALANCE

The hypothalamus has significant roles in fluid balance by regulating both the intake (by drinking) and output (through kidneys and sweat glands) of water. Evidence indicates that a "drinking" or "thirst" center is located in the lateral hypothalamus and a "thirst satiety" center in the medial hypothalamus. The *osmoreceptor neurons* in these hypothalamic centers respond to the osmolality of the blood passing through these nuclei. They set off events which stimulate or inhibit water intake. Other factors such as dryness of the oral mucosa from decreased salivary flow also influence intake of water.

The hypothalamus has a crucial role in the conservation and loss of body water through the regulation of urine flow in the kidneys by ADH, which is produced by the neurons of the supraoptic and paraventricular nuclei of the hypothalamus. ADH (vasopressin) is synthesized by the neurons in these nuclei and carried by axoplasmic transport in the supraopticohypophyseal tract to the neurohypophysis where it is stored or released into the systemic blood circulation. The ADH acts upon the kidney (distal convoluted and collecting tubules) to increase the reabsorption of water from the dilute glomerular filtrate in the tubules back into the bloodstream, thus concentrating the urine. Water is thereby conserved and is not excreted in the urine. Increases in osmolality in blood flowing through the hypothalamus stimulate the release of ADH; this results in antidiuresis and conservation of water. Decreases in osmolality inhibit the release of ADH; this results in diuresis and excretion of water in urine. Other factors may have a role; vascular receptors monitoring blood volume or flow in the body project input to the hypothalamus, in this way influencing the release of ADH.

A deficiency in the formation and release of ADH may result in *diabetes insipidus* (increased excretion of water without increase in sugar), in which as much as 10 to 12 liters of urine may be excreted per day.

Following an injury of the infundibular stem and the axons of its neurons, diabetes insipidus may result. This may be temporary, because the axons regenerate and a new functional neurohypophysis is established.

FOOD INTAKE AND ENERGY BALANCE

The hypothalamic region involved with feeding responses has been called the "appestat," with the ventral medial hypothalamic nucleus called the "satiety center" and the lateral hypothalamic nucleus called the "hunger" or "feeding" center. Stimulation of the ventral median nucleus inhibits the animal's urge to eat. Destruction of the pair of nuclei produces an animal exhibiting decreased physical activity and a voracious appetite (not true hunger) with a twofold to threefold increase in food intake. The animal becomes obese. Stimulation of the lateral hypothalamic nucleus induces the animal to eat, whereas its destruction produces an animal that refuses to eat until severe emaciation from starvation ensues.

Two theories have been proposed to explain how these centers are influenced. According to the *glucostat hypothesis*, hypothalamic neurons respond to blood glucose levels. According to the *thermostat hypothesis*, blood temperature is the causative factor, with an increase resulting from the specific dynamic action of ingested blood and with a decrease resulting from dissipation of heat through the skin.

EXPRESSIONS OF EMOTION AND BEHAVIOR

The behavioral patterns associated with emotional experiences are of two general types: (1) subjective "feelings" and (2) objective physical expressions. The subjective aspects of emotion, from depression to euphoria, are more intimately bound up with the cerebral cortex. Many of the objective physical expressions are largely mediated through the hypothalamus and are recognizable as the enhanced activity of the autonomic nervous system. They include alterations in heartbeat (palpitations) and blood pressure, blushing and pallor of the face, dryness of the mouth, clammy hands, dilatation of the pupil (glassy eye), cold sweat, tears of happiness or sadness, and changes in the concentration of blood sugar. Stimulation of the hypothalamus in man is said to evoke changes in blood pressure and rate of heartbeat without any psychic manifestations.

Sexual Expressions

The sympathetic and parasympathetic systems are integrated in sexual and reproductive activities. Commencing with sexual arousal elicited from either psychologic or genital stimulation, the subsequent phases are essentially similar in both male and female. In the next phase, the engorgement of the erectile tissue resulting in the erection of the clitoris or penis is a response to parasympathetic stimulation (nervus erigentes S3 and S4). Loss of parasympathetic activity, as in diabetic neuropathy, results in impotency in the male (failure of erection and ejaculation). In the female, the parasympathetic fibers stimulate the secretions from the cervical glands to further moisten the vagina and engorge the labia minora. Stimulation by sympathetic fibers produces peristaltic waves that propel semen along the ductus deferens and contractions that discharge emission secretions from the seminal vesicles and prostate gland to form the substance of the ejaculate. The phase of ejaculation through and out of the urethra involves the coordinated activity of the parasympathetic fibers and somatic motoneurons (pudendal nerves S2-S4). During orgasm, the motoneurons evoke the spasmodic contraction of the bulbocavernous, ischiocavernous, and pelvic floor voluntary muscles that eject the ejaculate from the penis. Weakness of erection or premature ejaculation may occur as the consequence of overactivity of the sympathetic system. Often this has an emotional basis. Depression of sympathetic activity, following treatment with certain drugs, may result in impaired ability to ejaculate.

"Pleasure Centers" and "Punishing Centers"

The hypothalamus is very closely linked to the limbic system and commonly is considered part of it. Stimulation of some parts of the hypothalamus elicit expressions of pleasure or of punishment (see Chap. 22).

Responses to Intense Stress and Trauma

The response of the brain to profound crises involving intense stress and trauma is to mobilize the resources that act to protect the organism. These resources include activating the neural circuits involved with the "fight, fright, and flight" activities (Chap. 20). Among these activities are (1) the release of catecholamines for the initial preparation for the emergency by the neurons of the locus ceruleus with their widespread distribution (Chap. 15); (2) the release of pain-blunting endorphins and enkephalins by the hypothalamus and other neural complexes (Chap. 9); and (3) the release of the stress-response hormones by the hypothalamus and pituitary gland, namely corticotropin-releasing hormone (CRH) and adrenocorticotropic hormone (ACTH).

SLEEP-WAKE CYCLE, CIRCADIAN RHYTHMS, AND THE SUPRACHIASMATIC NUCLEUS

Sleep-Wake Cycle

The hypothalamus is associated with the state of awakeness and is integrated somehow into the sleep-wake cycle. The *ascending reticular activating system* (ARAS), which projects to the hypothalamus, and the diffuse projections from the hypothalamus to the cerebral cortex are among the neural substrates for the sleep-wake cycle (Chap. 22). The bilateral ablation of the regions posterolateral and caudal to the mammillary bodies produces a tame, apathetic, and often somnolent monkey or cat. Stimulation of the hypothalamus may induce drowsiness and sleep.

Many mammalian physiologic activities are expressed in daily rhythms that are close to 24 hours. These circadian rhythms (circa—about, diem—a day) run exactly 24 hours in the presence of normal light-dark cycles of day and night. In humans, the core body temperature fluctuates about a degree, being highest in the afternoon and lowest early in the morning. Other circadian rhythms include the: secretions of certain hormones, such as release of corticosteroids; excretion of certain electrolytes, such as potassium and calcium; eating; drinking; and the sleep-wake cycle. A circadian rhythm is not absolutely controlled by light or dark. It persists as a slightly modified rhythm in individuals who have lived for months in a cave with a constant moderate level of illumination. These humans adjust to a circadian rhythm that is close to 25 hours.

Circadian Rhythms and the Suprachiasmatic Nucleus

The primary circadian clock (mind's clock, pacemaker, or oscillator) of the mammalian brain regulating the daily rhythms is the suprachiasmatic nucleus (SCN) located in the anterior hypothalamus immediately above the optic chiasma (Fig. 21.1). The SCN is a critical component of the neural system known as the *circadian timing system* (CTS) (Klein, Moore and Reppert, 1991). This is a system defined as the set of neural structures having a primary role in circadian rhythm generation and its regulation. Circadian rhythms have evolved as an adaptation to the solar cycle of light and dark. They have two principal features: (1) the rhythms are generated by endogenous pacemakers in the absence of the light-dark cycle and (2) the entrainment by the light-dark cycle necessitates the presence of photoreceptors (retina) and visual pathways and their linkages to the pacemakers. In turn, the latter project their influences to critical nuclei of the brain. In common with CTSs of other organisms, the human CTS has three components: (1) photoreceptors and the visual pathways to mediate entrainment, (2) circadian pacemakers, and (3) efferent projections that couple the pacemakers to the neural systems that express the circadian cycles. Thus, functional disorders of the CTS could reflect alterations in each or combinations of these components. At the present time, little is known relating these components to specific changes in the circadian cycles.

The two subdivisions of the SCN are characterized by the presence of neuroactive substances and by the source of their visual projections. (1) One division receives (a) a direct visual input from the retina via the retinohypothalamic tract (RHT), and (b) an indirect visual input from the retina (W cells in cat) via a projection to the intrageniculate leaflet within the lateral geniculate body of the thalamus (Chap. 19). Neurons of this leaflet project to the SCN via the geniculohypothalamic tract (GHT). This division contains VIP containing neurons. Evidence suggests that the RHT and GHT pathways act through intracellular receptor-second messenger systems upon pacemaker neurons (Chap. 3). It is through these systems that the

primary role of the SCN as the circadian pacemaker links its sensitivity to environmental light and dark cycle to the mechanism of entrainment. In turn, this integrates the SCN as an important member of the neuroendocrine system. (2) The second division of the SCN receives input primarily from the serotonergic neurons of the raphe nuclei of the brainstem. There are no terminations from the optic tract. Many SCN neurons contain vasopressin as well as other neuroactive substances.

Much evidence supports the concept that the SCN contains the pacemaker of fundamental importance to the expression of the circadian rhythms in mammals, including humans. Surprisingly, the efferent projections from the SCN are not extensive and mainly are restricted to parts of the hypothalamus and midline thalamus; modest projections to the lateral septal nucleus and periaqueductal gray also are present. With its relatively restricted distribution of SCN projections, it is difficult to conceive how these limited projections can regulate and modulate the vast array of behavioral and physiological expressions associated with the circadian rhythms.

The biological clock oscillates in the mammalian fetus. In turn, this fetal clock is entrained by redundant circadian signals from the mother. The entrainable circadian clock prepares the developing fetus to adapt more readily for adjusting to life following birth.

Although the rhythms within the SCN may be influenced by neural and endocrine activity, the SCN is considered to play the central role in the regulation of circadian rhythms; however, it is possible that it may be the primary pacemaker for all circadian rhythms. As yet, the mechanisms involved in the circadian oscillations of the SCN are still enigmatic.

The effects of light on emotion and behavior are thought to be influenced through three variables: intensity, predominant colors in the light spectrum, and the proportion of light and dark every 24 hours. The effect of light may be conveyed by alterations in the release of melatonin, which is released from the pineal body only during the day (see Pineal Body, later). Changes in the daily cycles of light and dark presumably play a part in the winter-long depressions afflicting some people. As the days grow shorter, such individuals become sad, anxious, sleepy, uninterested in work and play, and there is weight gain from increased craving for, and intake of, carbohydrates.

CIRCUMVENTRICULAR (CV) ORGANS

Adjacent to the median ventricular cavities (third ventricle, cerebral aqueduct, and fourth ventricle) are specialized areas called *circumventricular (CV) organs*. These include (1) the median eminence of the tuber cinereum, the neurohypophysis, and the pineal body which are sites of neuroendocrine activity and (2) the organum vasculosum of the lamina terminalis, subfornical organ, subcommissural organ, and the area postrema (AP)(Fig. 21.5) which are chemoreceptive areas whose functional roles are not fully understood. The common vascular, ependymal, and neural organization of these structures differs from that found in typical brain tissue. They are referred to as "being in the brain but not of it" and as leaky areas, primarily because they lack a blood brain barrier. All CV organs are unpaired and located along

the ventricular surface near the midline except for the paired AP of the medulla. These leaky areas are isolated from the brain by a lining of specialized ependymal cells, called tanacytes, that separate these organs from the ventricles. The tanacytes are linked to each other by tight junctions that prevent the free exchange between the CV organs and the cerebrospinal fluid.

Median Eminence of the Tuber Cinereum

The *median eminence* of the *tuber cinereum* is that portion of the floor of the hypothalamus where the releasing and inhibiting hormones are released from the axon terminal into the capillary loops of the hypophyseal portal system. In essence, it is the site of the neurovascular link between the CNS and the adenohypophysis.

Neurohypophysis

As previously noted, the *neurohypophysis* is the site for the storage and release of vasopressin and oxytocin, which are synthesized in the supraoptic and paraventricular nuclei. The nerve

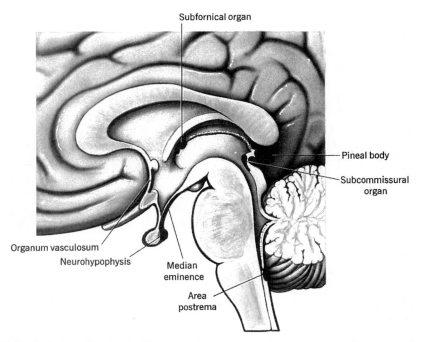

Subfornical organ

Pineal body

Subcommissural organ

Organum vasculosum
Neurohypophysis
Median eminence
Area postrema

Figure 21.5: Midsagittal view of the brain illustrating the location of the circumventricular organs. (After Weindl.)

terminals of the supraopticohypophyseal tract containing these neurohormones are intermingled among cells called pituicytes, which are modified glial cells.

Pineal Body (Figs. 1.8, 13.3, and 21.5)

The *pineal body (pineal gland* or *epiphysis cerebri)* is a midline cone-shaped structure located in the caudal epithalamus just above the midbrain. Descartes called it "the seat of the soul." It is a highly vascular structure of parenchymal cells (*pinealocytes*), astrocyte-like glial cells, and calcareous granules (corpora arenacea). The parenchymal cells have processes that terminate on the basal lamina of the perivascular space surrounding the fenestrated capillaries. The only innervation of the pineal body is by postganglionic sympathetic fibers from the superior cervical ganglia. Vesicles are present in the nerve endings and parenchymal cells. Pineal secretions include melatonin, serotonin, norepinephrine, and neuropeptides. Theories regarding the functional significance of the pineal body range from its being a vestigial structure to a significant endocrine gland. Evidence suggests that the pineal body has a neuroendocrine role in the modulation or regulation of rhythmic activities of the endocrine system as expressed, for example, in seasonal reproductive cycles. In turn, these rhythms are, in a large measure, influenced by the environmental light, diurnal cycles of night and day (circadian cycles) and their graded differences during the seasons.

Environmental light exerts its influences upon the pineal body through the following presumed circuitry. Photostimulation of the retinas is projected directly to the SCN of the hypothalamus. From this nucleus, a multineuronal pathway descends and terminates in the upper thoracic intermediolateral cell column—the site of the origin of preganglionic sympathetic neurons. The axons of these neurons course through the white rami and sympathetic trunk to terminate in the superior cervical ganglia with postganglionic neurons whose axons terminate in the pineal body (Chap. 20). In some way, the sympathetic influences modulate the release of melatonin from the pineal body into the vascular system. One of the targets for melatonin is the

serotonergic raphe nuclei of the brainstem (Chap. 13.), which, through their rostral projection, feed back to the SCN. In turn, this modulates influence upon the limbic system and the hypothalamus. Melatonin seems to have an active role in light-influenced reproductive cycles in many birds and mammals.

Organum Vasculosum of the Lamina Terminalis and Subfornical Organ

The *organum vasculosum* of the *lamina terminalis (supraoptic crest* and *"prechiasmatic gland")* is a highly vascular region of the lamina terminalis. Its loops of fenestrated capillaries are surrounded by wide, fluid-filled perivascular spaces.

The subfornical organ (*intercolumnar tubercle*) is an elevation located between the diverging columns of the fornix at the level of the interventricular foramina of Monro. It is partially covered by the choroid plexus. Its sinusoids and glomerular loops are supplied by adjacent blood vessels.

These two organs have nerve endings synapsing with their neurons. In addition, the messenger angiotensin II, the production of which is enhanced by a reduction in blood volume, binds to receptor sites of the neurons of these organs. The neurons have axons that project to the supraoptic and paraventricular nuclei of the hypothalamus. The interaction within these organs seems to provide the feedback information involved with the hypothalamic control of the posterior lobe of the hypophysis. This includes roles in drinking behavior (osmoregulation), release of ADH, and the physiological control of body fluid balance.

Subcommissural Organ

The *subcommissural organ* is located in the roof of the cerebral aqueduct just rostral and ventral to the posterior commissure. It is composed of specialized ependymal cells and glial cells in a capillary bed of nonfenestrated endothelium. The secretory ependymal cells release a neutral mucopolysaccharide compound product directly into the ventricular fluid. It condenses to form Reissner's fiber, which extends through the cerebral aqueduct, fourth ventricle, and central canal of the spinal cord to coccygeal levels. Its function is not known.

Area Postrema

The AP is a particularly interesting structure because of its function as a chemoreceptor trigger zone for emesis. The AP, located outside of the blood-brain barrier, is sensitive to circulating blood-borne toxins. Anatomically, it is a bilateral structure that forms a slight bulge into the IVth ventricle where this cavity joins the central canal at the level of the obex (Fig. 13.3). The AP is composed of small neurons, astrocyte-like cells, and a rich overlapping arterial and sinusoidal network that characterizes it. The main inputs to the AP are from the adjacent solitary nuclei with which it is reciprocally connected, and from the vagus and glossopharyngeal nerves. It also is connected with the parabrachial nucleus, hypothalamus, and amygdala (either directly or via the solitary complex). A host of substances are present within AP cells and/or afferent axon terminals including peptides, catecholamines, amino acid transmitters, hormone-releasing hormones, and receptors. Oxytocin, vasopressin, and TRH (generally associated with the hypothalamus) are among these.

Ablation of the AP in several patients with intractable nausea and vomiting provided total relief and rendered them resistant to apomorphine, the classic emetic agent. Experimentally, such ablations have been shown to block emesis elicited by apomorphine as well as to other agents circulating in the blood, but not to substances that cause stomach-induced emesis. In some species, emesis and, presumably, motion sickness can be blocked by removal of the AP.

SUGGESTED READINGS

Braak H, Braak E. The hypothalamus of the human adult: chiasmatic region. *Anat Embryol (Berl)*. 1987;175:315–330.

Carpenter D. Central nervous system mechanisms in deglutition and emesis. In: Handbook of Physiology. Section 6. The Gastrointestinal System. Vol I. Bethesda, Md: American Physiological Society; 1989:685–714.

Coleman R. *Wide Awake at 3:00 A.M. By Choice or By Chance?* New York, NY: WH Freeman; 1986.

Cooper P, Martin J. Neuroendocrinology and the brain peptides. *Trends Neurosci*. 1982;5:186–189.

Edmunds L. *Cellular and Molecular Bases of Biological Clocks. Models and Mechanisms for Circadian Timekeeping.* New York, NY: Springer-Verlag; 1987.

Johnson L, Colquhoun W, Tepas D, Colligan M, eds. Biological rhythms: sleep and shift work. *Advances in Sleep Research*. 1981;7:1–640.

Klein D, Moore R, Reppert S, eds. *Suprachiasmatic Nucleus: The Mind's Clock.* New York, NY: Oxford University Press; 1991.

McEwen B. Interactions between hormones and nerve tissue. *Sci Am*. 1976;235(1):48–59.

Nauta W, Haymaker W. Hypothalamic nuclei and fiber connections. In: Haymaker W, Anderson E, Nauta W, eds. *The Hypothalamus*. Springfield, Ill: Charles C Thomas; 1969:136–209.

Pfaff D. *Estrogens and Brain Function: Neural Analysis of a Hormone-Controlled Mammalian Reproductive Behavior.* New York, NY: Springer-Verlag; 1980.

Renaud L. Magnocellular neuroendocrine neurons: update on intrinsic properties, synaptic inputs and neuropharmacology. *Trends Neurosci*. 1987;10:489–502.

Rusak B, Bina K. Neurotransmitters in the mammalian circadian system. *Annu Rev Neurosci*. 1990;13:387–401.

Silverman A, Zimmerman E. Magnocellular neurosecretory system. *Annu Rev Neurosci*. 1983;6:357–380.

Swanson L, Sawchenko P. Hypothalamic integration: organization of the paraventricular and supraoptic nuclei. *Annu Rev Neurosci*. 1983;6:269–324.

Vertes R. Brainstem control of the events of REM sleep. *Prog Neurobiol*. 1984;22:241–288.

Weitzman E. Sleep and its disorders. *Annu Rev Neurosci*. 1981;4:381–417.

Reticular System and Limbic System

22

Reticular formation

Limbic system

Role of the limbic system

The limbic system and the reticular system are neural constructs that have at least two things in common: (1) their anatomic substrates are imprecise and (2) their actions are woven into the fabric of emotional and behavioral expressions in a way that makes it difficult to account for their individual roles.

The reticular system is an integrating system in which influences from the sensory inputs, via both spinal and cranial nerves, as well as from cerebral and cerebellar sources, converge and interact. The system's anatomic substrate is the *reticular formation* (RF). The neural networks of the RF convey and process influences which become associated with vaguely appreciated senses, such as poorly localized pain, with neural activities of the sleep-wake cycle, and with affective behavioral expressions.

The limbic system, really an assemblage of cerebral and midbrain structures, is active in emotions and the visceral and behavioral responses associated with them. It is integral to actions for self-preservation of the organism such as feeding, fight and fright, and to the preservation of the species, for example, mating, procreation, and care of offspring. There is reason to associate the limbic system with the drives behind motivation and to perception, thought, and self-awareness. Part of the system is involved in the mechanisms of memory formation.

RETICULAR FORMATION

Anatomy

The network of neurons comprising the substrate of the RF is present throughout the length of the neuraxis. Its extensive and widely distributed influences are involved with modulating many physiologic and behavioral activities. It is most prominent as the brainstem RF that forms the central core of the medulla, pons, and midbrain (**Fig. 22.1**; Chap. 13). The RF extends caudally throughout the spinal cord as a zone between the gray and white matter (zone labeled spinospinalis tract in **Fig. 7.6**). It extends rostrally in the region of the thalamus (**Fig. 24.2**) as the *zona incerta*, near the subthalamic nucleus (**Fig. 24.3**). The brainstem RF is conceptualized as a highly structured mosaic of discrete yet interactive subsystems with each having a distinctive circuitry. The neurons of the brainstem RF are organized with their extensively branched dendritic trees oriented in a transverse plane as "segments" (**Fig. 22.1**) and their long branching axons extending both rostrally and caudally (**Fig. 22.1**). These axons form a widespread network of connections with neurons of the hypothalamus, thalamus, cerebrum (including cerebral cortex), cerebellum, and spinal cord.

Ascending influences are processed and

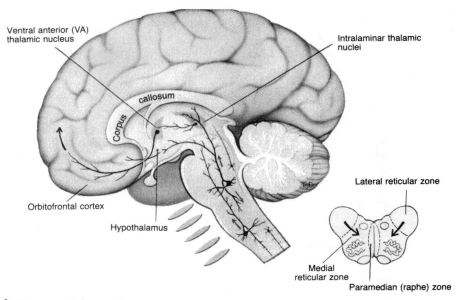

Figure 22.1: The central tegmental tract of the ascending reticular pathway system. In general, the multineuronal, multisynaptic relays of the brainstem reticular formation (RF)(located in the tegmentum) extend rostrally into two telencephalic regions: (1) posteriorly into the intralaminar, ventral anterior (VA), and dorsomedial thalamic nuclear complexes and (2) anteriorly into the hypothalamus. The thalamic component projects, via the VA thalamic nucleus, to the orbitofrontal cortex. The inset at the lower right should be considered as a series of neuropil "segments."

    The cross-section through the brainstem (medulla) illustrates the division of the brainstem RF into a midline raphe or paramedian zone, a medial reticular or "efferent" zone, and a lateral reticular or "sensory" zone. Arrows indicate the general direction of flow of neural influences.

conveyed by ascending reticular pathways such as the *central tegmental tract* (Chap. 13) and the spinoreticulothalamic pathway (Chap. 9), and by descending pathways such as the corticoreticulospinal pathways and those of the autonomic nervous system. The circuitry essential to the various behavioral states such as the sleep-wake cycle is known as the ascending reticular activating system (ARAS). The biochemically defined circuits within the ARAS include noradrenergic, serotonergic, and dopaminergic circuits described in Chapter 15.

    The brainstem RF is subdivided at all levels into three zones (Fig. 22.1): (1) midline raphe and paramedian zone, (2) medial zone (medial two-thirds of the tegmentum), and (3) lateral zone (lateral one-third).

    The lateral zone (also called the "sensory" zone) is composed of small cells with relatively short ascending and descending axons that terminate primarily in the medial reticular zone. The lateral zone is considered to be an afferent and association area because it receives multi-

ple "sensory" inputs from the spinal cord, cranial nerves, cerebellum, and cerebrum. The medial zone ("motor" or "efferent" zone) is characterized by the presence of many large neurons whose axons bifurcate into long ascending and long descending branches. These fibers, which have numerous collaterals, form the *central tegmental tract* of the brainstem tegmentum. The output from the motor zone is: rostrally to the hypothalamus and intralaminar nuclei of the thalamus, caudally to the spinal cord via rubrospinal and reticulospinal tracts, posteriorly to the cerebellum, and laterally to the cranial nerve nuclei.

    The central tegmental tract is integrated into (1) the ARAS; (2) the spinoreticulothalamic pain pathway (Chap. 9); and (3) the corticorubrospinal, corticoreticulospinal, corticobulbar, and corticoreticular pathways (Chap. 11).

Roles and Connections

The reticular system is the recipient of a continuous stream of multimodal "sensory" stimuli.

Its responsiveness to these inputs is expressed through fluctuations in the expressions of its output. These are revealed in the variety of nuances associated with such behavioral states of the sleep-wake cycle as drowsiness, attentiveness, awareness, and alertness. The monoaminergic neurons of the brainstem, especially those of the raphe nuclei and locus ceruleus, have a significant role in the neural activity that evokes these behavioral expressions (Chap. 15).

Sleep is not just an absence of wakefulness; rather, it is the product of active processes involving the brainstem ARAS that regulates the level of activation of the brain. The irreversible coma (loss of consciousness) resulting from severe head injury is associated with extensive damage to the cerebral cortex, or of the midbrain RF, or both. A large lesion of the midbrain RF produces an animal that is in a constant behavioral stupor or in a coma. In contrast, a lesion in the pontine RF results in an animal that is constantly awake (see "Locked-in" syndrome, Chap. 17).

The brainstem RF exerts powerful influences through specialized nuclear groups for carrying out vital functions. These include cardiovascular centers for the control of blood pressure and respiratory centers for regulation of breathing.

The bulbar RF contributes to postural control through influences exerted on the upper motoneuron pathways (reticulospinal and vestibulospinal tracts). This is also demonstrated in such tonic and phasic motor actions as expressed in relaxation and fidgeting.

The reticulothalamic projections influence the diffuse thalamocortical activating system. Stimulation of the core of the brainstem or of the sensory cranial nerves in sleeping animals results in the change of electroencephalogram (EEG) sleep pattern to that exhibited during arousal. The reticular system can activate the cerebral cortex through activity of the intralaminar and ventral anterior thalamic nuclei.

Different stimuli exert their influences differentially upon the ARAS. Acoustic stimuli are more effective than visual stimuli. Pain conveyed via the trigeminal nerve and spinal nerves has a fairly potent ability to evoke arousal. General anesthetics, including pentobarbital and volatile anesthetics, tend to block transmission through the ARAS but do not affect the specific lemniscal pathways. The latter continue to convey their influences. This is one basis for the belief that talk by surgeons during an operation may be "heard" by the cortex of the anesthetized patient.

LIMBIC SYSTEM

The limbic system consists of a complex of many neural structures with a long phylogenetic history. It is involved in memory (Chap. 25), control of visceral functions through the autonomic nervous system (Chap. 20), olfaction, and emotional behavior. The latter includes major roles in expressions of aggression, fear and sexual activity.

The anatomic substrate of the limbic system primarily consists of the limbic lobe and certain areas of gray matter deep to the lobe cortex. The limbic lobe (Fig. 1.7) includes the cingulate gyrus, isthmus, parahippocampal gyrus, hippocampal formation (which consists of the hippocampus and dentate gyrus), and the uncus (primary olfactory cortex). The gray matter areas of the limbic system are principally the amygdaloid and habenular nuclei, septal area, hypothalamus, and midbrain tegmentum. The septal area comprises the small septal nuclei and cortex just rostral to the anterior commissure. The midbrain component includes neurons of the RF. In a broader context, the prefrontal cortex of the frontal lobe is considered to be the neocortical representation of the limbic system (Chap. 25). The limbic system receives a vast range of inputs directly and indirectly from many sensory sources and is interrelated with the basal ganglia. Its output is sent along pathways (1) from the hypothalamus and midbrain tegmentum to the brainstem and spinal cord (by way of the autonomic pathways, descending reticular pathways, and the somatic nervous system) and (2) to the hypophysis and, thereby, to the endocrine system.

Connections and Circuits

The structures of the limbic system are organized into several complex linkages. The following circuits are to be seen as abstractions.

Circuit 1: Amygdala and Its Connections

The *amygdaloid nuclear complex* (*amygdala*) is located at the tip of the temporal lobe deep to the uncus and immediately in front of the hippocampal formation. The amygdala consists of several anatomically and functionally distinct parts: (1) a corticomedial nuclear group (CMN), (2) a basolateral group, and (3) a central (centromedial) group. Although separate, there are abundant reciprocal interconnections between the groups. The amygdala receives input from many areas of the cerebral cortex, the olfactory system, the thalamus, and from the brainstem RF. It projects its output to the hypothalamus along two pathways: (1) stria terminalis and (2) ventral amygdalofugal fibers (Fig. 22.2). Other fibers terminate in the brainstem RF and in the ventral striatum (Chap. 24).

The *CMN* receives major input from the olfactory system (via the olfactory tract) and some from other limbic centers (via the stria terminalis). The CMN projects its output through the stria terminalis to limbic structures (e.g., septal area) and the hypothalamus with which it is re-

ciprocally connected. The olfactory input does not involve the perception of smell, but rather the subtle emotional and motivational associations evoked by odoriferous stimuli (e.g., odor-related responses to the smell of food). The olfactory system is more than just a perceiver of odors; it is an activator and a sensitizer involved with the triggering of behavioral patterns. The perception and discrimination of smell is associated with the cortex of the uncus (area 28) (Fig. 1.7) which overlies the amygdala; scarring in the region of the uncus may cause epileptic seizures known as "uncinate fits" that are preceded by an olfactory aura. The amygdala may have a role in appetite and appetitive behavior through its projection to the ventromedial nucleus of the hypothalamus (see "appestat," Chap. 21).

The *basolateral nucleus* (BLN) is reciprocally connected with the cortex of the temporal lobe including higher ordered sensory and association areas involved with the visual, auditory, and tactile senses. It also is reciprocally connected with anterior parts of the cingulate gyrus, perhaps of importance in learning of emotion-

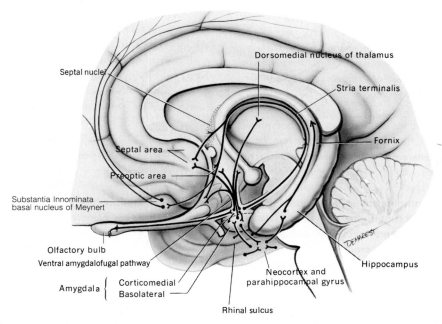

Figure 22.2: Some connections of the limbic system, with emphasis on the circuitry associated with the amygdala. Many of the circuits are reciprocal. Descending fibers terminating in the brainstem reticular formation are not illustrated.

ally driven motor skills and integration of emotional and cognitive processes. The BLN projects its output via ventral amygdalofugal fibers to the hypothalamus, dorsomedial (DM) nucleus of the thalamus, and nucleus accumbens (ventral striatum). The latter participates in the planning of movements (Chap. 24).

The *central nucleus* receives input from the brainstem, especially from the viscerosensory relay nuclei (e.g., solitary nucleus and parabrachial nucleus) and projects its output influences to the hypothalamus, locus ceruleus, brainstem viscerosensory nuclei, and various other nuclei of the autonomic nervous system, including the dorsal motor nucleus of the vagus. The central nucleus, in particular, appears to be involved in the mechanisms of fear, both its acquisition and display.

The amygdala has two output channels, namely (1) the stria terminalis and (2) amygdalofugal pathways (**Fig. 22.2**). The stria terminalis projects from the CMN group to the medial hypothalamus. The ventral amygdalofugal pathway projects its efferents (1) from the central nucleus via descending fibers to the brainstem and (2) from the BLN group to the lateral hypothalamus and the thalamus, particularly to the DM thalamic nucleus.

Experimental evidence indicates that, collectively, all the nuclear groups of the amygdaloid complex are critical processing centers involved with emotion and emotional expressions, olfaction, and control of visceral functions. Electric stimulation of the amygdala in the living subject can result in bradycardia, alteration in respiration, pupillary dilation, and urination—all influences mediated via the hypothalamus.

Substantia Innominata, Basal Nucleus of Meynert, and Extended Amygdala

Rostral to the hypothalamus and globus pallidus and below the anterior commissure is a region of gray matter called the *substantia innominata* in which is located the *basal nucleus of Meynert* (**Fig. 22.2**). The substantia innominata has reciprocal connections with the amygdala, hippocampus, and hypothalamus. The basal nucleus has reciprocal linkages with the hippocampus. Of significance are the projections from large

cholinergic neurons of the basal nucleus of Meynert to the entire neocortex with a relatively orderly and topographic distribution. These projections are considered to play a major role in neural processing associated with intellectual functions (Chap. 25). The nucleus may also play a role in modulating the amygdala and the neocortex. Some cells of the substantia innominata, together with cell groups of the bed nucleus of the stria terminalis (located in the basomedial forebrain bordering the anterior commissure), are regarded as a rostral extension of the central nucleus of the amygdala.

The continuum of central nucleus, substantia innominata, and bed nucleus of the stria terminalis is referred to as the *extended amygdala* which is juxtaposed to the ventral striatum and ventral pallidum. This emphasizes the close geographic relationship of limbic structures with parts of the basal ganglia concerned with motor activity related to emotional stimuli (Chap. 24). These may in part be reflected by alterations in facial expression displaying fear, happiness, sorrow, anger, etc., and in the connotations of posture such as stooped versus erect.

Circuit 2: Hippocampal Formation and the "Papez Circuit"

The hippocampal formation consists of the hippocampus proper and the dentate gyrus (**Fig. 22.3**). The subiculum is transitional between the hippocampus and entorhinal cortex (area 28) of the parahippocampal gyrus, and some consider it to be part of the hippocampal formation. The hippocampus forms the floor of the temporal (inferior) horn of the lateral ventricle. The ventricular surface is covered by a thin lamina of axons called the alveus. The fibers of the *alveus* arise from the hippocampus and from the adjacent *subiculum*. These fibers converge to form a flattened band called the *fimbria of the fornix* which continues as the fornix (**Fig. 22.3**). The *fornix* with its approximately 1.25 million fibers is the major output channel of the hippocampus; it also contains some fibers travelling in the opposite direction, particularly from the septal region, that terminate in the hippocampus. The alveus also forms a small fascicle called the longitudinal stria that courses around the posterior aspect of the corpus callo-

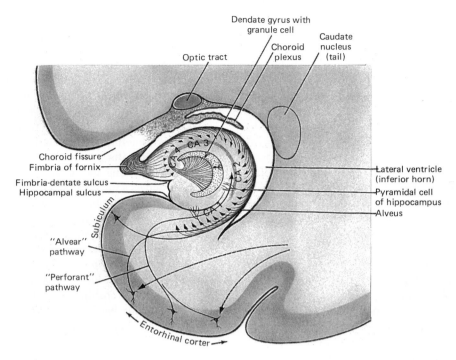

Figure 22.3: Diagram of a transverse section through the dentate gyrus, hippocampus, subiculum, and entorhinal cortex (area 28) of the parahippocampal gyrus. (1) Input to the entorhinal area and subiculum is derived from several areas of temporal lobe cortex; (2) output from the entorhinal area projects to the dentate gyrus and hippocampus via the alveus ("alvear path") or via the perforant path; (3) connections of the entorhinal area and subiculum with other cortical areas generally are reciprocal; (4) axons of pyramidal cells of the subiculum and hippocampus pass through the alveus and fimbria into the fornix; and (5) axons of the granule cells in the dentate gyrus terminate in the hippocampus. Cornus ammonis (CA) refers to the fields of the hippocampus.

sum to the supracollosal gyrus (induseum griseum), adherent to its dorsal surface (**Fig. 22.4**).

The hippocampal formation is composed of archicortex (Chap. 25) characterized by the presence of three layers—molecular, pyramidal (granular for the dentate gyrus), and polymorphic (**Fig. 22.3**). The *molecular layer* is synaptic and mainly consists of a meshwork of axonal, dendritic, and glial processes (neuropil). The *pyramidal layer* of the hippocampus contains several rows of relatively large triangular or pyramidal-shaped cell bodies with axons that enter the alveus and are the main output of the hippocampus. Pyramidal cell apical dendrites extend into the molecular layer along with axon collaterals. Interneurons also are present in the pyramidal layer. For the dentate gyrus, this middle layer is called the *granular layer* because of its dense aggregation of small stellate cells.

Dendrites of these cells extend into the molecular layer and their axons, called mossy fibers, terminate within the hippocampus near the base of pyramidal cell apical dendrites. The *polymorphic layer*, covered by the alveus, is composed mainly of neuropil, like the molecular layer that includes the extensive basal dendrites as well as axon collaterals of Purkinje cells. The hippocampal formation is divided into fields CA1, CA2, CA3, and CA4. CA1 is continuous with the subiculum. CA4, located at the hilus of the more or less V-shaped dentate gyrus with which it coalesces, is regarded as part of CA3 by some investigators. The designation CA comes from Cornu Ammonis (Ammon was an Egyptian god with a ram's head), another name for the hippocampus conferred because of its shape in the coronal plane. The hippocampal formation has reciprocal connections with the parahippocampal gyrus which, in turn, has widespread recip-

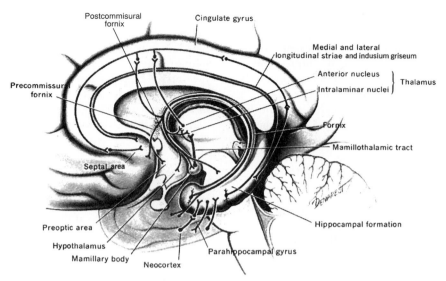

Figure 22.4: Some connections of the limbic system, primarily those of the parahippocampal gyrus and hippocampus. The "Papez circuit" includes the hippocampus via fornix → mamillary body via mamillothalamic tract → anterior thalamic nuclear group → cingulate gyrus → parahippocampal gyrus → hippocampus. The subiculum is a pivotal cortical area projecting to widespread regions of the cerebrum. Many connections are reciprocal.

rocal cortical interconnections. Afferents from the medial part of the entorhinal area (area 28) traverse the subiculum and alveus (*alvear pathway*) and terminate on basilar dendrites and cell bodies of pyramidal cells in the subiculum and CA1 (Fig. 22.3). Afferents from the lateral part of the entorhinal area pass through the alvear path as the *perforant pathway* and terminate on apical dendrites of pyramidal cells in CA1, CA2, and CA3 and granule cells of the dentate gyrus. The hippocampus receives monaminergic input from the raphe nuclei and the locus ceruleus. The output of the subiculum and hippocampus is conveyed via the fornix to the mamillary bodies, other hypothalamic nuclei, and nuclei in the vicinity of the septal region and the substantia innominata, including the basal nucleus of Meynert. The hippocampus is bilaterally interconnected via fibers that decussate in the fornical (hippocampal) commissure and turn back in the contralateral fornix; some postdecussational fibers continue rostrally in the opposite fornix. The fornix divides around the anterior commissure into precommissural and postcommissural fibers and it is the latter group, arising from the subiculum, that terminates in the mamillary body as well as to a lesser extent in the anterior, intralaminar, and lateral

dorsal nuclei of the thalamus. The precommissural fibers of the fornix mainly come from CA1 to CA3. The mamillothalamic tract projects from each mamillary body to the anterior thalamic nuclear group; the latter projects to the cortex of the cingulate gyrus (Chap. 25) as does field CA1 of the hippocampus and the subiculum. Commencing in the cingulate gyrus, multineuronal linkages terminate in the cortex of the parahippocampal gyrus.

The reciprocal connections of the hippocampus with the many areas of the neocortex are critical in its presumed role of receiving novel sensory inputs that are registered as short-term memory. Within a limited time span this memory may become a long-term memory (Chap. 25). Memory disorders are characteristic features of lesions of the hippocampus.

The classic *Papez circuit* for emotions (1937), comprises the sequence of hippocampus → fornix → mamillary body → mamillothalamic tract → anterior thalamic nuclear group → cingulate gyrus → parahippocampal gyrus and neural linkages back to the hippocampus. Input to the parahippocampal gyrus and hippocampus is derived from the cingulate cortex and from association areas of the cerebral cortex

(Chap. 25). Papez regarded the cingulate cortex "as the receptive region for the experiencing of emotion." This circuit is an important part of the limbic system; however, the hippocampus in particular appears to be much more involved with memory than with emotions per se.

Although described separately, it should be recognized that the hippocampal formation is interconnected with portions of the amygdala.

Circuit 3: Septal-Hypothalamus-Midbrain Continuum

This "continuum" encompasses the septal region of the forebrain, the hypothalamus, epithalamus (Chap. 1), and the medial midbrain tegmentum (**Fig. 22.5**). It is knit together largely by the *medial forebrain bundle*. This multineuronal, multisynaptic pathway is composed of neurons with short branching axons extending longitudinally within the continuum. It projects rostrally to the hypothalamus and septal region and caudally into the brainstem RF.

Within the medial forebrain bundle are the descending pathways of the autonomic nervous system from the hypothalamus together with the ascending projections of the reticular system. Another circuit associated with this continuum is the sequence from the septal region via the fibers of the stria medullaris thalami to the habenular nucleus, and from there via the habenulointerpeduncular tract (tractus retroflexus) to the interpeduncular nucleus of the midbrain. The latter projects to the medial midbrain tegmentum and into the medial forebrain bundle and, in addition, sends fibers back to the habenula.

Circuit 4: Dorsomedial Nucleus of the Thalamus and Prefrontal Cortex

The prefrontal cortex has been called the neocortical representative of the limbic system because of its role in emotional behavior and motivation (Chap. 25). The cortex is necessary for the experience or feeling of emotion. The DM thalamic nucleus serves as an intermediary in this circuitry; it has reciprocal connections with the prefrontal lobe (role in memory and cognition; Chap. 25), hypothalamus, and the medial midbrain tegmentum.

ROLE OF THE LIMBIC SYSTEM

The limbic system is involved with many of the expressions that make us human, namely, emo-

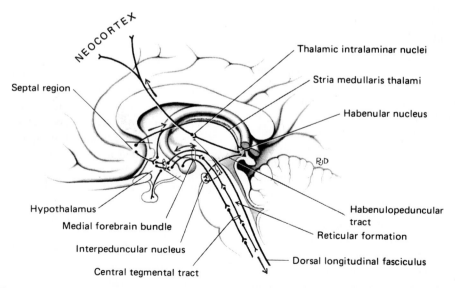

Figure 22.5: Some connections of the limbic system. The medial forebrain bundle is a multineuronal pathway extending from the septal area through the lateral hypothalamus to the brainstem tegmentum. Note the pathway system comprising the sequence of septal area and preoptic area → habenular nucleus → midbrain tegmentum and interpeduncular nucleus. The latter projects to the midbrain tegmentum.

tions, behavior, and states of feeling; however, the limbic system is not independent in this, rather, it interacts with sensory pathways and cortices, as well as association cortices regarded as playing a primary role in cognitive processes. Different feelings and emotions appear to involve more than one pathway and, for some, the right hemisphere is thought to be more important.

Stimulation of Structures Within the Limbic System

Electric stimulation of the amygdala and nearby regions in the unanesthetized monkey produces a number of actions. Activities associated with feeding and nutrition are elicited, including sniffing, licking, biting, swallowing, and retching movements. Monkeys exhibit *agonistic behavior patterns*—behavior manifested by animals in an attack-and-defense contest during fight or fright. The peaceful monkey becomes a furious and aggressive animal that attacks and bullies; once the stimulus is turned off, the peaceful monkey reappears. Similar observations have been made in man. The increase in the secretion of digestive juices in the alimentary canal after repeated acute stimulations of the amygdala may be followed by the appearance of gastric erosions similar to peptic ulcers in the stomachs of monkeys. The possibility of psychic factors in the production of peptic ulcers in man is implied. Although the role of the amygdala in aggressive behavior is striking, as described above, its role in the acquisition and expression of fear or emotional memories may be as important.

Stimulation of the hippocampal formation may result in respiratory and cardiovascular changes and in a generalized arousal response. In the expression of arousal, the formation acts as a supplemental motor area by inducing somatic movements such as facial grimaces, shoulder shrugging, and hand movements, which are considered to be normal behavioral gestures.

Responses indicative of activity of the autonomic nervous system are evoked by stimulation of the cingulate gyrus and septal area. These responses, observed even in man, include changes in the tone of the blood vascular system, in respiratory rhythms, and in the activity of the digestive system.

Aggressiveness can be inhibited or decreased in monkeys by stimulating the septal area. Stimulation of a "boss" monkey with implanted electrodes reduces its aggressive behavior. If stimulation is prolonged over a period of days, the other monkeys of the colony sense this change. They lose their fear of the "boss" and take new liberties, such as invading its territory and securing a larger share of food. The former situation returns after stimulations cease.

"Pleasure Centers" and "Punishing Centers"

Stimulation by implanted electrodes of certain regions of the limbic system drives an animal to seek further stimulation. The animal will trip a lever over and over again in order to continually restimulate itself—an expression of positive reinforcement on self-stimulation. Such nodal sites have been named "pleasure centers" or "rewarding centers." The stimulation of some regions excites the animal to avoid further stimulation—an expression of negative reinforcement on self-stimulation. Such sites have been named "punishing centers" or "aversion centers." The so-called pleasure centers have been located in the subcallosal area, cingulate cortex, hippocampal formation, amygdala, hypothalamus, midbrain tegmentum, and anterior nuclei of the thalamus. Sites of punishing centers are in the midbrain tegmentum, and certain thalamic and hypothalamic areas.

The several human subjects whose septal areas were stimulated had feelings of pleasure or a "brightening of their attitude." They giggled, talked more, and expressed themselves more freely when the current was on.

Shocks from electrodes within the "punishing centers" evoke behavioral patterns in which monkeys grimace, quiver, and shake. They bite and tear objects with their mouths, their eyes dilate, and their hair stands on end. If stimulated for hours, monkeys become irritable, refuse to eat, and may become ill. These effects can be eliminated by stimulating a "pleasure center."

Klüver-Bucy Syndrome

Monkeys with the anterior temporal lobes ablated bilaterally exhibit a constellation of activities and expressions associated with emotion known as the *Klüver-Bucy syndrome*. With the bilateral loss of the amygdala, uncus, anterior temporal cortex, and portions of the hippocampal formation, the animal is apparently released ("*release phenomenon*") from expressing fear. Wild and aggressive monkeys become tame and docile. The marked absence of emotional responses, such as anger, is accompanied by the loss of facial expressions and vocal protests usually noted during aggressive activities. Monkeys are normally afraid of snakes, but, with this syndrome, they will now pick up, handle, and examine a live snake with ease. The animal is able to see and to locate objects visually, but is apparently unable to recognize the objects fully by sight. This visual agnosia in humans, with a comparable ablation, is characterized by the loss of ability to recognize friends and familiar places (Chap. 25). Animals in this state probably have auditory and tactile agnosias. Such animals exhibit strong *oral tendencies*, expressed as a compulsion to examine objects repeatedly with their lips and mouth. These overreacting animals are said to be *stimulus-bound* with an irresistible impulse to touch, smell, and taste the object many times. An explanation for this behavior is that, because of the agnosia, the animal keeps trying to obtain additional clues in a concerted attempt to identify the familiar object that it cannot recall. Evidence suggests that the stimulus-bound behavior occurs with the removal of the amygdala only. Hypersexual behavior is marked with many manifestations of autosexual, homosexual, and heterosexual activities.

Korsakoff's Syndrome and Ablations of the Hippocampus

Patients with a form of amnesia, known as *Korsakoff's syndrome*, have pathologic changes in neural complexes associated with the limbic system—namely the mamillary bodies of the hypothalamus and the DM nucleus of the thalamus. This affliction is the consequence of chronic alcoholism and thiamine deficiency. The patient displays a profound memory loss and becomes easily confused. The symptoms are also exhibited by humans who have undergone bilateral removal of the anterior temporal lobe including the amygdala and the hippocampus. The patient forgets to answer a question just asked, or may reply with an irrelevant answer (called *compensatory confabulation*). Patients with this psychosis learn slowly, but once the subject matter is learned, they appear to forget at a normal rate. One concept suggests that the memory deficits are due, in some degree, to defective neural processing (encoding) at the time of learning rather than exclusively to a flaw in the retrieval from memory. Patients with bilateral lesions involving the uncus and amygdala, and sparing the hippocampus, do not have memory disturbances. Conversely, a bilateral lesion restricted merely to field CA1 of the hippocampus apparently suffices to impair memory without affecting other aspects of cognitive activity.

Medial Temporal Lobe and Schizophrenia

The term *schizophrenia* is used to describe a group of related disorders of cognition, personality, and behavior, among others, that affect about 1% of the population. Evidence is accumulating that indicates involvement of genetic and, perhaps, environmental factors of dysfunction of dopamine transmission (Chap. 15) in many cases. Anatomically, there is a high correlation with pathology in medial parts of the temporal lobe, particularly the hippocampus, adjacent parts of the parahippocampal gyrus, and, to a lesser extent, the amygdala. Alterations range from cell loss to cytoarchitectural reorganization and are attributed to early developmental disturbances. The cerebral ventricles, especially the temporal horns of the lateral ventricles, generally are enlarged accompanied by some tissue loss. It should be emphasized that other parts of the brain also exhibit pathological changes, but to a lesser extent. Given the complex circuity of the medial portion of the temporal lobes, widespread regions of the cerebrum, such as cingulate and prefrontal cortex, may be affected and contribute to the disease.

SUGGESTED READINGS

Amaral D, Insausti R. Hippocampal formation. In: Paxinos G, ed. *The Human Nervous System*. San Diego, Calif: Academic Press; 1990.

Bloom F, Lazerson A, Hofstadter L. *Brain, Mind and Behavior.* 2nd ed. New York, NY: W.H. Freeman; 1988.

Cartwright R. *A Primer on Sleep and Dreaming.* Reading, Mass: Addison-Wesley; 1978.

Carlsen J, Heimer L. The basolateral amygdaloid complex as a cortical-like structure. *Brain Res.* 1988;441:377–380.

Damasio A. Toward a neurobiology of emotion and feeling: Operational concepts and hypotheses. *The Neuroscientist.* 1995;1:19–25.

Davis M. The role of the amygdala in fear and anxiety. *Annu Rev Neurosci.* 1992;15:353–375.

De Olmos J. Amygdala. In: Paxinos G, ed. *The Human Nervous System.* San Diego, Calif: Academic Press; 1990.

Easter S Jr. Birth of olfactory neurons. Lifelong neurogenesis. *Trends Neurosci.* 1984;7:105–109.

Foster N, Chase T, Patronas N, Gillespie M, Fedio P. Cerebral mapping of apraxia in Alzheimer's disease by positron emission tomography. *Ann Neurol.* 1986;19:139–143.

Holmes E, Jacobson S, Stein B, Butters N. Ablations of the mammillary nuclei in monkeys: effects on postoperative memory. *Exp Neurol.* 1983;81:97–113.

Isaacson R. *The Limbic System.* 2nd ed. New York, NY: Plenum; 1982.

Kalivas P, Nemeroff C, eds. The mesocorticolimbic dopamine system. *Ann N Y Acad Sci.* 1988;537:1–540.

Klüver H, Bucy P. Preliminary analysis of functions of the temporal lobes in monkeys. *Archives of Neurology and Psychiatry.* 1939;42:979–1000.

LeDoux J. Emotion, memory and the brain. *Sci Am.* 1994;270:50–59.

Mesulum M, Mufson E. Neural inputs into the nucleus basalis of the substantia innominata (Ch 4) in the rhesus monkey. *Brain.* 1984;107:253–274.

Papez J. A proposed mechanism of emotion. *Archives of Neurology and Psychiatry.* 1937;38:725–743.

Roberts G. Schizophrenia: the cellular biology of a functional psychosis. *Trends Neurosci.* 1990;13:207–211.

Scoville W, Milner B. Loss of recent memory after bilateral hippocampal lesions. *J Neurol Neurosurg Psychiat.* 1957;20:11–21.

Vogt B, Gabriel M, eds. *Neurobiology of Cingulate Cortex and Limbic Thalamus.* Boston, Mass: Birkhäuser; 1993.

Zola-Morgan S, Squire L, Amaral D. Human amnesia and the medial temporal region: enduring memory impairment following a bilateral lesion limited to field CA-1 of the hippocampus. *J Neurosci.* 1986;6:2950–2967.

Thalamus

23

Major morphologic and functional aspects

Neurons and nuclei of the thalamus

Nuclei of the thalamus: major connections and functions

Limbic thalamus

Some transmitters of the thalamus

Extrathalamic modulatory pathways projecting to the cerebral cortex

Internal capsule

Functional considerations

Lesions of the thalamus

The *thalamus*, also called the *dorsal thalamus*, is a large paired egg-shaped mass of nuclei located in the diencephalon (**Figs. 23.1 to 23.3**). It extends rostrally to the interventricular foramen, superiorly to the transverse cerebral fissure, inferiorly to the hypothalamic sulcus, and posteriorly, it overlaps the midbrain (**Figs. 1.5, 5.1**). The thalamic nuclei process, integrate, and relay information for the sensory, motor, limbic, and motivational systems. Some have a critical role in sensation and motor control. The thalamus also regulates levels of alertness.

MAJOR MORPHOLOGIC AND FUNCTIONAL ASPECTS

The thalamus is located between the third ventricle medially and the posterior limb of the internal capsule laterally (**Fig. 23.3**). At its rostral end is the *reticular nucleus* (R in **Fig. 23.1**) which extends along its lateral aspect but is shown truncated in the figure. Its most caudal entity is the *pulvinar* (P). The diagonally oriented *internal medullary lamina*, a complex of nuclei and fibers, divides the thalamus into medial and lateral groups of nuclei. The lateral

group, in turn, is divided into a ventral tier and a dorsal tier of nuclei. The ventral tier includes the *ventral anterior nucleus* (VA), *ventral lateral nucleus* (VL), and *ventral posterior nucleus* (VP) (ventrolateral group in **Table 23.1**). The *medial geniculate body* (MGB) and *lateral genicu-*

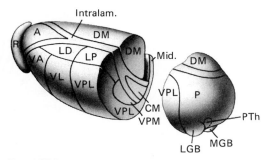

Figure 23.1: The left thalamus. The reticular nucleus (R) extends along the lateral aspect of the thalamus; only its rostral portion is shown. A = anterior nuclear group, CM = centromedianum, DM = dorsomedial nucleus, Intralam. = intralaminar nuclei, LD = lateral dorsal nucleus, LGB = lateral geniculate body, Mid. = midline nuclei, P = pulvinar, PTh = posterior thalamic nucleus, R = reticular nucleus, VA = ventral anterior nucleus, VL = ventral lateral nucleus, VPL = ventral posterior lateral nucleus, and VPM = ventral posterior medial nucleus. Not shown: ventral posterior inferior nucleus.

late body (LGB), collectively called the meta-thalamus, are classified by some authors as ventral tier nuclei. The dorsal tier comprises the *lateral dorsal nucleus* (LD), *lateral posterior nucleus* (LP), and the P. The medial group is the *dorsomedial nucleus* (DM) (or *mediodorsal nucleus*). In the rostral aspect of the thalamus between the bifurcated internal medullary lamina is the *anterior nuclear group* (A). Within the internal medullary lamina are the *intralaminar nuclei*; one of these, the *centromedian* (CM) is illustrated in **Fig. 23.1**. On the medial surface of the thalamus are *nuclei of the midline* also known as the *periventricular nuclei*.

All thalamic nuclei receive afferent input from at least one extrathalamic source. (1) *All nuclei, except the reticular nucleus, have reciprocal connections with the cerebral cortex.* (2) *All influences received by the cerebral cortex are derived from thalamic nuclei*, with some exceptions—pathways of the olfactory system (Chap. 14) and the extrathalamic modulatory pathways that project to the cortex (see later). (3) *Interconnections between the thalamic nuclei, if any,*

are scarce. Exceptions are the extensive interconnections between the *intralaminar thalamic nuclei and with the reticular nucleus*.

On a functional basis, the thalamic nuclei may be classified as *relay nuclei* and *diffuse-projecting nuclei* (**Table 23.1**). (1) Each relay nucleus is associated with a distinct sensory modality or with an input derived from a subdivision of the motor system. Projections from each relay nucleus terminate in a cytoarchitecturally or functionally defined region (field) of the cerebral cortex. Subdivisions of each relay nucleus terminate in small segments of each field. In turn, each thalamic nuclei receives a massive projection from the field of the cortex to which it projects. These recurrent projections are presumed to enable the cortex to modulate the input relevant to the ongoing activity. (2) The diffuse-projecting nuclei have widespread connections with neurons in other nuclei and the cortex. They exert influences that affect the activity of the neurons in the thalamus and the cerebral cortex. They have a role in governing the level of arousal. (3) Fibers projecting (a)

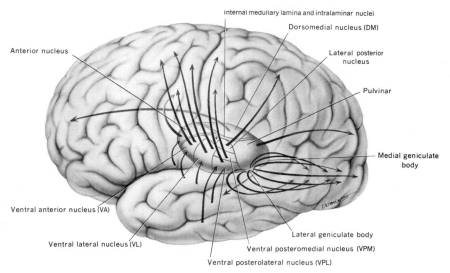

Figure 23.2: Major nuclei and some major cortical projections of the thalamus. Many nuclei have reciprocal connections (corticothalamic projections indicated by arrows) with the cortex. The medial geniculate body projects to auditory areas 41 and 42; the lateral geniculate body to visual area 17; the ventral posterior medial (VPM) nucleus to the sensory postcentral gyrus (face region of areas 1, 2, and 3) and secondary sensory area; the ventral posterior lateral (VPL) nucleus to the sensory postcentral gyrus (body region of areas 1, 2, and 3) and secondary sensory area; the ventral lateral (VL) nucleus to motor areas 4 and 6; the ventral anterior (VA) nucleus to motor areas 6 and 8 and the orbitofrontal cortex; the anterior nucleus to the limbic cortex; the lateral posterior nucleus (LP) and pulvinar (with reciprocal connections) to the association cortex of the parietal and occipitotemporal cortex; and the dorsomedial nucleus (with reciprocal connections) to the prefrontal cortex.

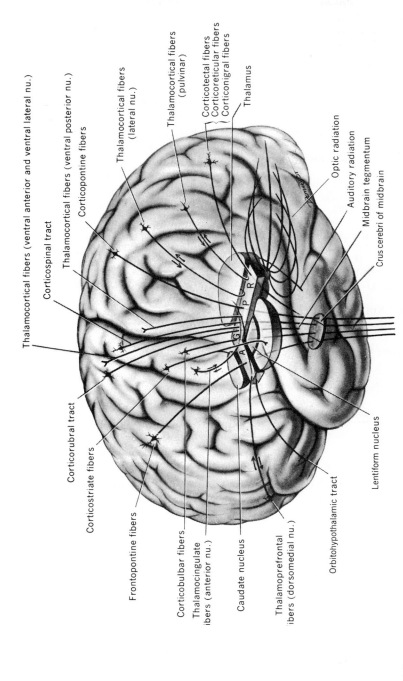

Figure 23.3: Some component fiber tracts of the internal capsule and their cortical connections. Reciprocal projections between a thalamic nucleus and a cortical area are indicated by arrows pointing in two directions. The nuclei refer to nuclei of the thalamus. A = anterior limb, G = genu, P = posterior limb, R = retrolenticular portion of posterior limb of internal capsule.

Table 23.1: Topographic Grouping of the Nuclei of the Thalamus (Fig. 23.1): Major Connections and Functions

RELAY NUCLEI
Anterior nuclear group (A)
   Anteroventral nucleus (AV, the principal nucleus)
   Anterodorsal nucleus (AD, an accessory nucleus)
   Anteromedial nucleus (AM, an accessory nucleus)
Medial Nuclear Group
   Dorsomedial Nucleus (DM, mediodorsal or medial nucleus)
Ventrolateral Nuclear Group
   Ventral anterior nucleus (VA)
   Ventral posterior nucleus (VP)
      Ventral posterolateral (posterior lateral) nucleus (VPL)
      Ventral posteromedial (posterior medial) nucleus (VPM)
      Ventral posteroinferior (posterior inferior) nucleus (VPI)
      Posterior thalamic nucleus (PTh)
Lateral Nuclear Group
   Lateral dorsal (LD, dorsal lateral) nucleus
   Lateral posterior nucleus (LP)
Posterior Nuclear Group
   Medial geniculate body (MGB)
   Lateral geniculate body (LGB)
   Pulvinar (P)
DIFFUSE PROJECTING NUCLEI
Intralaminar Nuclei (Intralam)
   Rostral Group
      Central medial, paracentral and central lateral nuclei
   Caudal Group
      Parafascicular (Pf) and Centromedian (CM) nuclei
Reticular Nucleus (R)
Midline (Periventricular) Nuclei (Mid)

from the thalamus to the cortex and (b) from the cortex to the thalamus pass through the internal capsule and corona radiata (**Figs. 23.3, 13.5**). Few, if any, interconnections exist between the relay nuclei of the thalamus.

NEURONS AND NUCLEI OF THE THALAMUS

The major thalamic nuclei contain two basic types of neurons: projection (relay) neurons and interneurons. The relay neurons have a large axon which projects to the cerebral cortex; each axon has some collaterals that terminate in the same nucleus and many that terminate in the reticular nucleus. In some major nuclei, the

axons of the large relay neurons terminate in lamina IV of the cortex and the smaller relay neurons in lamina VI. The interneurons have axons that terminate locally within the same nucleus of origin. They are concerned with information processing within the nucleus.

Functionally, thalamic nuclei are called specific or nonspecific. (1) *Specific thalamic nuclei* are characterized as having reciprocal connections with localized areas of the cerebral cortex. Depending upon the author, these are restricted to those nuclei associated with sensory and motor systems, or to all the relay nuclei. (2) *Nonspecific thalamic nuclei* are characterized as receiving input from the brainstem reticular formation, other thalamic and basal forebrain nuclei, and projecting their output widely to all areas of the cerebral cortex. These comprise the midline and intralaminar thalamic nuclei. The thalamic reticular nucleus also is classified as nonspecific, although it relays no projections to the cortex.

The thalamocortical fibers terminating in the cerebral cortex have been subdivided into specific projections and nonspecific projections. Specific projections originate from a specific thalamic nucleus. They terminate in a restricted area of the cortex in an ordered and defined pattern. These features are the hallmark of the relay nuclei. Nonspecific projections are diffuse and not restricted to a cortical area. To summarize, each cortical area receives both specific and nonspecific thalamocortical projections. The restricted specific projection arises from a thalamic relay nucleus and diffuse nonspecific projections from other thalamic (and even extrathalamic) sources. Nonspecific projections to the cerebral cortex may originate from several sources, including specific relay thalamic nuclei, nonspecific thalamic nuclei, and extrathalamic nuclei.

NUCLEI OF THE THALAMUS: MAJOR CONNECTIONS AND FUNCTIONS (FIGS. 23.2 AND 23.4)

Anterior Nuclear Group

The anterior group comprises the *anteroventral, anterodorsal,* and *anteromedial nuclei* which

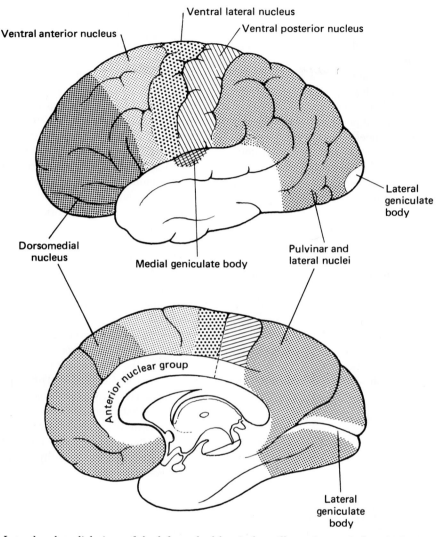

Figure 23.4: Lateral and medial views of the left cerebral hemisphere illustrating cortical projection areas of some thalamic nuclei. Much of the temporal lobe does not receive projections from the specific thalamic nuclei. Such an area is known as an athalamic cortex.

form the *anterior thalamic tubercle*. They are the major component of the *limbic thalamus* and are integrated in the *Papez circuit* and the limbic system (Chap. 22). The anterior nuclei contain the highest concentration of muscarinic receptors of the thalamus. They have reciprocal connections with the: (1) hypothalamus, particularly the mamillary body via the mamillothalamic tract, (2) parahippocampal gyrus of the temporal lobe via the fornix, (3) cingulate gyrus of the limbic lobe, and (4) the prefrontal cortex.

The latter is the neocortical component of the limbic system.

Dorsomedial Nucleus

The massive *dorsomedial nucleus* (DM) located between the internal medullary lamina and the third ventricle, is divided into a *magnocellular (large cell) portion* and a *parvocellular (small cell) portion*. Its principal inputs are from the amygdala, olfactory system, and hypothalamus and its primary output is to the prefrontal lobe. In primate evolution, the relative increase in size of this nucleus parallels that of the frontal lobe. The nucleus has rich connections with the intralaminar nuclei, nuclei of the midline, and the LP. The magnocellular portion has reciprocal connections with the amygdala, lateral hypothalamus, and the temporal and orbitofrontal neocortex. The parvocellular portion has massive topographically organized reciprocal connections with the prefrontal cortex (areas 9, 10, 11, and 12—all rostral to area 6, Chap. 25). A point-to-point relation exists among the areas in the amygdala, DM nucleus, and frontal lobe. The DM nucleus has massive reciprocal connections with the *frontal eye field* (area 8, **Fig. 25.5**).

The DM nucleus acts to integrate certain influences from somatic and visceral sources and, in conjunction with the prefrontal cortex, has roles in various expressions of affect, emotion, and behavior. Psychosurgical studies (such as following prefrontal lobotomy, leukotomy, Chap. 25) indicate that the DM nucleus and the frontal lobe cortex are involved with affective behavior.

Ventral Anterior Nucleus

The *ventral anterior* (VA) and the *ventral lateral* (VL) *thalamic nuclei* are motor relay nuclei associated with the somatic motor system. The VA nucleus is divided into two subdivisions: (1) a parvocellular (principal) part (VApc) and (2) a magnocellular part (VAmc). Each part receives input from different sources without overlap. VApc receives afferents from the medial segment of the globus pallidus and VAmc from the pars reticulata of the substantia nigra. VA projects selectively to the supplementary motor area (SMA, area 6) (**Figs. 25.3 and 25.4** and Chap. 25). Premotor cortical area 6 projects primarily to VApc and area 8 to VAmc. Fibers from the primary motor cortex do not terminate in the VA nucleus. Nonspecific input from the intralaminar nuclei to the "nonspecific portion" of VA are processed and projected to the orbitofrontal cortex.

Ventral Lateral Nucleus

The ventral lateral nucleus (VL) is an integral nucleus in the feedback circuits of (1) cerebral

cortex to cerebellar cortex back to cerebral cortex (**Fig. 18.3**) and (2) cerebral cortex to basal ganglia to cerebral cortex (**Figs. 24.1 to 24.5**) (Chaps. 18 and 24). The VL nucleus receives direct input from the contralateral cerebellar hemisphere via the dentatothalamic tract (specifically from globose, emboliform, and dentate nuclei) (Chap. 18). It also receives input from the medial segment of the ipsilateral globus pallidus. There is apparently no overlap of the termination of the input from the cerebellum and globus pallidus (Chap. 24). The portion of VL receiving input from the cerebellum projects to the premotor cortex (part of area 6) and to the primary motor cortex (area 4, Chap. 25). The connections with area 4 are *somatotopically* and *reciprocally organized* with (a) the medial region of VL interconnected with the cortical face area, (b) the intermediate region interconnected with the upper limb and body area, and (c) the lateral region interconnected with the pelvis and lower limb area. The portion of VL receiving input from the globus pallidus projects to the supplementary motor area (portion of area 6, Chap. 25). Through its projections to the cortex, VL exerts its role as a critical subcortical gateway to the cerebral cortex acting as a prime mover in the motor pathways (Chap. 24). Lesions in the VL may ameliorate the contralateral tremors and rigidity in patients with Parkinson's disease (Chap. 24).

Ventral Posterior Nucleus

The ventral posterior nucleus (VP) of the *ventrobasal complex* is a somatosensory relay nucleus comprised of the *ventral posterolateral* (VPL), *ventral posteromedial* (VPM), *ventral posteroinferior* (VPI), and *posterior thalamic* (PTh) *nuclei*. VP is highly organized with precise topographical representation and separation of the sensory modalities of the contralateral half of the head and body (Chaps. 9, 10).

VP is the nucleus of termination of somatosensory and gustatory pathways. VPL and VPI are nuclei of termination of the lateral spinothalamic tract (pain and thermal sense from the body), medial lemniscus ("pressure" touch and vibratory sense from the body), anterior spinothalamic tract (light touch from the body), and spinocervicothalamic tract (touch, proprioception, and vibratory sense from the body). In addition, VPI is a nucleus of the vestibular pathway (Chap. 16). VPM is the nucleus of termination of the trigeminothalamic tracts (general sensory modalities of the head) and of the gustatory pathways from the nucleus solitarius. A somatotopic distribution in VPL is represented as follows: the pathways from the lower extremity terminate posterolaterally and from the upper extremity anteromedially, with fibers from the body in between. The different modalities also are topographically localized within VPM: (a) taste is projected to the medial portion of the nucleus, (b) tactile sense to the lateral portion, and (c) thermal sense to the intermediate portion. The topographic and sensory modality organization are preserved in the thalamocortical projections. The projections terminate in the primary somatic sensory cortex (SI; areas 3, 1, and 2) and the secondary somatic sensory cortex (SII; Chap. 25).

Posterior Thalamic Nucleus (Fig. 23.1)

The input to PTh is derived from diverse sensory sources including from the spinothalamic tracts, trigeminothalamic tract, medial lemniscus, inferior colliculus, and ascending reticular pathways. Its neurons are multi-modal, rather than modality specific, in that they respond to combinations of pain, tactile (mechanoreceptive), vestibular, and auditory stimuli. Physiologically, the neurons of this nucleus respond to high threshold somatic sensory and auditory stimuli and have properties consistent with an involvement in central nervous system pain mechanisms. The PTh nucleus projects to the secondary somatic sensory area of the cerebral cortex (Chap. 25). It is thought to have a role in the perception of pain and noxious stimuli.

Lateral Dorsal Nucleus

The lateral dorsal nucleus (LD) is a part of the limbic thalamus; it is actually a caudal extension of the anterior nuclear group. The input to LD is derived from the septal areas. It has reciprocal connections with the posterior cingulate gyrus and parahippocampal gyrus. The LD may be involved in emotional expression exhibited by the limbic system.

Lateral Posterior Nucleus and the Pulvinar

The lateral posterior nucleus (LP) is considered to be a rostral extension of the massive pulvinar (P). The LP and P receive significant afferent input from nuclei associated with the visual system such as the superior colliculus and the pretectal nuclei. They are presumed to have a role in the processing of directed visual attention. Both nuclei have reciprocal connections with areas 5 and 7 of the posterior parietal cortex and the pulvinar with widespread portions of the temporal lobe as well. The projection field of the P sometimes is referred to as parietotemporo occipital association cortex.

Medial Geniculate Body

The medial geniculate body (MGB) is a nucleus in the auditory pathways that receives its main afferent input from the inferior colliculus via the brachium of the inferior colliculus. These ascending fibers terminate in the appropriate isofrequency laminae, resulting in a highly ordered bilateral tonotopic projection of the cochlea within the MGB. This tonotopic organization is projected via geniculocortical fibers to the tonotopically organized primary auditory cortex where high pitch tones are localized medially and low tones laterally (area 41 and 42, Chap. 16).

Lateral Geniculate Body

The lateral geniculate body (LGB) is a six-layered nucleus that (1) receives input from the retina of both eyes via the optic tract and (2) has reciprocal connections via the geniculocalcarine tract (optic radiations) with the primary visual cortex (VI, area 17). The LGB has two critical functional roles: (1) the precise transmission of visual input from the retina to the primary visual cortex and (2) the modulation and regulation of the flow of visual information to the primary visual cortex. The latter expressions involve the extensive corticogeniculate projections from area 17 to the LGB. These are integrated into feed-forward and feedback inhibitory circuits (Chap. 3) which process "visual" information and regulate its flow. These connections are thought to be involved in arousal, in regulating the level of visual attention, and in modulating the flow of information to area 17.

Intralaminar Nuclei

The intralaminar nuclei are structurally and functionally rostral extensions of the brainstem reticular formation into the diencephalon. They are extensively interconnected with each other.

Afferent input to the intralaminar nuclei is derived from the brainstem reticular formation, substantia nigra, superior colliculus, pretectum, and spinothalamic tract (pain). The deep cerebellar nuclei project to the intralaminar nuclei with the exception of the parafascicular nucleus (Pf). The central medial and Pf receive afferents from the globus pallidus of the basal ganglia.

The intralaminar nuclei have rich projections to both the putamen and caudate nucleus of the striatum and to widespread areas of the cerebral cortex. All intralaminar nuclei have reciprocal interconnections with the cerebral cortex. (1) A triangular relation exists between defined regions of the cerebral cortex, intralaminar nuclei, and striatal nuclei. From a common cortical area, corticothalamic fibers project to defined regions of the intralaminar nuclei and corticostriatal fibers to the striatum. To complete the triangle, intralaminar-striatal projections interconnect the same regions of the intralaminar nuclei and the striatum. (2) Each of the intralaminar nuclei has diffuse and reciprocal thalamocortical projections to wide areas of the cerebral cortex. The central medial nucleus projects to rostral portions of the frontal lobe including the limbic areas and cingulate gyrus. The Pf projects to the lateral and rostral areas of the frontal lobe. The CM nucleus has copious projections to the premotor and motor areas, and the central lateral nucleus to the somatic sensory areas, related parietal areas, and visual association areas of the occipital cortex.

The intralaminar nuclei have several roles. Their widespread cortical projections are involved with the maintenance of arousal which is integral to the general state of awareness. Their connections to the somatic sensory areas of the cortex indicate a role in sensorimotor integration. The direct spinothalamic, trigeminothalamic, and multisynaptic thalamic pain pathways do have some terminal connections in these nuclei and presumably have a role in arousal and/or in pain perception.

Reticular Nucleus

The *reticular nucleus of the thalamus* is a thin, two- to three- neuron thick shield located on the lateral, anterolateral, and posterolateral surfaces of the thalamus medial to the internal capsule (**Fig. 23.1**). This nucleus is thought to be derived from the ventral thalamus and is neither anatomically nor functionally related to the brainstem reticular formation (Chap. 13). The input to the reticular nucleus is derived from (1) collateral fibers of thalamocortical axons projecting from relay and intralaminar nuclei of the thalamus to the cortex and (2) axon collaterals of corticothalamic fibers projecting from the cortex to the relay nuclei of the thalamus. The outputs of its neurons are via (a) long axons that extend medially into the relay and intralaminar thalamic nuclei and (b) short axons terminating within the nucleus. Neurons in restricted locations in the reticular nucleus project back to the thalamic nucleus from which each receives its input. The neurons of the reticular nucleus do not project directly to the cerebral cortex. The neurons of the reticular nucleus are GABAergic. The nucleus has a high concentration of nicotinic cholinergic receptors, which are sensitive to acetylcholine.

The role of the inhibitory GABAergic neurons of the reticular nucleus is presumably to monitor, integrate, and "gate" activities and to regulate the level of activity of the thalamic nuclei, thereby indirectly influencing the cerebral cortex. This is accomplished through its connections that enable its neurons to sample the activity of the axons passing from the thalamus to the cortex and from the cortex to the thalamus. The thalamic reticular nucleus exerts some influence on the basal ganglia (Chap. 24). This occurs through the circuitry of collateral branches of both the thalamostriatal fibers from the intralaminar nuclei and the reciprocal pallidothalamic fibers from the globus pallidus; these collaterals interact with neurons of the reticular nucleus.

Midline (Periventricular) Nuclei

The midline nuclei are a thin band of nuclei adjacent to the third ventricle. Dorsal midline nuclei have connections with both the striatum and the limbic cortex (e.g., prefrontal lobe). Thus, the midline nuclei and intralaminar nuclei are similar in that they have topographic projections to both the cerebral cortex and striatum. Ventral nuclei have connections with the hippocampal region. Brainstem reticular neurons project ascending adrenergic and serotoninergic fibers to the midline nuclei. A role in visceral activities has been presumed.

LIMBIC THALAMUS

The limbic thalamus is generally defined as the nuclei of the thalamus having connections with the limbic lobe cortex and in particular with the cingulate gyrus (Chap. 22). These include the anterior nuclear group of the thalamus (VA) and portions of some other thalamic nuclei. Cortical areas 24, 25, and 29 of the cingulate gyrus receive major projections from the anterior nuclear group (**Fig. 25.6**). Other thalamic nuclei with some connections to the cingulate gyrus include the DM, LD, LP, P, and the intralaminar nuclei. The limbic thalamus is conceived as having a role in visceral emotions, the visceral aspects of behavior, and even in learning and memory.

SOME TRANSMITTERS OF THE THALAMUS

The inhibitory transmitter GABA and the excitatory transmitter glutamate and perhaps aspartate are associated with the thalamus (Chap. 15). GABAergic neurons include virtually all cells of the thalamic reticular nucleus and interneurons within the thalamic nuclei. In addition, GABA is released by axons of neurons of the globus pallidus and substantia nigra that terminate in the VA and VL nuclei of the thalamus. The inhibitory interneurons in the sensory relay nuclei presumably contribute to the enhancement of stimulus contrasts by lateral inhibition (Chap. 3) and thus, the selection of certain types of stimuli and the suppression of other types (Chaps. 9 and 10). The GABAergic neurons of the reticular nucleus, as noted above,

"gate" the thalamic activity projected to the cerebral cortex.

Glutamate is the major neurotransmitter released by the thalamic neurons projecting to the cortex as well as by the massive corticothalamic projections originating in lamina VI of the cortex. These include the reciprocal pathways involving (1) the VA and VL nuclei with roles in motor function (Chaps. 11, 18, and 24) and (2) the other thalamic nuclei with roles in the sensory and limbic systems (Chaps. 9, 10, 16, and 22).

EXTRATHALAMIC MODULATORY PATHWAYS PROJECTING TO THE CEREBRAL CORTEX

The *extrathalamic modulatory pathways* comprise systems that arise from cholinergic and monoaminergic nuclei located primarily in the brainstem and the basal forebrain. They project, without any relays in the thalamus, directly to the cerebral cortex where they exert modulatory control over the excitability level of the cortical neurons. They have roles in relation to wakefulness, arousal and the phases of sleep.

The *serotonergic pathway* originates in the raphe nuclei located in the midbrain and rostral pons (Chap. 15). They may be involved with sleep and pain control. The *noradrenergic pathway* originates in the locus ceruleus. These neurons are actively releasing norepinephrine during arousal and situations of attention and extreme vigilance. The *dopaminergic pathway* arises in neurons of the ventral tegmental area and terminates in all areas of the cortex. The densest projections are to the motor cortex. The *cholinergic* and *GABAergic pathways* originate respectively from the basal nucleus of Meynert and associated nuclei in the basal forebrain. The cholinergic neurons of the basal nucleus project to the cerebral cortex and the GABAergic nucleus from the basal forebrain to the hippocampus. Changes in these acetylcholine terminals of the cortex may contribute, in some degree, to the dementia of Alzheimer's disease. They have a role in cortical arousal. The *histaminergic pathway* (histamine) arises from neurons in the lateral hypothalamus and terminates in all areas of the cortex.

Nuclei of the brainstem reticular formation and basal forebrain have axons that terminate in the intralaminar thalamic nuclei; the latter in turn, have diffuse projections terminating in all areas of the cortex. Thus, the monoaminergic and cholinergic pathways exert continuous modulatory influences on thalamic and cortical neurons and the resultant behavioral state (sleep-wake) of the individual.

INTERNAL CAPSULE

The internal capsule is one portion of a continuous massive sheet of fibers projecting to and from the cerebral cortex. The sheet extends as the *crus cerebri* of the midbrain, the *internal capsule* of the diencephalon, and the *corona radiata* of the cerebral white matter to the cerebral cortex (Chap. 1 and **Figs. 1.8, 9.2, 10.3, 13.5, and 23.3**). The fibers of the internal capsule convey almost all the neural input to and output from neocortex (Chap. 25); they are the direct lines of communication with the subcortical nuclei, especially of the thalamus, brainstem, and spinal cord. The internal capsule is subdivided into an anterior limb located between the head of the caudate nucleus and the lenticular nucleus, the genu located at the bend (genu) between the anterior and posterior limbs, and a posterior limb located between the thalamus and the lenticular nucleus and extending behind it (retrolenticular portion of the posterior limb) (**Figs. 1.8 and 23.3**).

The fibers passing through the *anterior (caudatolenticular) limb* of the internal capsule include: (1) frontopontine fibers to nuclei in the pons, (2) corticostriate fibers to the striatum, and the following pathways composed of reciprocal connections of fibers between the (3) prefrontal cortex and DM, (4) cingulate gyrus and anterior thalamic nucleus, and (5) septal area and hypothalamus (medial forebrain bundle).

The *genu* of the internal capsule contains corticobulbar and corticoreticular fibers.

The *posterior (thalamolenticular) limb* is composed of both motor pathways and sensory pathways. Through the rostral half of this limb pass the corticospinal, corticorubral, and corticoreticular tracts. Through the caudal half of this limb pass thalamocortical projections from the VA, VL, and VP thalamic nuclei.

The *retrolenticular (postlenticular) portion* of the posterior limb is composed of the optic (geniculocalcarine) radiation, auditory (geniculotemporal) radiation, and corticopontine fibers from the temporal, parietal, and occipital cortices.

FUNCTIONAL CONSIDERATIONS

An axiom of thalamic organization is that the nuclei of the dorsal thalamus provide the last subcortical processing stations of the ascending pathways before the resultant information is projected to the neocortex. This may be the initial critical stage in generating each sensory modality into a sensation.

The thalamus is a major neural processor and integrator involved in essentially all activities of the forebrain. All general and special sensory systems, except for the olfactory system, project their major output to the thalamus before the processed information is relayed to the cerebral cortex. The intralaminar nuclei, nuclei of the midline, and part of the VA nucleus are essential components of the reticular system acting as linkages in the circuitry between the brainstem reticular pathways and the higher centers of the limbic lobe and the neocortex. Thalamic output is the chief source of input to the cerebral cortex; these connections are, to a large degree, integrated into circuits comprising (1) reciprocal connections between thalamic nuclei and the cerebral cortex and (2) circuits between the cortex, basal ganglia, thalamus, and cortex (Chap. 24). The thalamus has a critical role in somatic motor activity through its strategically located nuclei (VA and VL), which receive inputs from the cerebellum and basal ganglia and project influences to the motor cortex (Chaps. 18 and 24).

The thalamus is conceived as being essential for cognition and awareness and may also be critical for arousal. The neuropathological findings in the brain of Karen Ann Quinlan support this view; she was in a persistent vegetative state for 10 years (9 without a respirator)—a condition in which there is wakefulness (arousal) but neither cognition nor awareness.

In her case, the most severe damage was not in the cerebral cortex, but in the thalamus. Her brainstem reticular formation was relatively intact.

"Affect" in sensory appreciation is apparently mediated through the thalamic reticular system, DM, and anterior nuclear group. The *affect* of an individual relates to his emotional tone and somewhat to the phase of the sleep-wake cycle. Well-being, malaise, and a state of contentment are expressions of affect. The degree of agreeableness or disagreeableness of any stimulus depends on the state of an individual. The same objective degree of pain, temperature, or touch can evoke a remarkable variety of subjective degrees of reactivities. This variety is an expression of affective sensory mechanisms.

Through the interaction of the nonspecific nuclei and specific nuclei, the thalamus exerts a regulatory drive upon the cerebral cortex. These nuclei act as modulators and modifiers of thalamic processing. In addition, the synchronization and desynchronization of thalamic activity are considered to be dependent, in part, upon recurrent collateral branches of thalamic neurons feeding back on interneurons; in turn, these connections modulate the neurons projecting to the cortex. The thalamus is essential to such expressions of synchrony (or desynchrony) as (1) the rhythmic brain wave activity observed in an EEG and (2) the phasic and tonic movements mediated by the motor pathways. The thalamus is considered to be a "prime mover" of motor pathways. The modulatory effects are exerted in concert with the VL and VA nuclei through (1) the cerebellothalamocortical pathway (Chap. 18) and (2) the globus pallidus-thalamocortical pathway (Chap. 24). Through integrative, modulatory, and synchronizing activities, the thalamus exerts a major effect upon the motor expressions via the cerebral cortex and its projection pathways, including the corticospinal, corticorubrospinal, corticostriate, and corticoreticulospinal tracts, among others.

LESIONS OF THE THALAMUS

Lesions of the thalamus (as a consequence of vascular impairment) may produce signs known as the *thalamic syndrome*. All general somatic modalities may be diminished on the contralateral half of the head and body without complete anesthesia (lesion of VP nucleus), all general modalities from the face may be normal (VPM not damaged), tactile sense from the face may be intact (bilateral projections from principal trigeminal nucleus), and some pain and temperature sense on the contralateral side may be retained (these modalities may be bilaterally represented in the thalamus or some qualities of these modalities may be felt in the midbrain). In this syndrome, the threshold for pain, temperature and tactile sensations is usually raised on the side contralateral to the lesion. In addition to the diminution of sensations, mild stimuli may evoke disagreeable sensations (dysesthesias). The feelings elicited from a pinprick may be an intolerable burning and agonizing pain. Heat, cold, and pressure from one's clothes can be exceedingly uncomfortable. Intractable pain, which does not respond to analgesics, may be a consequence. In response to environmental stimulation, affect qualities are expressions of modified and exaggerated stimuli during emotional stress. For example, the application of a warm object to the hand may evoke a range of feelings from pain to pleasure.

These highly overactive sensory responses are probably the result of alterations in frequencies and patterns of input to the thalamus, irritation of injured neurons, and changes in the quality of the output to the cerebral cortex. In addition, the release from some cortical influences upon the thalamus may be contributory (release phenomena).

A neocerebellar lesion results in cerebellar dyskinesia. This is an expression of a release phenomenon, in which the VL nucleus is released from the normal cerebellar influences relayed rhythmically through the dentatothalamic pathway. Without these influences, the abnormal movements are expressed. The amelioration of cerebellar dyskinesias in humans may occur following a surgically placed lesion in the contralateral VL nucleus.

SUGGESTED READINGS

Albe-Fessard D, Berkley K, Kruger L, Ralston H III, Willis W Jr. Diencephalic mechanisms of pain sensation. *Brain Res Rev.* 1985;356:217–296.

Allendoerfer K, Schatz C. The subplate, a transient neocortical structure: its role in the development of connections between thalamus and cortex. *Annu Rev Neurosci.* 1994;17:185–218.

Bentivoglio M, Spreafico R, eds. *Cellular Thalamic Mechanisms.* Amsterdam: Excerpta Medica; 1988.

Bentivoglio M, Kultas-Ilinsky K, Ilinsky I. Limbic thalamus: structure, intrinsic organization and connections. In: Vogt B, Gabriel M, eds. Cingulate Gyrus and Limbic Thalamus. A Comprehensive Handbook. Boston, Mass: Birkhauser, Springer-Verlag; 1993:71–132.

Goldman-Rakic P, Porrino L. The primate mediodorsal (MD) nucleus and its projection to the frontal lobe. *J Comp Neurol.* 1985;242:535–560.

Hess W. *Diencephalon: Autonomic and Extrapyramidal Functions.* New York, NY: Grune & Stratton; 1954.

Jones E. *The Thalamus.* New York, NY: Plenum; 1985.

Kinney H, Korein J, Panigrahy A, Dikkes P, Goode R. Neurological findings in the brain of Karen Ann Quinlan. The role of the thalamus in the persistent vegetative state. *N Engl J Med.* 1994; 330:1469–1475.

Macchi G, Rustioni A, Spreafico R, eds. *Somatosensory Integration in the Thalamus: A Re-evaluation Based on the New Methodological Approaches.* Amsterdam: Elsevier; 1983.

Nauta W, Domesick V. Neural associations of limbic system. In: Beckman A, ed. *The Neural Basis of Behavior.* New York, NY: Spectrum; 1982: 175–206.

Papez J. A proposed mechanism for emotion. *Archives of Neurology and Psychiatry.* 1937;38:725–743.

Price J, Russchen F, Amaral D. The limbic region. II. The amygdaloid complex. In: Björklund A, Hökfelt T, Swanson L, eds. *Handbook of Chemical Neurochemistry. Integrated Systems of the CNS.* Vol. 5, part 1. New York, NY: Elsevier; 1987: 279–388.

Pritchard T, Hamilton R, Morse J, Norgren R. Projections of the thalamic gustatory and lingual areas in the monkey, Macaca fascicularis. *J Comp Neurol.* 1986;244:213–228.

Richardson R, DeLong M. A reappraisal of the functions of the nucleus basalis of Meynert. *Trends Neurosci.* 1988;11:264–267. Riss W, Koizumi K, Brooks C, eds. Basic thalamic structure and function. *Brain Behav Evol.* 1972;6:1–560.

Russchen F, Amaral D, Price J. The afferent input to the magnocellular division of the mediodorsal thalamic nucleus in the monkey, Macaca fascicularis. *J Comp Neurol.* 1987;256:175–210.

Schell G, Strick P. The origin of thalamic inputs to the arcuate, premotor and supplementary motor areas. *J Neurosci.* 1984;4:539–560.

Seifert W. *Neurobiology of the Hippocampus.* New York, NY: Academic Press; 1983.

Smith O, DeVito J. Central neural integration for the control of autonomic responses associated with emotion. *Annu Rev Neurosci.* 1984;7:43–65.

Stein B, Meredith M. *The Merging of the Senses.* Cambridge, Mass: Bradford Books, MIT Press; 1993.

Stephan H. Evolutionary trends in limbic structures. *Neurosci Biobehav Rev.* 1983;7:367–374.

Basal Ganglia and Extrapyramidal System 24

Basal ganglia

Schemata of the general circuitry associated with the basal ganglia

Parallel organization of functionally segregated circuits linking basal ganglia, thalamus, and cortex

Side circuits

Resume

Functional considerations

The brain influences somatic motor activity through groups of descending pathways designated in the early clinical literature as the *pyramidal* and *extrapyramidal* systems (Chap. 11). The rationale for this dichotomy was that all upper motoneuron tracts except the pyramidal tract should be lumped together as extrapyramidal tracts. The outflow through these systems is largely the product of interactions among the cerebral cortex, cerebellum, and basal ganglia. The pyramidal system constitutes a *direct link*, and the extrapyramidal system an *indirect link*, from the motor cortical areas to the lower motoneurons of the cranial and spinal nerves. The pyramidal system pathways include the corticospinal (pyramidal) and corticobulbar tracts. The extrapyramidal pathways are the corticorubral-rubrospinal and the corticoreticular-reticulospinal tracts. Because these two systems are so intertwined functionally, they should be regarded as partially different components of a single motor system.

BASAL GANGLIA

The *basal ganglia* are regarded as subcortical nuclear complexes that play a critical role in the integration of motor activity. Along with the cerebellum, the basal ganglia act at the interface between the sensory systems and many motor responses. In essence, the basal ganglia receive information from the cerebral cortex, integrate and process this input, and project to the thalamus, which relays the output to specific areas of the cerebral cortex. This affects motor, emotional, and cognitive behaviors. Although the functional organization of the basal ganglia circuitry is most complex, a conceptualization of its basic connections has been unraveled. Clinically, the terms *movement disorders* and *malfunctioning of the basal ganglia* are essentially synonymous. Such disorders as Parkinson's disease and Huntington's chorea are expressions of basal ganglia disturbances. As a basis of understanding these statements, a modern classification of the nuclei comprising the basal ganglia (**Table 24.1**) and fundamentals of the circuitry are presented.

The basal ganglia and their related neural centers are enumerated in Chapter 1, shown in **Figures 1.8, 23.3, 24.1 to 24.3**, and detailed in **Table 24.2**. The nuclear complexes classified as basal ganglia include the corpus striatum, substantia nigra, subthalamic nucleus, and ventral tegmental area (VTA). This classification is primarily based on the relation of these structures with somatic motor function.

Table 24.1: Classification of Basal Ganglia Nuclei

Input Nuclei	Caudate nucleus
	Putamen
	Nucleus accumbens
Intrinsic Nuclei	Globus pallidus (lateral segment)
	Subthalamic nucleus
	Substantia nigra (pars compacta)
	Ventral tegmental area (VTA)
Output Nuclei	Globus pallidus (medial segment)
	Substantia nigra (pars reticularis)
	Ventral pallidum

The corpus striatum is divided into the striatum (neostriatum) and the globus pallidus (pallidum or paleostriatum). The striatum is divided into the putamen (about 55% by volume), caudate nucleus (about 35% by volume), and nucleus accumbens (ventral striatum). The globus pallidus is divided into the medial segment, lateral segment, and ventral pallidum. The recently added ventral striatum and ventral pallidum are described subsequently. The substantia nigra consists of two parts, called the pars reticularis (SNr) and pars compacta (SNc). During development, the fibers of the internal capsule pass through the territory of the basal ganglia with the result that it separates the (1) putamen from the caudate nucleus and the (2) subthalamic nucleus and substantia nigra from the globus pallidus. The putamen and the globus pallidus are collectively called the lenticular (lentiform) nucleus. The caudate nucleus and putamen, though separated by the fibers of

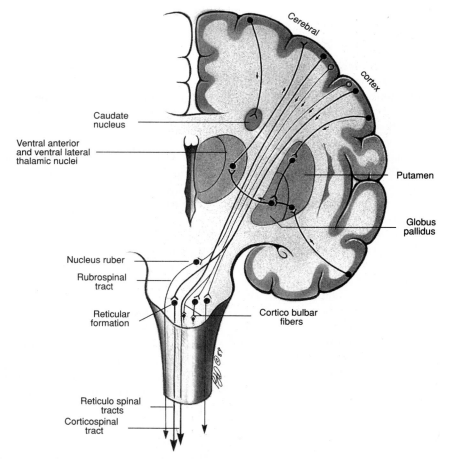

Figure 24.1: The core circuit linking the cerebral cortex, basal ganglia, thalamus, and motor cortex to the descending pathways. The sequence comprises (1) the cerebral cortex to (2) the striatum (putamen and caudate nucleus) to (3) the globus pallidus to (4) the thalamus (VA and VL nuclei) to (5) the supplementary, premotor, and motor cortices where (6) the corticospinal, corticorubrospinal, corticoreticulospinal, and corticobulbar pathways originate.

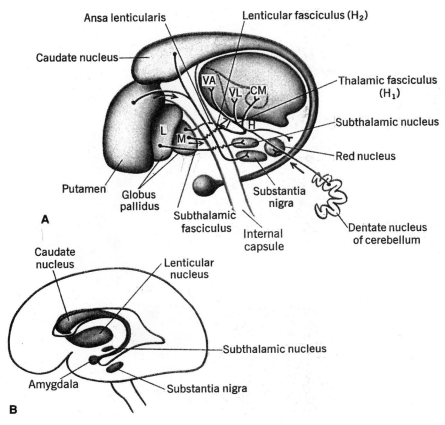

Figure 24.2: Structures involved in the circuitry of the basal ganglia. **A.** The location of the basal ganglia in relation to the lateral ventricle. **B.** Some efferent projections of the basal ganglia and cerebellum. The pallidofugal fibers from the globus pallidus form three bundles: ansa lenticularis, lenticular fasciculus, and subthalamic fasciculus. The former two bundles and the projections from the dentate nucleus of the cerebellum join to form the thalamic fasciculus that terminates in the thalamus. L and M refer to the medial and lateral segments of the globus pallidus. VA = ventral anterior thalamic nucleus; VL = ventral lateral thalamic nuclei; CM = centrum medianum; ZI = zona incerta.

Table 24.2: Basal Ganglia and Related Centers

Corpus striatum	Striatum (neostriatum)	Caudate nucleus Putamen	Dorsal striatum
		Nucleus accumbens	Ventral striatum
	Globus pallidus (pallidum, paleostriatum)	Medial (internal) segment Lateral (external) segment	Dorsal pallidum
		Ventral pallidum	
	Substantia nigra	Pars compacta Pars reticularis	
	Subthalamic nucleus Ventral tegmental area (VTA)		

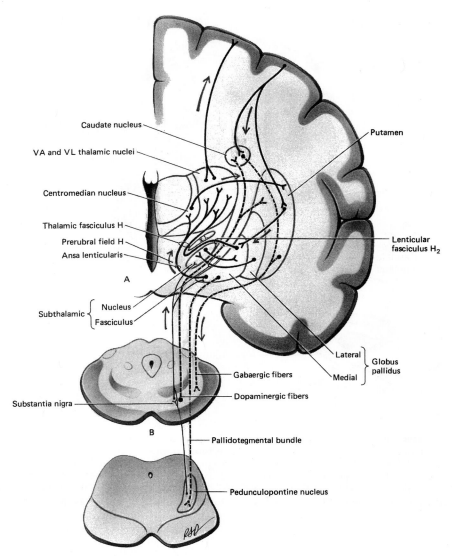

Figure 24.3: Main circuits associated with the basal ganglia illustrated in (**A**) a coronal section through the cerebrum and (**B** and **C**) transverse sections through the upper and lower midbrain. Note (1) circuit 1—cerebral cortex to striatum to globus pallidus to VA and VL of thalamus (via ansa lenticularis, lenticular fasciculus, and thalamic fasciculus) to motor cortex; (2) circuit 2—striatum via gabaergic fibers to substantia nigra to striatum via dopaminergic fibers; (3) circuit 3—globus pallidus to subthalamic nucleus and back via subthalamic fasciculus, and (4) circuit 4—striatum to globus pallidus to centrum medianum to striatum. ZI = zona incerta.

the internal capsule, are paired in the sense that they have similar inputs and outputs (Fig. 24.2). The medial segment of the globus pallidus and the SNr are similarly coupled. The VTA is a cluster of neurons in the midbrain tegmentum located just medial to the substantia nigra, pars compacta. The SNc and VTA may have similar roles.

Ventral Striatum and Ventral Pallidum (Table 24.2)

The nucleus accumbens, called the ventral striatum, is located ventral to the anterior limb of the internal capsule where it is continuous with both the caudate nucleus and putamen. Its cyto-architecture and histochemistry are similar to

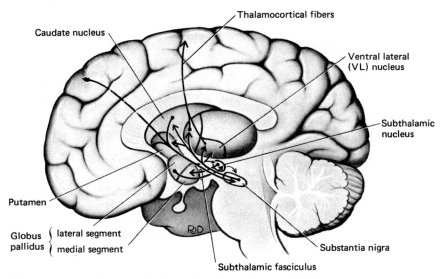

Figure 24.4: Circuits associated with the basal ganglia. Note circuit 2—striatum (caudate nucleus and putamen) to substantia nigra to striatum and to VA and VL thalamic nuclei to motor cortex, and circuit 3—globus pallidus to subthalamic nucleus to globus pallidus.

that of the striatum. The ventral striatum projects to the ventral pallidum. It serves as a link with the limbic system through input from the amygdala and hippocampal formation, and output via the ventral pallidum to the dorsomedial thalamic nucleus.

The substantia innominata (Fig. 22.2) is an area located ventral to and extending rostrally from the basal ganglia. Associated with the substantia innominata is the basal nucleus of Meynert (Chap. 25) and some neurons considered to be a ventral extension of the globus pallidus. The latter, called the *ventral pallidum*, has projections that eventually affect descending motor systems. Through these connections, the ventral pallidum, together with the ventral striatum, exert a role in planning and integrating movements that are related to motivational and emotional stimuli.

SCHEMATA OF THE GENERAL CIRCUITRY ASSOCIATED WITH THE BASAL GANGLIA

The cerebral cortex, basal ganglia, and thalamus are organized into a complex of neural circuits. Until recently, the role of the basal ganglia was conceived as being primarily to integrate and process diverse inputs from wide areas of the neocortex, and relay influences to the ventral lateral (VL) and ventral anterior (VA) thalamic nuclei. Portions of these nuclei, known as the "motor nuclei" of the thalamus, that receive input from the basal ganglia, project to supplementary and premotor regions of area 6, as well as to the motor cortex (area 4). The following schemata are abstracted from a most complex circuitry.

These consist of a core circuit, divisible into four or more parallel segregated circuits, and two side loops—one with the subthalamic nucleus, and the other with the substantia nigra. These are outlined as six circuits.

Generalized Core Circuit

The basic generalized core circuit comprises cerebral cortex → striatum → globus pallidus → thalamus → cerebral cortex. Processed information then is transmitted via upper motoneuronal pathways (e.g., the corticospinal tract) to the lower motoneurons (Fig. 24.1). Some structures associated with this circuit are illustrated in Figure 24.2. A generalized feedback circuit goes back to the striatum via thalamostriate fibers from the intralaminar nuclei.

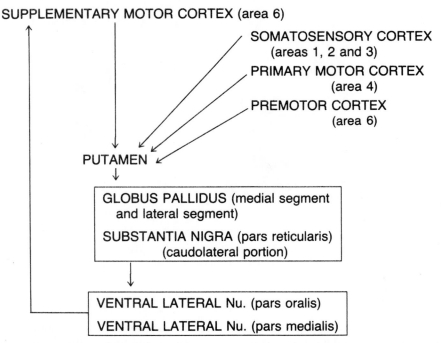

Figure 24.5: Sensory-motor loops. The closed loop starts in the supplementary motor cortex (area 6) and terminates in the supplementary motor cortex. The open loop involves input to the closed loop from the somatosensory cortex (areas 1, 2, and 3), primary motor cortex (area 4), and premotor cortex (area 6). (Adapted from Alexander, DeLong, and Strick, 1986.)

Anatomic and physiologic data indicate that the general core circuit serves as a template for at least four segregated cerebral cortex → basal ganglia → thalamocortical loops (Figs. 24.5 to 24.8). These circuits are organized in parallel, but convey functionally separate information from different cortical regions. Each of the four circuits described later receives its input from a given cortical region and sends impulses through the circuit back to a restricted target area within the original cortical region. Each circuit combines a "closed loop" and an "open loop." The "closed loop" portion comprises the input from a specific cortical area (e.g., supplementary motor cortex) back to the cortical area of origin (e.g., supplementary motor cortex). The "open loop" component comprises input to the loop from other cortical areas (e.g., premotor area, primary motor cortex, and primary somatosensory cortex) and terminates in the cortical area of origin of the closed loop (e.g., supplementary motor cortex).

PARALLEL ORGANIZATION OF FUNCTIONALLY SEGREGATED CIRCUITS LINKING BASAL GANGLIA, THALAMUS, AND CORTEX

The proposed basal ganglia-thalamocortical circuits include (1) a "motor circuit" (Fig. 24.5), (2) an "association circuit" (Fig. 24.6), (3) an "oculomotor" circuit (Fig. 24.7), and (4) a limbic circuit (Fig. 24.8). Several features are presumed to characterize each circuit. (1) The basic design of each circuit is similar in terms of having a central "closed loop." (2) Each circuit appears to receive corticostriate input from several partially overlapping functionally related cortical areas. These multiple inputs are progressively integrated by processing them in their passage through the pallidum and thalamus and back to one specific cortical area. (3) None of these loops is a rigid self-contained pathway; each receives diverse influences from the nuclei of the circuit.

ASSOCIATION LOOPS

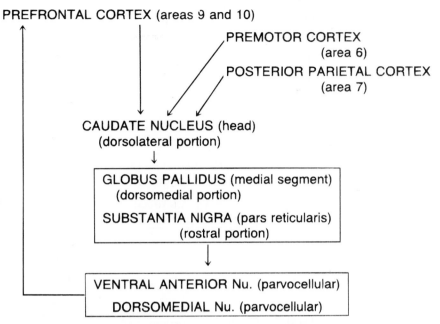

Figure 24.6: Association loops. The closed loop commences with the prefrontal cortex (areas 9, 10) and terminates in the frontal cortex. The open loop involves input from the premotor cortex (area 6) and posterior parietal cortex (area 7). (Adapted from Alexander, DeLong, and Strick, 1986.)

The significance of these parallel circuits is that they express another level of organization and functional specificity itself. Subsidiary inputs and circuits appear to modify and modulate the flow of information that passes through the major basal ganglia-thalamocortical circuits, and, thus, provide additional routes for influences to be exerted on these processing centers. There are other sources of input to the striatum, including from the VTA and the midbrain raphe nuclei.

Circuit 1: Motor

Widespread areas of the cerebral cortex, including the motor areas (Fig. 24.5), project corticostriate fibers in a topographically organized arrangement to the ipsilateral striatum (putamen and caudate nucleus). The motor cortices (areas 4 and 6) and primary somatosensory cortex (areas 3, 1, and 2) have preferential and bilateral projections to the putamen. The closed loop portion of the motor circuit begins and ends in the supplementary motor cortex. The open loop portion involves the other areas.

Striatopallidal fibers arising from all parts of the striatum terminate in both the medial and lateral segments of the globus pallidus. The medial segment is the origin of two fiber bundles, both of which terminate in the thalamus. Fibers from the ventral portion of the globus pallidus form the *ansa lenticularis*, which loops under the internal capsule, whereas fibers from the dorsal portion enter the *lenticular fasciculus*, which passes across the internal capsule and appears as a prominent band as it continues medially along the dorsal and rostral surfaces of the subthalamic nucleus (Figs. 24.2 and 24.3). In this location, the lenticular fasciculus forms the ventral border of the zona incerta, which is an extension of the brainstem reticular formation into the diencephalon. Fibers of the lenticular fasciculus and ansa lenticularis coalesce medial to the zona incerta and subthalamic nucleus where they are just rostral to the red nucleus in what is referred to as the prerubral field. The combined fascicles pass laterally and rostrally along the ventral border of the thalamus (dorsal to the zona incerta) as the *thalamic fasciculus* (Figs. 24.2 and

OCULOMOTOR LOOPS

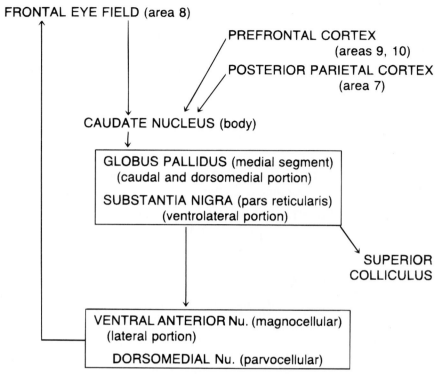

Figure 24.7: Oculomotor loops. The closed loop begins in frontal eye field (area 8) and terminates in the frontal eye field. The open loop involves input from the prefrontal cortex (areas 9, 10) and posterior parietal cortex (area 7). The projection to the superior colliculus may have a role in the control of saccadic eye movements to remembered visual targets. (Adapted from Alexander, DeLong, and Strick, 1986.)

24.3). It should be noted that dentatothalamic fibers from the cerebellum, as well as fibers of the medial lemniscus, also pass through the prerubral field and join the thalamic fasciculus. Pallidal efferent fibers turn dorsally and terminate in the VA, VL, and centrum medianum (CM) nuclei of the thalamus. The VA and VL nuclei project somatotopically to the supplementary motor cortex (area 6), premotor cortex (area 6), frontal eye field (area 8), and prefrontal cortex (areas 9 and 10). These projections terminate on neurons of lamina IV of the cortex.

Other connections of this circuit add to the complexity of interactions involving the nuclei of the basal ganglia (**Fig. 24.3**). The globus pallidus, for example, projects to the CM and other intralaminar thalamic nuclei; the former, in turn, projects to the putamen of the striatum, as well as diffusely to the cortex Chap. 23). In a

sense, the intralaminar nuclei are incorporated into a circuit of striatum to globus pallidus to intralaminar nuclei and back (**Fig. 24.2**). In addition, the globus pallidus has reciprocal connections with the pedunculopontine nucleus of the midbrain (**Fig. 24.3**). The latter nucleus does not project caudally. *This is consistent with the evidence that none of the basal ganglia has fibers projecting to the lower brainstem and spinal cord. Rather, the output from the basal ganglia, which acts to influence cerebral cortical activities, is directed rostrally to cortical areas.* Several neurotransmitters have been identified with these circuits (**Fig. 24.9**).

Circuit 2: Association

The association circuit (**Fig. 24.6**) is different from the motor and oculomotor circuits in that

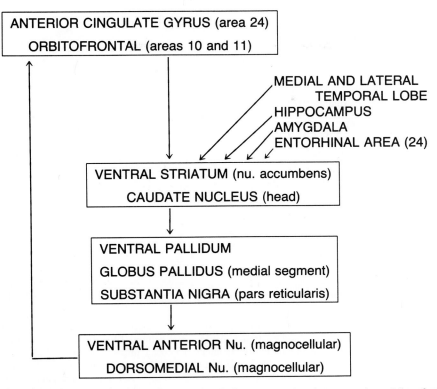

Figure 24.8: Limbic loops. The closed loop commences with the anterior cingulate gyrus (area 24) and orbitofrontal cortex (areas 10, 11) and terminates in these same areas. The open loop involves input from the medial and lateral temporal lobe, hippocampus, amygdala, and entorhinal area (area 24). (Adapted and modified from Alexander, DeLong, and Strick, 1986.)

the widespread association areas of the frontal, parietal, occipital, and temporal lobes have ipsilateral projections primarily to the caudate nucleus. The closed loop commences and ends in the prefrontal region (areas 9 and 10). Further, striatopallidal connections to the medial segment of the globus pallidus terminate in portions of the nucleus that project preferentially to intralaminar nuclei other than CM, as well as to VA and VL. In addition to diffuse cortical collaterals, these other intralaminar nuclei project back to the caudate. Also, the parts of VA and VL receiving input in this circuit forward the information to the prefrontal cortex (areas 9 and 10). Other features of this circuit are similar to those of the motor circuit.

Circuit 3: Oculomotor

The closed loop component of the oculomotor circuit (Fig. 24.7) begins and ends in the fron-

tal eye field (area 8). The open loop receives input from the prefrontal cortex (areas 9 and 10) and from the posterior parietal region (area 7). Fibers arising from these cortical areas project preferentially to the body of the caudate nucleus, whence, after processing, information is sent to the globus pallidus and the SNr. In addition to projections from these nuclei to the thalamus (VL, VA, intralaminar) as in the other circuits, nigral efferents also go to the frontal eye field (area 8) via relays in the dorsomedial nucleus of the thalamus, and directly to the superior colliculus to influence control of saccadic eye movements.

Circuit 4: Limbic

There are several circuits that can be described as limbic (Fig. 24.8), but they have been combined into one for simplification. The closed loop portion of a limbic circuit begins and ends

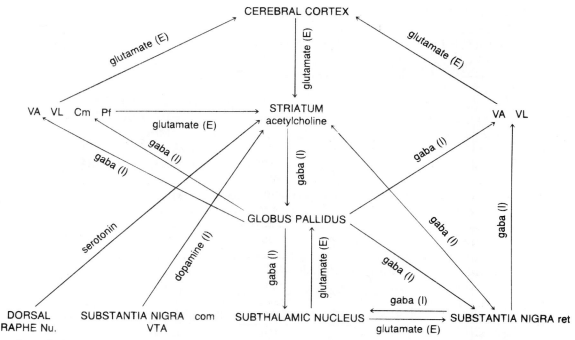

Figure 24.9: Some neurotransmitters associated with the cerebral cortex-basal ganglia-thalamocortical circuitry. The nuclei are represented by capital letters and the transmitters in small letters. (E) and (I) indicate that the transmitter has either an excitatory (E) effect or an inhibitory (I) effect. The VTA projects to the ventral striatum (nucleus accumbens). Note that dopamine differentially inhibits D_2 striatal projection neurons and excites D_1 neurons. Substantia nigra com. = substantia nigra pars compacta; substantia nigra ret. = substantia nigra pars reticularis; CM = centrum medianum; Pf = parafascicular nucleus; VA = ventral anterior nucleus; and VL = ventral lateral nucleus. (Adapted in part from Haber, 1986.)

in the anterior part of the cingulate gyrus (area 24) and orbitofrontal cortex (areas 10 and 11). The open loop component receives input from medial and lateral temporal lobe cortex including the entorhinal area (area 24), the amygdala, and hippocampus. These regions project to the ventral striatum (nucleus accumbens) and part of the head of the caudate nucleus, whence after processing, information is forwarded to the ventral pallidum, globus pallidus, and reticular part of the substantia nigra. Fibers from these nuclei go to the magnocellular divisions of the VA and dorsomedial thalamic nuclei which project to the cortex of the closed loop.

SIDE CIRCUITS

Circuit 5: Substantia Nigra

Striatum → substantia nigra → thalamus (VA and VL nuclei) → portions of the motor cortex (Figs. 24.3 and 24.4).

This circuit involves the substantia nigra. In brief, the substantia nigra (1) receives input from the ipsilateral striatum, subthalamic nucleus, and globus pallidus and (2) projects to the ipsilateral VL and VA thalamic nuclei (Fig. 24.5) as well as back to the striatum (Fig. 24.3).

The substantia nigra is divided into the ventrally located pars reticularis (adjacent to the crus cerebri) and the dorsally located pars compacta (Fig. 13.15). The *pars reticularis* has iron-containing glial cells, serotonin, and gamma aminobutyric acid (GABA). The *pars compacta* has dopaminergic neurons which contain neuromelanin (hence, its dark appearance). This neuromelanin pigment is a polymer of the catecholamine precursor Dopa (dihydrophenylalanine) and is absent in patients with Parkinson's disease, as well as in infants. There is linkage between the two parts of the nigra via dendrites of SNc neurons which extend into the SNr. The striatonigral fibers project almost entirely to the pars reticularis, although there are some terminals in ventral parts of the pars compacta. The projections from the substantia nigra are directed rostrally via (1) nigrostriatal fibers from the pars compacta to the striatum and (2) nigrothalamic fibers from the pars reticularis to the VA and VL thalamic nuclei. These thalamic nuclei project to portions of the motor cortical areas. The nigral efferent projections to the VA and VL nuclei terminate in different regions of these thalamic nuclei than do projections from the globus pallidus and from the cerebellum (dentatothalamic fibers); current evidence indicates that no overlap occurs among these three projections.

The SNr and the globus pallidus are sources of descending fibers to the *pedunculopontine nucleus* in the caudal midbrain (Fig. 24.3). These fibers are the most caudal projections from the basal ganglia. This tegmental nucleus is not a motor nucleus with linkages to the pons and medulla, or to any descending motor tracts originating in the brainstem. Rather, efferents from the pedunculopontine nucleus mainly go to the SNr, with some to the subthalamic nucleus and to the medial segment of the globus pallidus.

The nigrostriatal fibers from the pars compacta form the *dopamine neuronal system*, which releases dopamine in the striatum. The serotonin in the pars reticularis is derived from the dorsal tegmental nucleus of the midbrain raphe. The striatonigral fibers and the nigrothalamic fibers release the transmitter GABA. (Fig. 24.9 and section entitled, *Functional Considerations*.)

Circuit 6: Subthalamic Nucleus

Globus pallidus (lateral segment) → subthalamic nucleus → globus pallidus (both segments)(Figs. 24.3 and 24.4).

The subthalamic nucleus receives input from the ipsilateral globus pallidus (lateral segment), motor cortex, and pedunculopontine nucleus. It projects output to both segments of the ipsilateral globus pallidus, but mainly the larger lateral segment, and to the pars reticularis of the substantia nigra, with which it is reciprocally interconnected; this is another side circuit. The

fibers that reciprocally interconnect the globus pallidus and the subthalamic nucleus form the *subthalamic fasciculus*, which passes through the posterior limb of the internal capsule. Although previously it was thought that the output neurons of the subthalamic nucleus release the putative inhibitory transmitter glycine (or GABA), recent evidence indicates that they release glutamate which is an excitatory transmitter. Thus, the presumed role of the subthalamic nucleus is to act as the driving force regulating the output of the globus pallidus and substantia nigra (see later).

General Organization of Nuclei of Basal Ganglia

On the basis of their neural connections, the nuclei of the basal ganglia are organized as *input nuclei*, *intrinsic nuclei*, and *output nuclei* (Table 24.1). The input nuclei receive significant afferent information from non-basal ganglion sources and project their output to the intrinsic nuclei. The *intrinsic nuclei* interact and have connections with both input nuclei and output nuclei. After neural processing within the basal ganglia, the *output nuclei* project their influences to nuclei outside the basal ganglia.

The striatum (caudate nucleus, putamen, and nucleus accumbens) comprises the input nuclei. It receives its major input from the cerebral cortex; these inputs are *excitatory* (Fig. 24.9). The globus pallidus (lateral segment), subthalamic nucleus, SNc, and VTA (area of midbrain tegmentum located adjacent to the pars reticularis) comprise the intrinsic nuclei. The circuitry linking these nuclei together, and with the input and output nuclei, mainly consists of *inhibitory neurons*; an important exception are those of the subthalamic nucleus (Fig. 24.9). The globus pallidus (medial segment), SNr, and ventral pallidum comprise the output nuclei. The projections from these nuclei are largely directed to certain thalamic nuclei. These outputs are *inhibitory* (Fig. 24.9).

Cytoarchitectural and Compartmental Organization of the Striatum

Cell Types

The striatum contains two major neuronal populations, projection neurons whose axons terminate in other nuclei and intrinsic cells whose axons remain within the striatum.

The medium spiny neuron, which receives most of the extrastriatal input, is by far the most numerous type, constituting over 90% of the total population. These cells have axons that project out of the striatum and have GABA as the major neurotransmitter. Two classes of this cell type, with different projections, are recognized. Striatonigral neurons, including those with collaterals to the medial pallidal segment, mainly have D_1 dopamine receptors (see later) and release substance P and dynorphin. Striatopallidal neurons to the lateral segment primarily have D_2 dopamine receptors and release enkephalin. The dopaminergic input to these neurons from the substantia nigra presumably differentially modulates these cells and provides the basis for explaining various forms of basal ganglia induced motor disturbances (see below). Intrinsic neurons, whose axons do not leave the striatum, are of several types. *Large aspiny neurons,* which use acetylcholine as a neurotransmitter, have been clearly identified. They have excitatory effects on the projection neurons. Separate classes of intrinsic medium aspiny neurons contain somatostatin and neuropeptide y, among other substances.

Patch-Matrix Compartments

Based upon differences in neurochemical markers and connectivity, the striatum has been divided into smaller patch compartments (15% of the total) embedded in larger matrix ones. The concentration of acetylcholine is much higher in the matrix and there are other histochemical differences between the compartments as well. Neocortical projections from cells in more superficial parts of lamina V as well as the deep part of lamina III, go principally to the matrix compartment. Patch compartments receive terminals from neurons in deep parts of cortical lamina V which are well developed in cortex related to the limbic system. The functional significance of the patch-matrix compartmentalization, and the discontinuous distribution of acetylcholine and other transmitters in the striatum, is incompletely understood (see later), but appears to be related to regulating the balance

of output by the striatonigral and striatopallidal neurons.

RESUME

The basal ganglia are subcortical nuclei that play a primary role in the integration of somatic motor activity. The amygdala and hippocampus, nuclear complexes of the limbic system (Chap. 22) with connections to the ventral striatum, involve the basal ganglia in somatic movements associated with responses to motivational and emotional stimuli (see *Ventral Pallidum* and *Ventral Striatum*).

The striatum is the receptive complex of the corpus striatum (Table 24.2); its input is derived from widespread areas of the neocortex, intralaminar nuclei (CM and parafascicular nucleus) of the thalamus, substantia nigra, VTA, and dorsal raphe nucleus of the midbrain. The afferent corticostriate influences are mediated by the excitatory transmitter glutamate (**Fig. 24.9**). The intrinsic local circuit neurons of the striatum are cholinergic interneurons. The striatum is not a homogeneous structure; about 85% consists of a "matrix" and 15% of small "patches." The concentration of acetylcholine is much lower in the patches than in the matrix. The functional significance of this discontinuous distribution of acetylcholine and other transmitters has yet to be determined. The striatum projects its output via fibers that terminate in both segments of the globus pallidus and the SNr. The transmitter of both the striatopallidal and striatonigral pathways is GABA, but there are different comodulators in some neurons including the neuropeptides enkephalin, substance P, and dynorphin. Moreover, neurons projecting to the medial segment of the globus pallidus and the SNr have D_1 dopamine receptors whereas those going to the lateral segment of the pallidum have D_2 receptors. It should be noted that D_1 and D_2 dopamine receptors are among several types of dopamine receptors. They are associated with second messenger systems (Chap. 3). The D_1 receptors act to increase cAMP formation. They are located postsynaptic to dopamine neuron terminals in the striatum, nucleus accumbens, and substantia nigra. The D_2 receptors act to decrease cAMP formation.

They are located postsynaptic to dopamine neuron terminals in the striatum, nucleus accumbens, substantia nigra, and VTA.

The output of the basal ganglia is derived from neurons of the medial segment of the GP, the substantia nigra (pars reticularis), and ventral pallidum. The projections from these sources to VL and VA thalamic nuclei are distinct and their terminations do not overlap. The thalamic neurons receiving these inputs do not exert major effects on the primary motor cortex (area 4), but rather mainly project their outputs to premotor and supplementary motor areas (Chap. 25). The pallidothalamic and nigrothalamic fibers primarily exert inhibitory effects on the thalamus.

The substantia nigra receives input from both the striatum and globus pallidus of the corpus striatum, subthalamic nucleus, pedunculopontine nucleus, and dorsal nucleus of the midbrain raphe. A major output from the substantia nigra (pars compacta) terminates as dopaminergic endings in the striatum. The subthalamic nucleus receives input from the lateral segment of the globus pallidus and the motor cortex. The subthalamic nucleus projects its output to both segments of the globus pallidus, the substantia nigra (pars reticularis), and ventral pallidum. Recent evidence indicates that the excitatory neurotransmitter glutamate probably is the transmitter of the fibers projecting from the subthalamic nucleus to the globus pallidus. On the basis of this information, the suggestion has validity that the output of the subthalamic nucleus through excitatory influences on the medial segment of the pallidum and on the SNr, is the driving force regulating the output of the basal ganglia.

The basal ganglia, along with the cerebellum, act as the interface between our sensory systems and many motor responses. The pallidothalamic projections in the thalamus do not overlap the cerebellar projections from the deep cerebellar nuclei. No convergence from the pallidal and cerebellar inputs has been demonstrated on a single thalamic neuron.

The precise role of the basal ganglia in the regulation of normal movements is still a matter of speculation. They are thought to be involved in the regulation of background muscle tone and posture and in the initiation, control, and cessation of automatic movements such as in locomotion (running) and in athletics (throwing a ball). The basal ganglia are apparently involved in the transfer and modification of information from widespread neocortical areas to the motor cortex, especially the premotor and supplementary motor areas.

Both the basal ganglia and cerebellum have roles in cognitive processes such as working memory, rule-based learning, and in planning of future behavior. This is accomplished through connections of these structures with the prefrontal lobes. The GPm and a restricted region of the dentate nucleus project to parts of the thalamus that project to the prefrontal cortex, which is presumed to be involved in cognition.

FUNCTIONAL CONSIDERATIONS

Formerly the cerebral cortex, especially the motor cortex, was hierarchically placed at the highest level for orchestrating motor integration, and the subcortical structures were placed at another level and thought to function solely in a feedback capacity. The newer view states that both the basal ganglia and the cerebellum are crucial in the initial and early processing stages resulting in motor activity. The circuitry involving the sensory cortical areas, basal ganglia, and cerebellum act through the VA and VL nuclei, known as the *motor nuclei of the thalamus.* They serve as the main gateway through which these circuits become involved in generating activity in the motor cortical areas; they fire well in advance of and during each volitional movement. In addition, these circuits act as bridges between the sensory cortical areas and the motor cortical areas. In a real sense, these circuits are active participants during all phases of a movement from initiation to completion.

As we have seen, the role of the basal ganglia, cerebellum, and associated nuclei is to modulate motor activities through circuits which directly and indirectly feed back to the cerebral cortex. In turn, the cortex projects its influences to the brainstem and spinal levels through the descending motor pathways, upon the local circuitry influencing the alpha and gamma motor neurons. The malfunction of various nuclear complexes results in an imbalance in the interactions within the circuitry of the "extrapyramidal system." This is a plausible explanation for the variety and assortment of symptoms and signs noted in the disorders involving control of posture and movements. In some disorders there is an increase in muscle tone to a similar degree in the agonists and antagonists of a muscle group without an accompanying increase in reflex activity; this is called *rigidity*. Rigidity (Chap. 8) is a form of hypertonus in which the muscles are continuously or intermittently tense, and is associated with hyperactive static fusiform gamma motoneurons. In contrast, spasticity (Chap. 12) is a form of hypertonus in which the muscles are in phasic hyperactive activity when the muscles are on stretch. This is associated with hyperactive dynamic fusiform gamma motoneurons.

The abnormal involuntary movements, called *dyskinesias*, may be rhythmic or arrhythmic, generally without paralysis of the muscles. The motor disorders resulting from the improper functioning of the "extrapyramidal system," the basal ganglia, and associated nuclei include paralysis agitans (Parkinson's disease), athetosis, choreas, and ballism.

Parkinson's disease (paralysis agitans, parkinsonism) is characterized by rigidity and tremor. The rigidity is essentially the same in all muscles; it is accompanied by poverty of movements and *cogwheel rigidity*. Cogwheel rigidity is expressed when the examiner flexes and extends a limb joint of the patient; during the movement, an increased resistance suddenly gives way, and as the movement continues, this sequence is repeated, as in a cogwheel. From a standing position, the patient has difficulty in taking initial steps. The subject also has the same problem in arresting the movement. During forward locomotion, short, shuffling steps are taken. The "masked" face has a fixed expression, accompanied by no overt spontaneous emotional response. The tremor, with its regular frequency (3–6 per second) and amplitude, occurs while the subject is at rest; it is lost or reduced during a movement. Degenerative changes in the nigrostriatal pathway, raphe nuclei, locus ceruleus, and motor nucleus of the vagus nerve are present in parkinsonian patients; in addition, there is a marked reduction to absence of dopamine, serotonin, and norepi-

nephrine. It has been shown that Parkinson-like symptoms may be elicited by toxins, such as MPTP (1-methyl-4-phenyl-1,2,3,6-tetrahydropyridine), that selectively destroy nigrostriatal dopamine neurons while sparing other dopamine neurons. Administration of L-dopa (L-dihydroxyphenylalanine) in low doses may ameliorate the rigidity, and in high doses, the tremors. L-dopa is a common precursor of melanin and dopamine.

Beginning in the 1940s, a therapeutic approach for parkinsonism was to place small lesions in the globus pallidus and VL nucleus of the thalamus. In some patients, pallidal lesions alleviated the symptoms of rigidity and dyskinesia, and thalamic lesions reduced the tremor; however, the symptoms often recurred a few years after surgery. This approach fell into disfavor in the 1960s following the demonstration of the existence of the dopaminergic nigrostriatal pathway correlated with a depletion of striatal dopamine in patients with parkinsonism. Modern therapy includes administration of L-dopa (L-dihydroxyphenylalanine), a precursor of dopamine, together with a dopa decarboxylase inhibitor to block formation of dopamine outside of the brain. This drug does not stop the inexorable course of degeneration of the nigrostriatal neurons and eventually the treatment becomes ineffective. Dopamine receptor agonists, certain anticholinergics, and/or other agents also are used.

With the development of neuroimaging techniques, it has become possible to place lesions in the brain with much more precision than heretofore possible. As has received considerable attention in the public press, a striking amelioration of tremor, rigidity, and hypokinesia can be achieved by unilateral stereotactic lesions placed in the posteroventral part of the globus pallidus. Nonetheless, long term improvement has yet to be established and there has been a small percentage of cases with bad outcomes. Another strategy being explored is transplantation of fetal midbrain tissue including the substantia nigra into the striatum. In primate models of Parkinson's disease, caused by injecting MPTP, subsequent lesions produced in the subthalamic nucleus have been shown to reverse the signs. This, presumably, is due to reestablishing the appropriate balance of activity within the circuit of the basal ganglia (see later); however, this procedure is not feasible for clinical use.

Tardive dyskinesia is a form of dyskinesia that occurs in some patients following the chronic administration of phenothiazines (antipsychotic and tranquilizing drugs) as therapy for such psychoses as schizophrenia. The symptoms may include facial grimacing, lip smacking, and choreoathetotic movements of the limbs and trunk. Treatment is to stop giving the drug. Suggested causes include alteration of the dopaminergic receptors resulting in their hypersensitivity to dopamine. The consequential alteration in the balance among the dopaminergic, intrastriatal, cholinergic, and gabaergic agents results in the involuntary movements.

The movements of *athetosis* are slow and are exaggerated by voluntary movement. The slow, writhing character of the involuntary movements of the neck, trunk, and extremities appear wormlike. The alternating adduction and abduction of the shoulder joint is accompanied by flexion and extension of the wrist and fingers. Usually the wrist is flexed, and the fingers hyperextended. Grimaces of the face may occur during the limb movements. This dyskinesia may be due to a lesion in the striatum, mainly in the putamen. Such injury suggests that the striatum has an inhibitory role. Athetosis is frequently associated with cerebral palsy. It occurs as the result of brain lesions during or prior to birth.

Choreas (dances) are characterized by jerky, irregular, brisk, graceful movements of the limbs accompanied by involuntary grimacing twitching of the face. These movements are expressed primarily by the distal segments of the extremities. In advanced cases, the patient is almost always in motion when awake. There is no reduction in muscle power.

Huntington's Disease (Chorea) is a hereditary autosomal dominant disorder (chromosome 4). From its initial subtle symptoms that may not commence until a person is in their thirties, the affliction features progressive increases in the severity of chorea (choreiform movements) and dementia. Death generally occurs 15 to 20 years after onset. The early stages of the disease have been correlated with a preferential loss, mainly in the caudate nucleus, of the D_2 receptor and enkephalin containing neurons that project to the lateral segment of the globus pallidus, with a relative sparing of the D_1 neurons that project to the substantia nigra and to the medial pallidal segment. The latter are affected in later stages. Although not markedly degenerated, the cholinergic interneurons clearly are damaged in later stages as evidenced by a significant reduction in the amount of striatal cholinesterase. A reduction in substance P and enkephalin in the globus pallidus and substantia nigra also occur. The involuntary choreiform movements are presumed to result from the imbalance in the neuronal loop of gabaergic striatonigral, dopaminergic nigrostriatal, and cholinergic intrastriatal neurons. The impaired cognitive function is attributed to the concomitant loss of neocortical neurons.

Ballism ("throwing") is characterized by violent, high-amplitude, flail-like movements originating mainly from the activity of the proximal appendicular muscles of the shoulder and pelvis. There is a reduction of muscle tone. The movements cease during sleep. These symptoms are exhibited unilaterally with a lesion in the contralateral subthalamic nucleus. Because, clinically, ballism almost always occurs on one side only and is usually due to a vascular accident, it is also known as *hemiballism*.

Symptoms associated with the malfunctioning of the basal ganglia are usually observed bilaterally; however, symptoms on one side result from lesions in the contralateral basal ganglia. This is a consequence of the circuits by which the basal ganglia project to the ipsilateral cerebral cortex, which, in turn, relays its influences via the motor pathways to the contralateral side (i.e., see *ballism* above). The abnormal movements resulting from lesions in the basal ganglia circuitry are an expression of release phenomena, in which the inhibitory influences on such structures as the globus pallidus or VL nucleus of the thalamus are lost or reduced. Surgical lesions of these "released structures" (globus pallidus and VL) are known to ameliorate the symptoms in many patients. In this context, the loss of dopamine, noted in patients with parkinsonism, is presumed to account for the reduction or loss of inhibitory influences upon the striatum. A likely underlying cause of disorders of the basal ganglia is that the disruption of

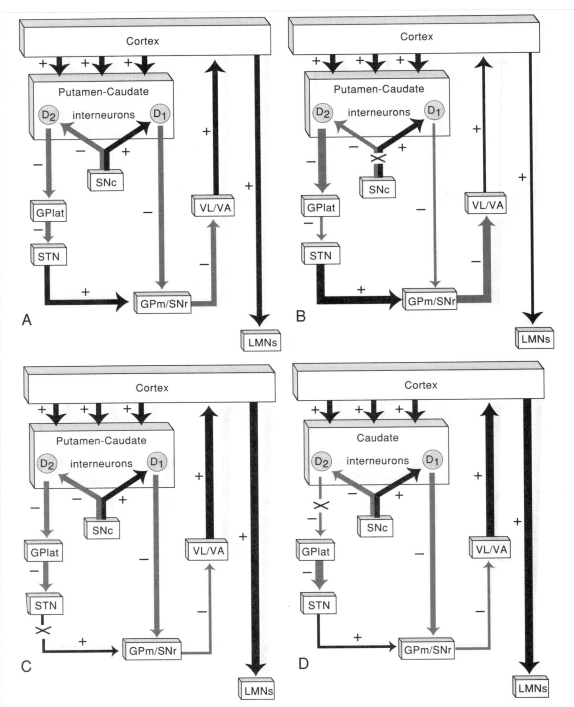

Figure 24.10: Functional connections of the basal ganglia with the thalamus and cortex illustrating relative balance of activity in different parts of the circuitry in normal and various pathological states. Black arrows = excitatory connections; gray arrows = inhibitory connections; thick arrows = increased influence; thin arrows = diminished effect. (**A**) normal; (**B**) destruction of the substantia nigra, pars compacta (SNc), as in Parkinson's disease; (**C**) destruction of the subthalamic nucleus (STN), as in ballism; and (**D**) selective loss of gabaergic striatal projection neurons to the lateral segment of the globus pallidus (GPl), as in early stage Huntington's chorea. D_1, striatal projection neuron with D_1 receptors, and expressing GABA, dynorphin, and substance P as neurotransmitters; D_2, striatal projection neuron with D_2 receptors, and expressing GABA and enkephalin as neurotransmitters; GPm/SNr = globus pallidus, medial segment, and substantia nigra pars reticularis (these are the output nuclei of the basal ganglia); LMNs = lower motoneurons; ($-$) = inhibitory link; and ($+$) = excitatory link. (Adapted and modified from Bergman, Wichman, and DeLong, 1990, and Gerfen, 1992.)

transmitter metabolism results in an abnormal output from the circuitry of the basal ganglia.

Alterations of Inhibitory/Excitatory Activity in Movement Disorders

As indicated earlier, motor activity is modulated by the basal ganglia via their inhibitory output to the thalamus and excitatory thalamocortical-upper motoneuronal pathways. Smooth, coordinated 'normal' movements require a proper balance of excitatory and inhibitory activity throughout the basal ganglia (**Fig. 24.10A**). Anything that alters the usual pattern of inhibition exerted upon the thalamus is in a position to disrupt normal motor function. Therefore, increased inhibition of the thalamus might be expected to diminish excitatory activity of the thalamocortical-upper motoneuronal pathways and reduce, or otherwise impoverish, motor activity. Conversely, decreased inhibition of the thalamus might be expected to increase excitation of the thalamocortical-upper motoneuronal pathways and produce an excess of motor activity.

Based upon the circuitry of the basal ganglia and the interplay of inhibitory and excitatory neurotransmitters (**Fig. 24.9**), the bradykinesis characteristic of parkinsonism is attributed to the increased activity of the basal ganglia output nuclei (GPm and SNr), which inhibit the VA and VL nuclei of the thalamus (**Fig. 44.10B**). Loss of dopaminergic nigrostriatal neurons, an attribute of this disease, presumably causes reduced inhibition selectively of the D_2 striatopallidal fibers to the lateral segment (GPl). Thus, the Gpl has greater inhibitory input than usual with resultant diminished activity; in turn, its inhibitory influence on the subthalamic nucleus is reduced. As a consequence, the excitatory influence of the subthalamic nucleus upon GPm/SNr is increased. These output nuclei inhibit the VL and VA to a greater than customary degree, ultimately reducing the activity of the lower motoneurons. Diminished excitation of the D_1 striatal neurons simultaneously occurs. This is because dopamine excites the D_1 neurons that project directly to the GPm/SNr, whereas it inhibits the D_2 striatopallidal neurons. In this situation, destruction of the nigrostriatal dopaminergic input would therefore simultaneously reduce inhibition on the

GPm/SNr by the D_1 cells and increase the former's inhibition of the thalamus, via the indirect D_2 striatopallidal pathway.

Conversely, lesions of the subthalamic nucleus decrease excitation of GPm/SNr, resulting in diminished inhibition of the thalamocortical part of the circuit (**Fig. 24.10C**). Thus, activity of the lower motoneurons is increased above usual levels. Following this line of reasoning, lesions of the subthalamic nucleus produced in MPTP-induced models of parkinsonism should restore the balance of activity in the internal circuitry of the basal ganglia. This has been demonstrated to occur. With lesions of the substantia nigra, there is excessive activity in the subthalamic nucleus, which is regarded as an important factor in generation of Parkinson's disease. In the primate model, this excessive activity is eliminated with the secondary lesion.

As noted, Huntington's chorea in the early stages is associated with lesions of the striatum (mainly caudate) selectively involving the enkephalin expressing gabaergic projection neurons whose axons terminate in the lateral segment of the pallidum. Reduced inhibition upon the GPl would cause greater inhibition of the subthalamic nucleus (**Fig. 24.10D**). In turn, excitation of GPm/SNr would be reduced, causing less inhibition of VL and VA as after lesions of the subthalamic nucleus directly. The end result would be increased activity of the lower motoneurons that is expressed as a hyperkinetic movement disorder. The pattern, as well as amount of activity, might be expected to be different from that elicited by other pathologies, accounting for the dissimilarities in movement disorders.

SUGGESTED READINGS

Alexander G, DeLong M, Strick P. Parallel organization of functionally segregated circuits linking basal ganglia and cortex. *Annu Rev Neurosci.* 1986;9:357–381.

Bergman H, Wichmann T, DeLong M. Reversal of experimental parkinsonism by lesions of the subthalamic nucleus. *Science.* 1990;249:1436–1438.

Brooks V. *The Neural Basis of Motor Control.* New York, NY: Oxford University Press; 1986.

Carpenter M. The basal ganglia: structure and function. In: McKenzie J, Kemm R, Wilcock L, eds. The Basal Ganglia: Structure and Function. Adv Behav Biol. New York, NY: Plenum; 1984;27: 1–66.

Carpenter M, Jayaraman A, eds. The Basal Ganglia. Structure and Function—Current Concepts. Adv Behav Biol. New York, NY: Plenum, 1987;32: 1–560.

Côté L, Crutcher M. The basal ganglia. In: Kandel E, Schwartz J, Jessell T, eds. *Principles of Neural Science.* 3rd ed. New York, NY: Elsevier; 1991: 647–659.

Evarts E. Brain mechanisms of movement. *Sci Am.* 1979;241(3):164–179.

Gerfen C. The neostriatal mosaic: multiple levels of compartmental organization in the basal ganglia. *Annu Rev Neurosci.* 1992;15:285–320.

Gusella J, Wexler N, Conneally P, et al. A polymorphic DNA marker genetically linked to Huntington's disease. *Nature.* 1983;306:234–238.

Haber S. Neurotransmitters in the human and nonhuman primate basal ganglia. *Hum Neurobiol.* 1986; 5:159–168.

Hallett M. Physiology of basal ganglia disorders: an overview. *Can J Neurol Sci.* 1993;20:177–183.

Heimer L, Switzer R, VanHoesen G. Ventral striatum and ventral pallidum. Components of the motor system. *Trends Neurosci.* 1982;5:83–87.

Kots Y. *The Organization of Voluntary Movement: Neurophysiological Mechanisms.* New York, NY: Plenum; 1977.

Marsden C, Rothwell J, Day B. The use of peripheral feedback in the control of movement. *Trends Neurosci.* 1984;7:253–257.

McKenzie J, Kemm R, Wilcock L. The Basal Ganglia: Structure and Function. Adv Behav Biol. New York, NY: Plenum; 1984;27:1–576.

Middleton F, Strick P. Anatomical evidence for cerebellar and basal ganglia involvement in higher cognitive function. *Science.* 1994:458–461

Pearson K. The control of walking. *Sci Am.* 1976; 235:72–86.

Phillips C, Porter R. *Corticospinal Neurones: Their Role in Movement.* New York, NY: Academic Press; 1977.

Sandler M, Feuerstein C, Scatton B. *Neurotransmitter Interactions in the Basal Ganglia.* New York, NY: Raven Press; 1987.

Schell G, Strick P. The origin of thalamic inputs to the arcuate, premotor and supplementary motor areas. *J Neurosci.* 1984;4:539–560.

Selemon L, Goldman-Rakic P. Longitudinal topography and interdigitation of corticostriatal projections in the rhesus monkey. *J Neurosci.* 1985;5: 776–794.

Stein P. Motor systems, with specific reference to the control of locomotion. *Annu Rev Neurosci.* 1978; 1:61–81.

Wexler N. Molecular approaches to hereditary diseases of the nervous system: Huntington's disease as a paradigm. *Annu Rev Neurosci.* 1991;14: 503–529.

Cerebral Cortex

Organization of the neocortex

Sensory areas of the neocortex

Higher cortical association areas

Motor areas of the neocortex

Blood flow in the cortex

Split-brain man and cerebral dominance

Memory

Many of the highest functions of humans reside in the intricate circuitry of the cerebral cortex. It has crucial roles in conceptual thinking, creativity, planning, and the ways in which we give form and substance to our thoughts. The cortex is essential to our abilities to appreciate the fine qualities of sensation and to organize skilled motor activities. Our multifaceted patterns of response require a continuous stream of sensory input and interactions of the cortex with subcortical nuclei such as the basal ganglia. Our conscious awareness of self, and of ourselves within the environment, are cortical expressions.

The cerebral cortex (pallium) is the 600 g gray mantle of the cerebrum, constituting about 40% of the brain by weight and containing 100 billion or more neurons of several types (Figs. 25.1 and 25.2). Of the total mass, the neurons weigh about 180 g and the glial cells and blood vessels weigh about 420 g.

The cerebral cortex is divided into the phylogenetically older *allocortex*, about 10% of the total, and the more recently evolved six-layered *neocortex (isocortex, neopallium)*, about 90% of the cortex. The *allocortex* consists of (1) the 3-layered *archicortex (archipallium)*, including the hippocampal formation (hippocampus and dentate gyrus); (2) the *paleocortex (paleopallium)*, including the parahippocampal gyrus and olfactory cortex (cortex of uncus); and (3) the *mesocortex*, including the cingulate gyrus,

fasciolar gyrus, and isthmus (Fig. 1.7). The allocortex incorporates the *limbic lobe* (Chap. 1), an artificial construct located on the medial aspect of the hemisphere where it forms a ring around the corpus callosum and rostral brainstem. The neocortex consists of the cortex of the frontal, parietal, occipital, temporal, and central lobes, excluding the limbic components (Chap. 1; Figs. 1.1 to 1.6).

The neocortex has been parceled (1) into functional areas (Figs. 25.3 and 25.4) and (2) into the commonly used scheme of Brodmann who numbered areas consecutively, based upon the arrangement of neurons as visualized in Nissl-stained preparations. More than 40 areas are discernable on the lateral and medial surfaces of the brain (Figs. 25.5 and 25.6). These areas of neocortex can be categorized into a continuum of five different cytoarchitectural types. The two extremes are referred to as *heterotypic* and include the primary sensory cortices and motor cortex. The former is the thinnest cortex (about 2 mm from pial surface to white matter), and because of a large population of small stellate shaped perikarya (see below) in a particularly well developed layer IV, it is called *hypergranular*. The heterotypic motor cortex is more than twice as thick and is called *agranular* because of the lack of a well defined layer IV. In addition, layer IV of this region is characterized by the presence of pyramidal cells, and layer V is enlarged. The great majority of cortex, comprising the association areas, is referred to as *homotypic* and includes the middle three gradations. The six layers are more readily differentiated in this type cortex.

ORGANIZATION OF THE NEOCORTEX

The neocortex is conventionally described as being organized in six horizontal laminae oriented parallel to the cortical surface (**Fig. 25.1**). The individual laminae are somewhat

obscured in heterotypic cortex where some of the laminae are highly developed and others are attenuated. In some areas, different laminae are subdivided. Although the lamination is the most conspicuous feature, the basic functional units of the cerebral cortex are physiologically defined vertical columns extending from the pial surface to the white matter (**Fig. 25.2**). These are not columns in the architectural sense, but rather are long three-dimensional slabs up to 0.5 mm in width and variable in length. Every column of each primary sensory cortex is concerned with a submodality (e.g., ocular domi-

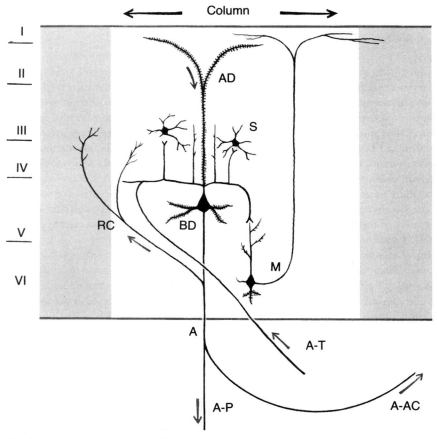

Figure 25.1: Vertical columnar organization of the neocortex. Roman numerals indicate the six horizontal laminae. The cell bodies of the pyramidal neurons and stellate (granule) neurons are present in laminae II through VI. Each pyramidal neuron is oriented in a vertical plane with its apical dendrite extending to lamina I, and its basilar dendrites extending horizontally. Its axon extends out of the cortex into the white matter and has recurrent branches projecting back to the cortex. The dendrites and axon of each stellate neuron (S) arborize and terminate within the immediate column. The axon of each Martinotti neuron (M) has an axon that extends from lamina VI to laminae I and II. A = axon of a pyramidal neuron, A-AC = axon of an association or commissural neuron, AD = apical dendrite of pyramidal neuron, A-P = axon of projection neuron, A-T = axon of a neuron of a specific thalamic nucleus, BD = basilar dendrites of a pyramidal neuron, and RC = recurrent collateral branch.

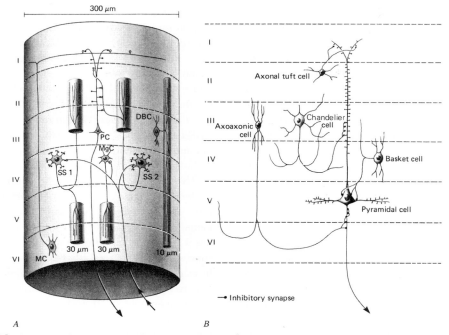

Figure 25.2: A. Modular organization of the neocortex as formed by its inputs from specific, commissural, and association afferent fibers. Note the (1) vertical cylindrical distribution of the axons of the intrinsic neocortical interneurons and (2) all neurons and fibers illustrated have putative excitatory synaptic connections that excite the pyramidal neurons. **B.** Cortical interneurons that have putative inhibitory synaptic connections that inhibit the pyramidal neurons. Different interneurons inhibit various segments of the pyramidal neurons; the inhibitory axoaxonic synapses of the axoaxonic cells just distal to the axon hillock of the pyramidal cell may act as the final processing mechanism regulating the discharge of the pyramidal neuron (see the Dendrite-Cell Body Unit and Neuron as an Integrator, Chap. 3). The processing also includes the disinhibition of interneurons by inhibitory synapses from other interneurons (not illustrated). Fibers from the pyramidal neurons of (1) lamina VI project to the thalamus, (2) lamina V project to subcortical structures (e.g., striatum, brainstem, and spinal cord), and (3) laminae II and III project to other areas of the cerebral cortex. DBC = double bouquet cell, MgC = microgliaform cell, MC = Martinotti cell, PC = pyramidal cell, and SS = stellate cell. Adapted from Szentagothai J. The neuron network of the cerebral cortex: a functional interpretation. *Proc R Soc Lond B Biol Sci.* 1978;201:219–248.

nance). Each of the cortical columns is (1) the terminus for afferent fibers from other cortical areas and the thalamus and (2) the source of efferent fibers terminating in other cortical columns of the same hemisphere (*association fibers*); in the same cortical area of the contralateral hemisphere (*commissural fibers passing through the corpus callosum and anterior commissure*); and in subcortical nuclei of the cerebrum, brainstem, and spinal cord (*projection fibers*). In general, the main receptive layers (input) of the cortex are laminae I through IV. The main efferent layers (output) are laminae V and VI.

The input to the neocortex, aside from association and commissural fibers, is derived primar-

ily from the thalamus. The output from the neocortex to subcortical regions is relayed via the following projection fibers: corticobulbar, corticoreticular, corticopontine, corticothalamic, corticostriate, corticorubral, corticonuclear, and corticospinal.

Neurons of the Neocortex (Figs. 25.1 and 25.2)

Five basic neuronal cell types (pyramidal, stellate, stellate [star] pyramidal, Martinotti, and horizontal) are representative of the numerous cortical neurons. The shape of the cell body and course taken by its axon are among the criteria used to characterize a cell. Pyramidal cells constitute the majority of cortical neurons. Each *pyramidal cell* has a pyramid-shaped cell body, a single branched *apical dendrite* extending toward the cortical surface, and several horizontally directed branched *basilar dendrites*. The *axon* typically arises from the base and enters the subcortical white matter; usually there is a collateral branch (*recurrent collateral*) going back to the cortex. The main axonal branches of the pyramidal cells form the association fibers, commissural fibers, and projection fibers listed above. Pyramidal cells, depending upon the size of the soma, are described as small, medium, large, or giant. The latter, called *Betz cells*, are about 100 μm high and are restricted to cortical lamina V of area 4 (Chap. 11). The designations external (III) and internal (V) pyramidal layers are derived from the neurons that characterize them. Although layer II is called the external granular layer, it is actually populated by small pyramidal neurons. *Stellate cells* are multipolar interneurons with a star-shaped body, short branched dendrites, and a short axon that arborizes and synapses with other cortical neurons in the immediate vicinity. Stellate cells that are local circuit neurons comprise two distinct morphological and functional populations, namely excitatory and inhibitory neurons. The latter, referred to as *aspiny neurons* because of a lack of dendritic spines, are mainly gabaergic. GABA is the major inhibitory neurotransmitter. *Spiny stellate cells* are glutamatergic. Glutamate is regarded as the major excitatory neurotransmitter of the cerebral cortex as indicated in the previous chapter. Many cortical neurons have comodulators, i.e., neuropeptides. Stellate cells are particularly conspicuous in lamina IV, and, because of their appearance in the Nissl stain, this lamina is called the internal granular layer. *Stellate pyramidal neurons* are large cells that combine the features of both stellate and pyramidal cells. These neurons have a stellate shape with an apical dendrite, together with numerous dendrites, radiating from the cell body. Stellate pyramidal neurons are characteristic of lamina VI and have an axon that enters the subcortical white matter. Each *cell of Martinotti* is a multipolar interneuron with short branched dendrites and a branching axon extending toward the cortical surface, that synapses with other cortical neurons. The *horizontal cell (of Cajal)*

is a small neuron of the most superficial cortical lamina that is absent or rare in adults; its axon is oriented parallel to the cortical surface. Lamina I is referred to as the molecular layer because it mainly consists of neuronal processes and contains relatively few cell bodies. Other neuronal types that mainly are inhibitory include *double bouquet cells*, *chandelier cells*, and *basket cells* (Fig. 25.2). Except for the pyramidal and the stellate pyramidal cells, all cortical cells are intracortical interneurons.

The input to the columns of the neocortex is derived primarily from other cortical areas (largest), thalamus, substantia innominata, locus ceruleus, brainstem raphe nuclei, and basal nucleus of Meynert; there are other sources of corticopedal fibers. In general, fibers from the primary thalamic relay nuclei terminate in a rich arborization within lamina IV and the adjacent part of III, while the efferent fibers from other cortical areas terminate in each of the cortical laminae. The axon collaterals of the pyramidal cells and the axons of many interneurons are oriented vertically. The lateral spread of the axons and dendrites is minimal. These neurons are interconnected into numerous chains of small and long loops. The locus ceruleus and possibly the raphe nuclei are excited by novel stimuli in the environment; each adrenergic fiber from the locus ceruleus arborizes widely in the output cortical laminae V and VI, while each serotoninergic fiber from the raphe nuclei arborizes widely in the input cortical laminae I to IV. The result is that the diffuse projections from these nuclei have global effects upon both the limbic system and cerebral cortex (see Prefrontal Cortex, later).

Functional Aspects

The cerebral cortex has been subdivided into areas described in terms of several structural and functional criteria. The functions of the cortex are inferred from subjective accounts and objectively observed responses of subjects (1) who have areas of cortex damaged by lesions or surgical ablation, (2) in whom cortical sites were stimulated electrically, and (3) who have irritative lesions resulting in epileptic seizures. An enormous amount of information concerning the function of different areas of the cortex has been generated in recent years using positron emission tomography (see later; also Chap. 5).

Functionally defined areas of the neocortex comprise the (1) sensory areas including primary sensory areas, secondary sensory areas, and association areas; (2) motor areas including primary motor area, premotor areas, and supplementary motor area; and (3) "psychical" and prefrontal areas.

SENSORY AREAS OF THE NEOCORTEX

General Somesthetic Senses

The primary somatic sensory (somatosensory) cortex (SI) includes the postcentral gyrus and its medial extension in the paracentral gyrus (areas 3, 1, and 2 of the parietal lobe) (Figs. 25.3 and 25.5). Area 3 is subdivided into 3a (located within the posterior bank of the central

sulcus in continuity with area 4 on the anterior bank) and 3b. This region receives input from the ventral posterior nucleus of the thalamus that conveys influences mostly from the opposite side of the head and body.

The projection to this area can be represented somatotopically as an upside down sensory homunculus with the head located ventrally near the lateral sulcus and the lower extremity in the paracentral gyrus (Fig. 25.4). It is clear from the drawing that the greatest representation is given to input from the face, tongue, lips, and hand, especially the thumb and index finger.

The cortical map of areas 3, 1, and 2 (postcentral gyrus) comprises detailed somatotopically organized modality-specific columns that represent various submodalities. Area 3a receives information from muscle spindle afferents and is closely related to the adjacent motor cortex. Somatosensory cortex is hierarchically organized. Area 3b gets input from both rapidly

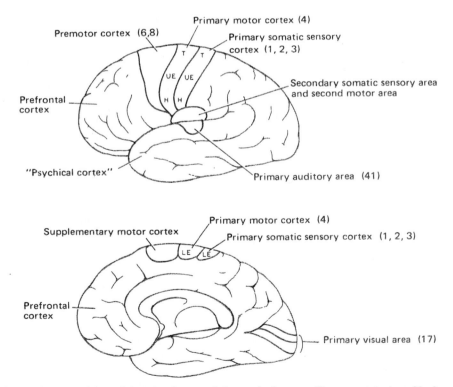

Figure 25.3: The location of several functional areas of the cerebral cortex. The representation of body parts of the primary motor and somatic sensory (somatosensory) cortices includes the head (H), upper extremity (UE), trunk (T), and lower extremity (LE). Numbers represent areas of Brodmann.

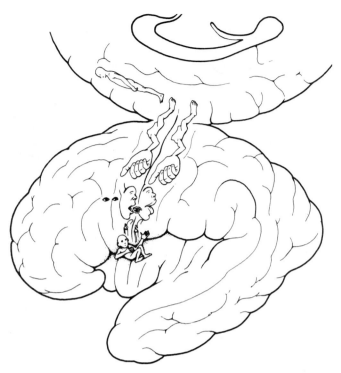

Figure 25.4: The homunculi in the cortex include those in the primary somatic sensory cortex (SI), primary motor cortex, supplementary motor cortex, and combined secondary somatic sensory cortex (SII) and second motor area.

and slowly adapting cutaneous receptors important for determining features such as size, shape, and texture and distributes this information to areas 1 and 2 for further processing. Thus, area 1 receives input from area 3, as well as from cutaneous receptors, and mediates perception of textures. The input to area 2 is from area 3 and deep pressure receptors; it serves to differentiate size and shape of objects and position of joints. In essence, each of these areas has a complete sensory homunculus, reflecting different response properties. The postcentral gyrus also is associated with the characterization of pain and temperature, but these modalities have only a slight representation here. Following unilateral lesions to the primary somatic sensory cortex, sensations of touch, position sense, and pressure are impaired on the contralateral side of the body, but pain and temperature, except for their localization, are, at most, minimally affected.

The secondary somatic sensory area (SII) is located on the superior tip of the lateral fissure

below the primary motor and sensory areas. SII is topographically organized with respect to such general sensory modalities as touch, position sense, pressure, and pain. This area receives input from SI as well as bilateral inputs from the ascending pathways (Chap. 23).

Further neural processing of the multisensory somesthetic input takes place before being integrated into the levels where perception of shape, size, texture, and the identification of objects by contact occur (e.g., stereognosis—recognition of an object, such as a coin or key, after handling it). This occurs in the association areas of the superior parietal lobule (sensory areas 5 and 7) and in the supramarginal gyrus (area 40). These areas have well-developed reciprocal connections with the pulvinar of the thalamus. Lesions in area 40 may result in tactile agnosia (see below). Functional activity of this area is essential for perception of the general senses. Areas 5, 7, and 40 of the parietal lobe comprise the *somatosensory association cortex.*

Electrical stimulation of SI can evoke paresthesias (numbness and tingling) and pressure sense from the corresponding part of the body. A lesion of SI results in deficits in position sense and in the ability to discriminate size, shape, and roughness by touch on the contralateral side of the body.

Taste and Vestibular Sensations

Taste is represented in area 43, located just above the lateral fissure. Two areas are associated with the vestibular system: one located adjacent to the face area of SI, and the other on the superior temporal gyrus adjacent to the primary auditory cortex. The feelings of dizziness and rotation occur during direct electrical stimulation of these areas.

Visual Sense

The primary visual cortex (area 17), also known as visual area I, is the striate area of the occipital lobe (**Figs. 25.5 and 25.6**). It occupies both banks of the calcarine sulcus, and is the cortical terminus of the optic radiations from the lateral geniculate body of the thalamus

(Chap. 19). The two principal roles of the striate cortex are (1) to perform the act of fusion of the inputs from both eyes into one image for binocular vision and (2) to analyze the visual world with respect to the orientation of stimuli in the visual fields. Simple and complex cells are localized within the striate cortex—they are detectors of straight lines, each having a specific orientation and position in the retina. The visuotopically organized striate cortex contains ocular dominance columns and orientation preference columns (Chap. 19).

The extrastriate association cortex includes area 18 (visual areas 2 and 3), area 19 (visual areas 4 and 5), angular gyrus (area 39), and inferotemporal cortex (areas 20 and 21) (**Figs. 25.5 and 25.6**). Actually, almost 40 separate visual areas have been identified. The complex and hypercomplex cells are found within visual areas 18 and 19 (Chap. 19). Complex cells respond optimally to linear environmental stimuli, whereas hypercomplex cells respond optimally to curvatures or angular changes in the direction of a line. Lesions in area 39 of the dominant hemisphere may result in patients being unable to comprehend the symbols of language and ex-

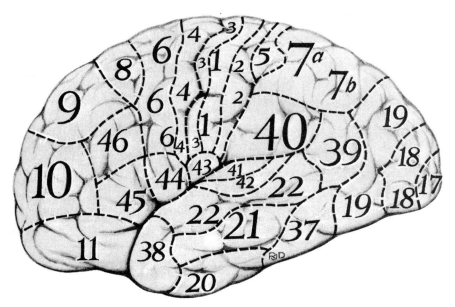

Figure 25.5: Cytoarchitectural map of the lateral surface of the human cerebral cortex. (Numbers represent the areas of Brodmann.)

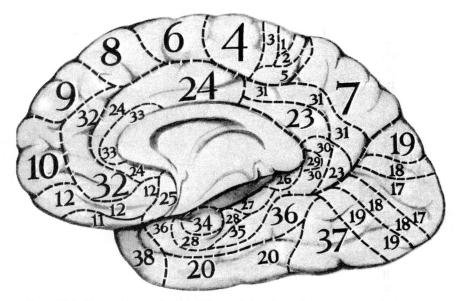

Figure 25.6: Cytoarchitectural map of the medial surface of the human cerebral cortex.

press themselves through them. This area is essential to the comprehension of a visual image. These association areas are integrated with the "psychical cortex" (see below) and the thalamus (pulvinar) through reciprocal connections. As yet, the manner in which visual images are perceived is unknown, but clearly different areas are important for perception of different kinds of visual information. Through corticotectal fibers, the so-called occipital eye field of areas 18 and 19 mediate slow pursuit and vergence eye movements (Chap. 19). Electrical stimulation of the former results in a conjugate eye movement to the opposite side.

The *inferotemporal cortex* of the tectal system (Chap. 19) has a role in higher visual functions. It reacts to such stimulus features as size, shape, contrast, and color. Monkeys with inferotemporal cortical lesions demonstrate a deficit in the performance of some visual discrimination tasks.

Auditory Sense

The primary auditory cortex (area 41) is located in the temporal lobe in the transverse gyri of Heschl on the floor of the lateral fissure (Fig. 25.3). It is the cortical terminus of the auditory radiations from the medial geniculate body

(Chap. 16). Neurons in this area respond to broad bands of the audible spectrum; it is tonotopically organized. The primary cortex is essential for the detection of changes in pattern and in the location of the source of a sound. Auditory area II (area 42) has a higher threshold to sound intensity than the primary cortex. There are at least five auditory cortical areas in the temporal lobe including area 22 of the superior temporal gyrus. Patients with lesions of area 22 on the dominant side have profound difficulty in the interpretation of sounds; the spoken language may be meaningless or extremely difficult for them to comprehend.

Claustrum

Evidence indicates that the claustrum (Fig. 1.8) is involved in sensory systems at the cortical level. The claustrum has reciprocal connections with the visual cortex (areas 17, 18, and 19), auditory cortex (areas 41 and 42), and somatosensory cortex (areas 1, 2, 3, 5, and 7). Its only known subcortical inputs are from the hypothalamus, intralaminar thalamic nuclei, and locus ceruleus, and it gives rise to no subcortical projections. Insight into its functional significance awaits future studies.

Plasticity in the Structure of Cortical Columns

A basic question in neurobiology concerns whether synaptic connections in the adult nervous system are static or dynamic. There is direct evidence that neural connections are dynamic in response to functional circumstances. It has been amply demonstrated that the organization of the neocortex in perinatal animals is determined in part by its input from peripheral receptors. For example, Woolsey and his collaborators showed that removal of a mystacial vibrissa (whisker) from a neonatal rodent prevents development of a cortical structure referred to as a barrel in a specific location. A barrel is a circular aggregation of neurons in lamina IV that forms part of a column representing a particular receptive field. Similarly, evidence indicates that the structural organization of adult primate neocortex exhibits changes in response to alterations in its input. Merzenich has shown electrophysiologically that the cortical receptive field of adjacent fingers, which is spatially completely separated under normal circumstances, in time becomes overlapping after the two fingers are surgically joined together (syndactyly). If the fingers are subsequently separated, the cortical representation ultimately reverts to the original discontinuous condition. Merzenich also has demonstrated in monkeys that the cortical representation of a single digit expands with repeated use of that finger. Evidence from human amputees suggests an even more extensive cortical reorganization in which the area representing the face expands to include the adjacent area that had represented the missing limb (Ramachandran, 1992). A competitive balance is continually taking place within and between cortical columns in which changing cortical inputs are associated with collateral sprouting and the loss, additions, rearrangement, and alterations of the synaptic connections.

Plasticity, at the cortical level, may in part explain the increased functional capability of the feet and toes in performing complex motor acts in cases where the arms fail to develop, or the enhanced acuity in one sensory system when another is rendered dysfunctional. In this context, it deserves mention that brain damage at an early age is less deleterious than similar lesions in adulthood.

HIGHER CORTICAL ASSOCIATION AREAS

Language Neural Circuitry

Conceptual Model for Language and Speech

The cerebral cortical areas associated with language are conceived as being organized following a model proposed by Geschwind which elaborated on circuitry diagramed in 1874 by Wernicke (**Fig. 25.7**). According to this scheme, neural channels originating in the sensory association cortical areas (visual, somatic sensory, and auditory) converge to *Wernicke's area (posterior language area)* located in the posterior portion of area 22 which occupies parts of the superior and middle temporal gyri. Some authors also include the supramarginal (area 40) and angular gyri (area 39). This entire region is part of the parieto-temporal-occipital association cortex. Area 22 is critical for the processing of the basic elements for the production of language. Representations visualized as words or images are conveyed from the visual cortex (occipital lobe) to the *angular gyrus (area 39)*. Constructs of form, size, and body image are projected from the somatosensory cortex (parietal lobe) to the *supramarginal gyrus (area 40)*. Auditory information of sounds and words is thought to be conveyed from the auditory cortex (temporal lobe) to the *angular gyrus (area 39)*. Information then is conducted to area 22. In essence, sensory systems converge on Wernicke's area for further processing.

The words to be spoken originate and are generated in *Wernicke's area*, and then are transmitted via the arcuate fasciculus to Broca's speech area *(anterior language area; areas 44 and 45 of the inferior frontal gyrus)*. Within Broca's area, a detailed coordinated program for vocalization is formulated and activated for controlling articulation through the sequencing of the musculature of the vocal cords, pharynx, tongue, and lips. This information is then transmitted to the motor areas (areas 4 and 6) where the appropriate motor pathways are activated for the production of the spoken language. Key elements of this circuitry have been demonstrated with positron emission tomography which also shows that the scheme is oversimpli-

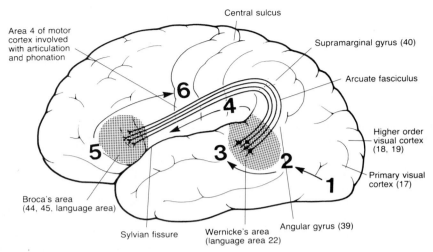

Figure 25.7: Probable sequence of neural transmission within the neocortex that occurs from the perception of an object within the visual areas to the formulation of the spoken language (i.e., naming an object seen). The presumed sequence comprises (1) the visual cortex—areas 17, 18, and 19, to (2) the angular gyrus—area 39, to (3) to Wernicke's area—area 22, via (4) the arcuate fasciculus, to (5) Broca's speech area 43 and 44, and, finally, (6) to the motor area 4 where the descending motor pathways involved with vocalization originate.

fied **(Fig. 25.8)**. With regard to language and speech, the left hemisphere of the brain assumes the critical role in about 95% of individuals (left hemisphere dominance) while the remaining 5% have either a right hemisphere dominance or a mixed right and left dominance (see Split-Brain Man and Cerebral Dominance later).

Aphasias

Aphasia, or the disruption of language or speech, may occur following a stroke in the cortex of the left (major) hemisphere **(Fig. 25.7)**. *Language* is the body of words and systems and their combinations used and understood by groups of people, while *speech* refers to facility in the formulation of language. There are several forms of aphasias.

Wernicke's or receptive aphasia results from a lesion of Wernicke's area. Although hearing and vision are normal, individuals with this disability show an essentially total failure to comprehend either the spoken and/or written language. Their speech is fluent but meaningless. Their conversations sound normal but are actually devoid of content and full of nonexistent words. Speech of such patients has the correct rhythms and sounds of normal speech. They

speak rapidly and have the normal nuances of articulation. Key words are omitted. They are replaced by empty senseless words, related words ("knife" for "fork"), or unrelated words ("hammer" for "book"). Afflicted subjects seem unaware of their meaningless speech. In essence, *Wernicke's area* has a role in language and, in addition, a significant role in reading and writing and in the production and comprehension of the spoken word (language).

Conduction aphasia results from lesions in the lower parietal lobe that damage the fibers of the *arcuate fasciculus* that connect Wernicke's area to Broca's area. In individuals with this *disconnection syndrome*, speech is fluent but quite meaningless. They show a poor ability to repeat phrases and the spoken language.

Anomia aphasia occurs following a lesion of the posterior portion of the left superior temporal gyrus near the angular gyrus. Patients demonstrate an inability to think of a specific word or the name of a person or an object. In a lesion limited to the angular gyrus, patients may lose the ability to read (called *alexia*) or to write (*agraphia*) even though they can understand the spoken language and can speak. These lesions interfere with the transfer of information from visual (occipital lobe) and general

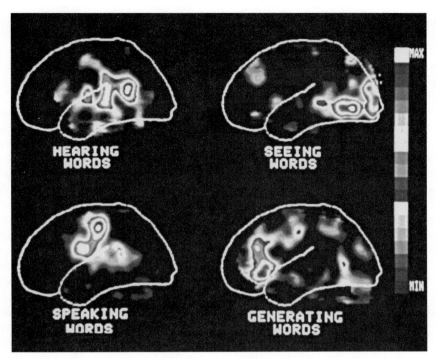

Figure 25.8: Positron emission tomographs (PET) show areas with increased blood flow elicited by language related activities. Note the relationships between these areas and those illustrated in Figure 25.7, including Wernicke's area. (Cotesy of Drs. Steve Petersen and Marcus Raichle, Washington University.)

somatic sensory (parietal lobe) cortex to Wernicke's area.

Global or *total aphasia* is associated with widespread damage of the cortex on either side of the lateral (Sylvian) sulcus, damaging Wernicke's and Broca's areas and the arcuate fasciculus. Such patients are unable to speak or comprehend language. In addition, they have severe impairment of language-related functions in that they cannot read, write, or name an object seen.

When *Broca's area* on the left side is damaged by a stroke, Broca's aphasia *(expressive aphasia)* may result. It is primarily a failure in the formulation of speech, which is labored, slow, and poorly articulated. Patients express themselves with faulty grammar and with great difficulty. They are fully aware of the disability. The muscles involved with speech are not paralyzed; this is demonstrated by the fact that these muscles operate normally in other tasks such as chewing, swallowing, and laughing. Many patients can often sing a formerly known song rapidly, correctly, and even with feeling. In re-

sponding to a question, the patient gives an understandable answer, but it is expressed with difficulty and with the omission of small words ("a" and "the") and endings. It is delivered in a telegraphic style, as for example in response to the question about the intention of going to a football game "Yes . . .Saturday one o'clock . . .Joe and Mary . . .baseball . . . .pitch . . .curve . . .and . . .run." The comprehension of reading and the ability to write are unimpaired.

Agnosias

Agnosia (lack of knowledge in Greek) refers to the inability to recognize or to be aware of an object when using a given sense (sight) even though this sense is essentially intact functionally.

A *tactile agnosia (astereognosis)*, the inability to recognize familiar objects through the senses of touch and proprioception, may result from lesions of the *supramarginal gyrus (area 40)* of the major hemisphere. Patients with tactile agnosia may have a disturbance of the body image; for example, they may not recognize their individual fingers and may confuse the left from the right side of the body.

A *visual agnosia*, the inability to recognize objects by sight, may result from a lesion in areas 18 and 19 of the major hemisphere. These individuals are able to characterize the objects by the use of other senses such as touch.

An *auditory agnosia*, the inability of an individual with unimpaired hearing to recognize familiar sounds, music, and words results from bilateral lesions in the posterior parts of the superior temporal gyrus (area 22). Such patients have reasonable ability to comprehend the spoken language and show good reading ability.

Apraxia

Apraxia is the inability to perform certain skilled and complex movements, even though there is no paralysis or disturbance in motor coordination and the sensory pathways are functioning normally. Lesions in various cortical areas (supramarginal gyrus, other regions of the parietal and occipital lobes, premotor cortex, and Broca's speech areas 44 and 45), in the association fibers interconnecting many of these cortical areas, and in the corpus callosum may result in several types of apraxias. Among these are: (1) an inability to perform skilled learned movements, ranging from the clumsy execution of writing and drawing to *agraphia*, a condition in which the subject cannot write; (2) an inability to carry out a sequence of complex motor acts (often called *transmissive apraxia*), e.g., subjects who are able to brush their teeth, comb their hair, wash their face, and tie their shoes automatically are unable, upon command, to perform the same tasks in that specific sequence (lesion in the supramarginal gyrus); and (3) the loss of articulate speech (sometimes called *oral aphasia*) with otherwise normal musculature of the tongue, lips, larynx, and palate. Subjects have use of only a few words in conversation and mispronounce common words or repeat the same word over and over again (lesion in Broca's areas 44 and 45 and in other regions).

Prefrontal Cortex

The prefrontal cortex (areas 9 through 12) and its rich reciprocal connections with the dor-

somedial nucleus of the thalamus, hypothalamus, and limbic system are well developed in man. The prefrontal lobe has been conceived as being a regulator of the depth of feeling of an individual. It is not involved in the perception of sensations, but rather in the "affect" associated with the sensation. The complex responses of an individual, from calmness to ecstasy, from gloom to elation, from friendliness to disagreeableness, have their roots in areas 9 to 12. Some evidence suggests that the prefrontal lobe has a role in memory and cognitive function (Goldman-Rakic, 1995).

The bilateral ablation of areas of the prefrontal cortex or interruption of the subcortical white matter (*prefrontal lobotomy, leukotomy*) may produce subjects who are less excitable but also less creative. Relief from anxiety is accompanied by a change in the patient's outlook and disposition. Drive, not intelligence as measured by I.Q. tests, is altered. Goal-directed activity and planning for the future are disturbed and generally neglected. The ability to remember information such as a sequence of numbers for a short period ("*working memory*") is impaired, particularly when lesions involve dorsolateral parts of the frontal lobes. The landmark case of Phineas Gage exemplifies the above. Gage was a foreman working on a project to lay track for the Rutland and Burlington Railroad in Vermont in 1848 when a tamping iron was blown through his head, producing a prefrontal lobotomy. Only transiently stunned, he survived for some 12 years. Although his brain was not recovered, the skull was preserved and recent reconstructions with neuroimaging techniques have confirmed that the prefrontal areas were damaged bilaterally, particularly medial and ventral parts; other parts of the frontal lobes, i.e., Broca's area, and areas 6 and 4 were spared. His personality changes were so profound that friends said "Gage was no longer Gage." Whereas he was physically as before and showed no apparent changes in memory, learning, or intellect, he became profane and irresponsible to the point of being unable to hold down a job.

A current view suggests that some of the expressions are, at least in part, associated with the interactions among the locus ceruleus, prefrontal lobe, and limbic system. The locus ceruleus, with adrenergic projections, imposes excitatory influences on both the prefrontal cortex and the limbic system. In turn, the prefrontal cortex, through its inhibitory influences, modulates the activity of the limbic system. Thus, following prefrontal lobotomy the limbic system, now released from some prefrontal constraints, has freer rein for its expression.

The perception of pain includes both the sensation of pain and the emotional reaction to the sensation. The neospinothalamic or fast pain pathway, involving the somatosensory cortex, is the warning system informing the individual of the presence, extent, and location of an injury causing the pain. The paleospinothalamic or slow pain pathway involves the unpleasant and nagging qualities, and signals that normal activity should be curtailed and attention should be paid to the pain. The "fast" system is relatively "free of emotional content," whereas the slow system contributes to the emotional quality of the insult. Both the limbic system and the prefrontal lobes contribute to the emotional coloration of the pain.

Relief from intractable pain may be obtained following prefrontal lobotomy. Although the pain persists, the patient is unconcerned about it because the psychic feeling associated with its intensity is lost. A modern concept suggests that the prefrontal cortex is the neocortical representative of the limbic system.

MOTOR AREAS OF THE NEOCORTEX

Primary Motor Cortex

This cortex is located in area 4 of the precentral gyrus (Fig. 25.3). Direct electric stimulation of this region evokes movements of the voluntary muscles on the opposite side. A map of this electrically excitable motor cortex produces a motor homunculus. Figure 25.4 depicts both the motor and sensory homunculi. The homunculus is upside down, with the head region near the lateral fissure and with the lower extremity on the medial surface in the paracentral lobule. The amount of the motor cortex devoted to specific regions is roughly proportional to the delicacy of control and innervation density of that region (e.g., large areas for fingers, thumb, lips

and tongue). Ablation of this cortex results in marked contralateral paresis, flaccidity, hyperactive deep tendon reflexes, and positive Babinski reflex and is followed by moderate motor recovery. (Note similarities to and differences from upper motoneuron paralysis; Chap. 12.)

Premotor Cortex and Supplementary Motor Area

The premotor cortex consists of areas 6 and 8. The supplementary motor area is in area 6 on the medial aspect of the frontal lobe (Figs. 25.3 and 25.4). Stimulation of this supplemental area elicits responses that outline a small homunculus with its head located rostrally. These responses are largely bilateral synergistic movements of a tonic or postural nature, affecting primarily the axial muscles and proximal muscles of the extremities. Stimulation of area 6 on the lateral cerebral surface produces adverse movements—these "orientation" movements are generalized actions, such as turning of the head and eyes, twisting movements of the trunk, and general flexion or extension of the limbs. Bilateral ablation of the supplementary motor area in the monkey results in hypertonus of flexor muscles and increased resistance to passive movements in the limbs, but it does not cause paresis.

Note that the symptoms of an upper motoneuron paralysis may be produced by lesions of both the primary motor cortex and supplementary cortex, but not of either separately. This suggests that the symptoms of upper motoneuron paralysis are probably the result of interruption of fibers from the primary motor cortex, supplementary motor cortex, and premotor cortex as they pass through the internal capsule. This is a frequent site for the location of a lesion resulting in the classical upper motor neuron paralysis in a "stroke" (Chaps. 4 and 12).

The role of *primary motor cortex* is to participate in the initiation of skilled, delicate, and agile voluntary movements. Although the primary motor cortex does contribute to the regulation of axial and proximal limb musculature, it has a critical role in the control of the distal limb muscles on the contralateral side of the body. The *premotor cortex* on the lateral surface of the frontal lobe has (1) a primary role in the control of proximal limb and axial musculature and (2) an essential role in the initial phases of orientation movements of the body and upper limb directed toward a target (e.g., tennis player's adjustments prior to the stroke). The *supplementary motor cortex* has a significant role in the programming of patterns and sequences of movements. For example, electrical stimulation of this area activates complex patterns of movements not only of the contralateral limbs, but of the ipsilateral limbs as well. The premotor cortex and the supplementary motor cortex project some fibers to the primary motor cortex.

Two additional coextensive motor and somatic sensory areas are present. In both, direct stimulation produces a somatotopic arrangement of motor responses as well as somatic sensations. These are the *second motor area* and *secondary somatic sensory area* located at the base of the pre- and postcentral gyri (**Fig. 25.3**). The functional significance of the motor representation of this area is not known. All four of the motor areas contribute fibers to the descending motor pathways, including the pyramidal tract.

Stimulation of area 8 results in conjugate saccadic movements of the eyes to the opposite side. This *frontal eye field* mediates voluntary eye movements (called *eye movements on command*; Chap. 19).

Motivation and Control of Movement

In a broad context, the initiation and regulation of volitional movements comprise (1) motivation and (2) control. Although how and where movements are initiated is, as yet, unknown, it is probable that *motivation-related* ones are generated within the limbic system, and that *control* is in the province of the basal ganglia and their circuitry (extrapyramidal system). In this concept, the drive and behavioral states, expressed as motivation, trigger the neural circuits involved with the actual control of motor activity (Chap. 24). The processing centers where the linkage between the limbic system and the striatal system is thought to occur is in the basal region of the forebrain, probably the *ventral striatum* (nucleus accumbens) and *ventral pallidum*. These components of the basal ganglia (Chap. 24) have ties with the limbic system

(Chap. 22) through their connections with the amygdala, hippocampus, ventral anterior, and dorsomedial thalamic nuclei. Functionally, this distinction between motivation and control is expressed in patients with abnormal movement disorders (i.e., choreas and Parkinson's disease). In these individuals, the motivation is intact and intense, but the execution is faulty.

BLOOD FLOW IN THE CORTEX

The mean blood flow in the brain of normal individuals is 50 mL per 100 g of tissue per minute; however, at any given moment the blood flow through a specific region may be greater or less than the mean as illustrated in **Figure 25.8**. The brain is similar to other body tissues in that the blood flow varies with the level of metabolism and functional activity within the tissue. An increase in blood flow takes place, for example, in the primary and association auditory cortices (areas 41 and 42) in both hemispheres and in Wernicke's areas in the left hemisphere during a conversation. Dynamic movements of the hand evoke blood flow increases in several cortical areas involved with hand movements and with sensory signals in the skin, joints, and muscles associated with the movements. Blood flow increases occur in the contralateral "hand" region of the motor cortex (area 4) and postcentral gyrus (somatosensory cortex) and of both ipsilateral and contralateral premotor and supplementary motor cortices (areas 6 and 8). The motor and sensory activities involved with the acts of reading aloud and listening result in an increase of blood flow in both the ipsilateral and contralateral auditory cortices, motor and somatosensory cortices ("face" and "mouth" areas), premotor and supplementary motor cortices, Broca's speech area, frontal eye fields (area 8), and visual association cortices of both sides.

SPLIT-BRAIN MAN AND CEREBRAL DOMINANCE

The presence in the cerebrum of the corpus callosum with its 300 million fibers in humans, and of the anterior commissure, suggests that interhemispheric commissural fiber pathways are of crucial significance to the functioning of the brain. Most of the callosal fibers interconnect with mirror image sites of both hemispheres. In addition, many fibers terminate in cortical areas different from the areas of origin (e.g., area 17 of one hemisphere projects to areas 18 and 19 of the other). Several areas do not receive callosal fibers; these include the hand and foot areas of the primary motor cortex (area 4), second motor area, somatosensory cortex (SI and II) and primary visual cortex (area 17). The commissural fibers to and from the temporal cortex, particularly the middle and inferior temporal gyri, pass through the anterior commissure (Fig. 1.7). In essence, the cortices of the two hemispheres are in continuous communication with each other through the fibers of the corpus callosum and anterior commissure.

Yet, when the corpus callosum is completely transected, even in humans, no functional alterations can be detected by the usual neurologic and psychologic examinations. Complex activities, such as playing musical instruments and writing, are performed with the same dexterity as prior to sectioning of the corpus callosum.

An experimental animal or human being with the corpus callosum and other commissures (anterior and hippocampal commissures) transected has, in a way, two brains; such individuals are called *twin-brain* or *split-brain* people. They behave normally, are alert and curious, perceive, learn, and retain learned activities, as do normal animals and human beings.

Studies of split-brain monkeys and human beings have been conducted so that the input from the periphery has been projected to only one hemisphere. The memories of perceptually learned information and of learned motor activities are apparently confined to the hemisphere to which the sensory information was relayed and from which the motor output was projected. If the corpus callosum is intact, this memory is utilized for motor expression by both hemispheres. Apparently the *engram*, or *memory trace*, laid down in the directly trained hemisphere is transferred via the callosal fibers to the opposite hemisphere, and a second engram is laid down in the contralateral hemisphere.

In common usage, dominance as applied to a hemisphere is imprecise, as each hemisphere is dominant for certain functions (Fig. 25.9). For example, the left hemisphere is dominant for language and the right hemisphere for spatial construction (stereognosis). Neither hemisphere should be regarded as subordinate overall. The "dominant" hemisphere is also called the *major hemisphere* and the "nondominant" hemisphere the *minor hemisphere*. In most individuals the major hemisphere is the left hemisphere and the minor hemisphere is the right hemisphere.

In human beings, speech and the language symbolisms of the written and spoken word are lateralized in the major hemisphere. Both the major (or "talking") hemisphere and the minor ("mute") hemisphere can comprehend, but normally only the major hemisphere "talks." Linguistic expression resides exclusively within the major hemisphere, whereas the comprehension of both the written and spoken language is represented in both hemispheres.

The minor hemisphere can perceive tactile, auditory, and visual information, but is unable to communicate through verbal language; however, it can respond and communicate by gestures (e.g., pointing) or emotional activity (e.g., fidgeting or blushing). The minor hemisphere is specialized to appreciate spatial dimensions, to grasp the totality of a scene, and to recognize the faces of people better than the major hemisphere. This mute hemisphere is presumed to have an essential role in creative acts associated with musical, poetic, and imaginative expressions.

Human split-brain subjects exhibit some interesting and curious disturbances of higher brain function. When these result from lesions of the corpus callosum, or of cortical association areas giving rise to commissural fibers, they are known as *disconnection syndromes*. The ultimate expression of the general sensory information which is conveyed from the right hand to the left or major hemisphere may differ dramatically from that which is conveyed from the left hand to the right or minor hemisphere. The right hand may be "unaware" of what the left hand is doing; for example, the right hand may be buttoning the patient's shirt while the left hand is unbuttoning it. The subject can name an object held in the right hand, but cannot name an object held in the left hand; the act of naming

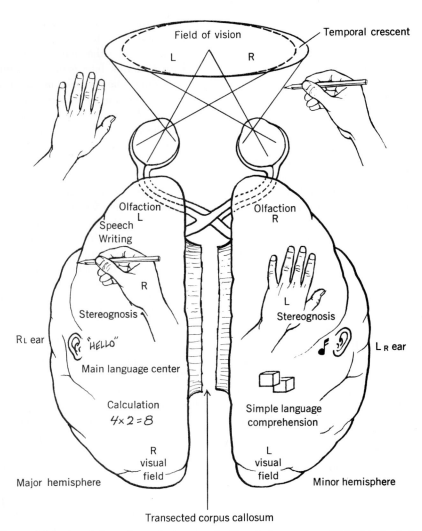

Figure 25.9: Some of the roles of the major and minor cerebral hemispheres as established in "twin-brain" humans. General senses from one hand and from half of the visual field are projected to the contralateral hemisphere. The olfactory sense is conveyed to the ipsilateral hemisphere. Hearing is largely projected to the contralateral hemisphere. (Adapted from Sperry, 1985.)

is a function of the major hemisphere. These patients can perform certain tasks better with the left hand than with the right hand. This indicates that the minor hemisphere does have some superior roles over the major hemisphere. For example, better performances are executed by the left hand than by the right hand in tasks involving spatial relations such as arranging blocks, drawing simple three-dimensional objects (cubes), and matching up designs.

Several basic conclusions concerning the roles of the cerebral hemispheres obtained from

studies of "twin-brain" subjects (**Fig. 25.9**) are: (1) perception and memory can be performed independently in both hemispheres, (2) language and speech are almost exclusively the roles of the major hemisphere, (3) the minor hemisphere is superior to the major hemisphere in the recognition and appreciation of spatial dimensions, (4) the primary role of the cerebral commissures is in the bilateral integration of the two hemispheres for linguistic functions, (5) it is through the major hemisphere that humans can express thoughts and knowledge through language, and (6) the commissures are essential for maintaining the unity of the higher sensory and motor functions of the cerebrum. The following is a rather simplistic summary of roles of the two hemispheres. The left (major) hemisphere may be considered to be the analytical, rational, and verbal half of the cerebrum. It is analytic as used in language recognition. The right (minor) hemisphere is the synthetic, intuitive, and nonverbal half. It is nonanalytical and used in perceptive recognition.

The lateralization of Broca's speech area is not causally related to handedness. Actually, speech functions are lateralized to the left hemisphere in most adults regardless of hand preference. Roughly 80% of adults are right-handed, 10% are left-handed, and 10% are ambidextrous. In right-handers, the left cortical motor areas control the right hand, while in left-handers the right cortical motor areas control the left hand. About 90% of right-handers have speech centers in the left hemisphere, while the other 10% have speech centers in the right hemisphere. About 65% of left-handers also have speech centers in the left hemisphere, 20% in the right hemisphere, and the remaining 15% have speech centers located bilaterally. Naturally ambidextrous subjects have their speech centers located as follows: 60% in the left hemisphere, 10% in the right hemisphere, and 30% in both hemispheres.

In general, injuries of the brain in infants and children are often accompanied by less severe neurological impairment and greater recovery of function (expression of more plasticity) than seen following similar injuries in the adult. This "infant lesion effect" is dramatically demonstrated following unilateral damage to the cerebrum. In a child, after extensive cerebral damage as a consequence of a cerebral infarction or hemispherectomy for relief from intractable seizures, there is marked compensatory recovery of functional deficiencies. The intact hemisphere can assume the ability to perform many of the impaired skilled movements and language functions.

MEMORY

Learning and memory are expressions of neuronal processing. *Learning* is the means by which we realize new knowledge and perceptions about events and experience. *Memory* is characterized as the consequence of the acquisition, storage, and recall of previous experiences that have been learned.

A general framework of neuronal circuitry of both parallel and hierarchical components relevant to memory in the primates including humans was proposed by Mishkin and Appenzeller (1987). The presence and presumed roles of different parts are based on studies of neurologic patients with impaired memories, and of primates with selectively placed lesions (Squire and Zola-Morgan, 1988). In essence, the sequence of feed-forward processing connections and their functional correlates in the cerebral cortical and subcortical circuits leading to memory (1) commences with sensory association cortical areas, (2) proceeds through channels converging to the neocortex of each anterior temporal lobe, (3) continues to the parahippocampal cortex and its projections to the amygdala and hippocampus, (4) proceeds via their diffusely distributed circuits including the basal forebrain area, and finally (5) completes the "circle" with projections from the basal nucleus of Meynert to broad areas of the neocortex (Fig. 25.10).

Neuronal channels comprise pathways from the visual, auditory, and somatic sensory association areas (including the angular and supramarginal gyri) that converge to the cortex of the anterior temporal lobe (Fig. 25.10). Each of these pathways consists of a number of converging and diverging processing channels and subsets of neuronal pools. Each subset is involved with a specific visual, auditory, or somatic sensory feature or combination of features.

On the basis of documented evidence, two visual pathways are likely. (1) One visual pathway consists of processing sequences directed toward the temporal lobe. It is involved with the "broader context" of the visual world. Its neurons respond to such environmental stimuli as shape and color basic to "object vision." A portion of the superior temporal gyrus has a role in analyzing visual motion related to the subjective perception of movement during a visual task. (2) Another visual pathway directed toward the posterior temporal lobe is involved with visual attention and the spatial relations of the object or the scene observed. This "spatial

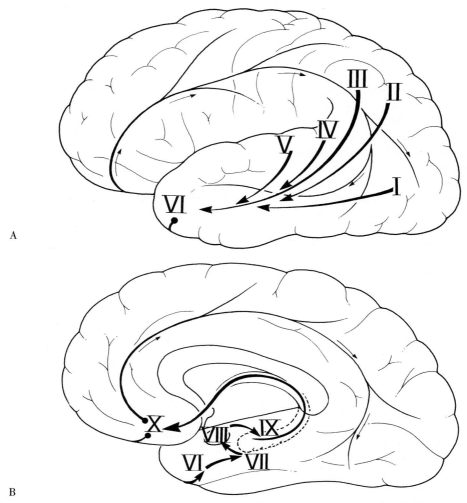

Figure 25.10: Possible sequence of neural transmission that is involved with the formulation of memory. **A.** Neocortical pathways converge from the sensory association areas via several neural circuits to the neocortex of the anterior temporal lobe. These circuits include the (I) "broader concept" visual pathway from the occipital lobe, (II) "spatial" visual pathways from the posterior parietal lobe, (III) somatosensory pathways from the parietal lobe, (IV) auditory pathways from the temporal lobe, and (V) the gustatory pathways from the superior temporal lobe cortex. These pathways converge to the anterior temporal lobe cortex (VI). **B.** From the anterior temporal lobe cortex, information is conveyed (VI) to the subiculum and parahippocampal gyrus of the paleocortex (VII). From this paleocortex, circuits project to the amygdala (VIII) and hippocampus (IX), both of which project widely (Chap. 22), including to the basal forebrain area including basal nucleus of Meynert (X). In turn, projections from the basal area "complete" the overall circuitry via fibers from the basal nucleus of Meynert back to the neocortical sensory association areas somehow to fix a new memory or to elicit an old memory. The "working memory" (memory retrieved and temporarily held) is extracted from "long term memory" that is consolidated and stored at multiple sites in the cerebrum.

system" is associated with the perception of an object in context with the other landmarks in the visual field—so-called object and pattern discrimination. This pathway is thought to interact with the tactile channels from the parietal lobe cortex (cross modality interactions). Other cortical pathways conveying information from the auditory, somatosensory, and gustatory association areas converge to the anterior temporal neocortex.

In essence, neurons in this temporal lobe cortex are responsive to a wide variety of features of the visual, auditory, tactile, and taste spheres—the highly processed inputs from the world bombarding stimuli upon the individual. Some confirmatory evidence has been obtained from electrical stimulation of this cortex in conscious patients (Penfield and Roberts, 1959). Such stimulation can evoke associations relative to "experiences." It may also elicit the recall of objects seen, music heard, or objects felt. Visual and auditory hallucinations may be produced, such as a clear reenactment, of an experience of the recent or distant past. The evoked experiences may be a symphonic melody that the subject thinks is being played on a phonograph or on a radio. The patient with temporal lobe tumors may have auditory or visual hallucinations and may see vivid scenes and friends not present and hear songs not being sung. The patient is cognizant of these hallucinations that are consistent with experiences seen or heard in the past (deja vu). In a sense, a neuron or small group of neurons in this area are "windows to our internal and external worlds."

Channels project from this temporal lobe cortex to limbic lobe cortex on the medial aspect of the temporal lobe (parahippocampal gyrus and subiculum). Reciprocal circuits project to and from this medial cortex to two major processing structures, namely the amygdala and the hippocampus that communicate with the limbic system. The amygdala also receives direct input from the olfactory system.

Bilateral removal of the medial portions of the temporal lobes including the amygdala and hippocampus results in severe memory deficits (even total amnesia) but specifically with the loss of the capacity to consolidate or retain short-term (recent) memory. These patients lose the capacity to form and to store new long-term memories; however, the long-term memories, acquired before the removal, remain essentially intact and can be recalled, often vividly, many years later. As generally used, short-term memory comprises the information and awareness that one retains for only a short time span. Unilateral removal of the amygdala and hippocampus does not result in impairments of memory (see Klüver-Bucy syndrome, Chap. 22).

The medial part of the temporal lobe has great importance in learning and memory functions. The hippocampus is an essential component in establishing memory; amnesia results following bilateral lesions of the hippocampus and the surrounding cortical regions, but sparing the amygdala. These observations indicate that the ablated structures are, in some way, involved with the consolidation of memory, but not with the actual storage of memory.

Bilateral ablation limited to the amygdala (monkey) has no detectable effect on memory. The widespread connections that the amygdala has with the neocortex and its strategic location as a major processing center suggest that the amygdala plays a role in the modulation of incoming sensory information. In addition, it may be important in establishing associations to events and in correlating information from different modalities. Another view is that both the amygdala and the hippocampus are essential for recognition memory (recognizing an object such as a glass) and associative memory (the glass can be associated with a glass of wine, water, or milk, or a bark with the image of a barking dog). The connections of the amygdala with the limbic system, including the hypothalamus, enables sensory events and perceptions to develop emotional associations and expressions (the latter through the autonomic nervous system). Thus, the amygdala may act as an intermediary between the sensory system and the emotions.

As to neural connections, the amygdala has reciprocal circuits with the cerebral cortex, striatum, hypothalamus, brainstem, thalamus, and hippocampus. The hippocampus projects its output via two major efferent circuits (1) via the fornix to the mammillary body and other sites (Chap. 22) and (2) reciprocally to the medial temporal lobe and hence via association bundles to the neocortical association areas of the four lobes including the prefrontal cortex (Chap. 22 for other connections). The evidence indicates that the hippocampus is implicated in memory mechanisms so as to make it possible for humans to compare the present circumstance with the previous experienced events. Lesions of the fornix or of the mammillary bodies (formerly thought to result in amnesia) results in a negligible and transient loss of memory.

Some evidence suggests that the medial thalamus, possibly the medial (dorsomedial) thalamic nucleus, is also involved in the formulation of memory. Bilateral damage of the midline diencephalon can result in profound amnesia in humans and severe memory impairment in monkeys. In essence, the reciprocal neural linkages between the hippocampus and the neocortex are conceived to have a role in the dynamics of memory. They are involved in the initial phase of learning (e.g., impression of novel image—namely, short-term memory). Then, followed by a limited period, the image, if retained, gradually becomes independent of the hippocampus into the long-term memory domain.

In general, the hippocampus seems to be more involved with registering cognitive information than emotion, whereas the amygdala has an essential role in the expression of emotion rather than cognition.

Another link in the memory channels involves the substantia innominata and the *basal nucleus of Meynert* (Chap. 22; Fig. 22.2). This region receives afferent input from the amygdala, insula, and parts of the parahippocampal gyrus; it projects output through diffuse connections with such centers as the amygdala, hippocampus, hypothalamus, and some brainstem nuclei. In addition, the basal nucleus has cholinergic neurons whose fibers are distributed widely to the entire neocortex in a quite orderly and topographic manner and are regarded as a major source of cortical acetylcholine. Its neurons have excitatory synapses with muscarinic receptors of cortical neurons. This nucleus is conceived of as acting as the final linkage (along with the output of the hippocampus to many areas of the neocortex) to close the loop that is involved with the processing and storage of acquired information—the "stored memories in the neocortex." One concept postulates that this link in the loop evokes changes in the neurons and local circuits of the sensory areas that fix a perception so that it is stored in the *memory* and, in addition, possibly releases previously stored memories in the neocortex to our conscious self.

Alzheimer's disease (presenile dementia), as well as senile dementia which is the same entity except for age of onset, is an affliction with initial signs of forgetfulness leading to progressively more severe mental deterioration. Pa-

tients exhibit a loss of memory and become confused and disoriented. They are incapable of abstract thought. In advanced stages, they cannot recognize even close friends and relatives. Diffuse cerebral atrophy, particularly involving the frontal and temporal lobes, is a constant attribute. Characteristic features include the presence of extracellular plaques of β-amyloid protein surrounded by degenerated axon terminals and of intracellular neurofibrillary tangles involving association cortex, hippocampus, and parts of the parahippocampal gyrus. Additionally, in this disease there is a selective loss of the cholinergic neurons of the basal nucleus of Meynert (Chap. 24). The symptoms may be due, in part, to the massive destruction of these neurons. Alzheimer patients have reduced neocortical acetylcholine and its precursor enzyme, acetylcholine transferase.

Modular Organization of the Brain

"An emerging view is that the brain is structurally and functionally organized into discrete units or 'modules' and that these components interact to produce mental activities" (Gazzaniga, 1989). In a broad sense the major sensory systems, are complexes of modular systems. This is expressed in the visual system where several anatomically and physiologically documented modules including cortical areas are embedded within the system. Each of these modules process such different dimensions of visual information as color, depth perception, and motion (Chap. 19; Hubel, 1987; Kaas, 1987). Higher degrees of processing within the functional specific anatomic modules of the cerebral cortex involved with memory have been demonstrated in the monkey (noted in this chapter; Mishkin and Apenzeller, 1987). Another complex of modules present in the human brain are those involved with a variety of language processes.

At higher levels, the human brain appears to have a modular organization consisting of identifiable component processes that participate in the generation of the cognitive state, including the appreciation of the surrounding world and past events, perception, reasoning, and the unitary experience of conscious awareness (Gazzaniga, 1989).

Dynamic Maintenance of Cortical Areas

Cortical areas (such as the V4 color area; Chap. 19) are functionally distinct divisions that are precisely localized. The circuitry of the neuronal organization within each area is (1) nurtured during development by "self-organization" and active neural activity patterns generated by inputs and (2) maintained during adulthood by active dynamic inputs (Kaas, 1987). Hence, cortical maps are shaped and sustained by neural activity.

The microorganization (local circuitry) of the cortex is in a constant state of flux depending upon a variety of competitive inputs. Stability in a cortical area results from a balance of these inputs. Increased input from greater usage tends to increase cortical space of a specific modality, whereas decreased usage tends to decrease each cortical space (Chap. 6). In essence, mental activity and physical exercise associated with stimulation derived from sensory receptors and the activation of reflexes and movements exert positive roles in sustaining and maintaining the integrity of cortical areas throughout life, including old age.

SUGGESTED READINGS

Amaral D. Memory: anatomical organization of candidate brain regions. In: *Handbook of Physiology.* Section I. *The Nervous System.* Vol. V. *Higher Functions of the Brain.* Bethesda, Md: American Physiological Society; 1987:211–294.

Beaton A. *Left Side, Right Side. A Review of Laterality Research.* New Haven, Conn: Yale University Press; 1986.

Benson D, Zaidel E, eds. *The Dual Brain: Hemispheric Specialization in Humans.* New York, NY: Guilford Press; 1985.

Chudler E, Dong W, Kawakami Y. Cortical nociceptive responses and behavioral correlates in the monkey. *Brain Res.* 1986;397:47–60.

Damasio A, Geschwind N. The neural basis of language. *Annu Rev Neurosci.* 1984;7:127–147.

Damasio H, Grabowski T, Frank R, Galaburda A, Damasio A. The return of Phineas Gage: clues about the brain from the skull of a famous patient. *Science.* 1994;264:1102–1105.

Freund H-J, Hummelsheim H. Lesions of premotor cortex in man. *Brain.* 1985;108:697–733.

Gazzaniga M. *The Social Brain: Discovering the Networks of the Mind.* New York, NY: Basic Books; 1985.

Gazzaniga M. Organization of the human brain. *Science.* 1989;245:947–952.

Geschwind N. Disconnexion syndromes in animals and man. I and II. *Brain.* 1965;88:237–294, 585–644.

Geschwind N. Specialization of the human brain. *Sci Am.* 1979;241:180–199.

Geschwind N, Singer W, eds. *Cerebral Dominance.* Cambridge, Mass: Harvard University Press; 1984.

Goldman-Rakic P. The issue of memory in the study of prefrontal function. In: Thierry A, Glowinski J, Goldman-Rakic P, Christen Y, eds. *Motor and Cognitive Functions of the Prefrontal Lobe.* Berlin: Springer-Verlag; 1995.

Grillner S, Wallén P. Central pattern generators for locomotion, with special reference to vertebrates. *Annu Rev Neurosci.* 1985;8:233–261.

Jones E, Peters A, eds. *Cerebral Cortex.* Vol. 2. *Functional Properties of Cortical Cells.* New York, NY: Plenum; 1984:1–354.

Jones E, Peters A, eds. *Cerebral Cortex. Vol. 5. Sensory-Motor Areas and Aspects of Cortical Connectivity.* New York, NY: Plenum; 1986:1–510.

Kaas J. The organization of neocortex in mammals: implications for theories of brain function. *Annu Rev Psychol.* 1987;38:129–151.

Lassen N, Ingvar D, Skinhøj E. Brain function and blood flow. *Sci Am.* 1978;239(4):62–71.

Lepore F, Ptito M, Jasper H, eds. *Two Hemispheres—One Brain: Functions of the Corpus Callosum.* New York, NY: Alan R. Liss; 1984.

LeVay S, Sherk H. The visual claustrum of the cat. *J Neurosci.* 1981;1:956–992.

Merzenich M, Nelson R, Stryker M, Cynader M, Schoppmann A, Zook J. Somatosensory cortical map changes following digit amputation in adult monkeys. *J Comp Neurol.* 1984;224:591–605.

Merzenich M. Sources in intraspecies and interspecies cortical map variability in mammals: conclusions and hypotheses. In: Cohen M, Strumwasser F, eds. *Comparative Neurobiology: Modes of Communication in the Nervous System.* New York, NY: Wiley; 1985.

Mesulum M. *Principles of Behavioral Neurology.* Philadelphia: F.A. Davis; 1985.

Mishkin M, Appenzeller T. The anatomy of memory. *Sci Am.* 1987;256(6):80–89.

Mishkin M, Ungerleider L, Macko K. Object vision and spatial vision: two cortical pathways. *Trends Neurosci.* 1983;6:414–417.

Olton D, Gamzu E, Corkin S, eds. Memory dysfunctions: an integration of animal and human research from preclinical and clinical perspectives. *Ann N Y Acad Sci.* 1985;444:1–553.

Rakic P, Singer W. *Neurobiology of Neocortex.* New York, NY: Wiley; 1988.

Ramachandran V, Stewart M, Rogers-Ramachandran D. Perceptual correlates of massive cortical reorganization. *Neuroreport.* 1992;3:583–586.

Rowland L. *Merritt's Textbook of Neurology.* 9th ed. Media, Pa: Williams & Wilkins; 1995.

Scientific American. Special Issue: Mind and Brain. 1992;267(3).

Sperry R. Some aspects of disconnecting the cerebral hemispheres (Nobel Lecture). In: *Les Prix Nobel.* Stockholm: Almquist & Wiksell International; 1982.

Sperry R. Some effects of disconnecting the cerebral hemispheres. In: Abelson P, Butz E, Snyder S, eds. *Neuroscience.* Washington, DC: American Association for Advancement of Science. 1985: 372–380.

Springer S, Deutsch G. *Left Brain, Right Brain.* 4th ed. New York, NY: W.H. Freeman; 1993.

Squire L. *Memory and Brain.* New York, NY: Oxford University Press; 1987.

Squire L, Zola-Morgan S. Memory: brain systems and behavior. *Trends Neurosci.* 1988;11:170–175.

Szentágothai J. The modular architectonic principle of neural centers. *Rev Physiol Biochem Pharmacol.* 1983;98:11–61.

Thompson R. The neurobiology of learning and memory. *Science.* 1986;233:941–947.

Van der Loos H, Woolsey T. Somatosensory cortex: structural alterations following early injury to sense organs. *Science.* 1973;179:395–398.

Wise S, Evarts E. The role of the cerebral cortex in movement. *Trends Neurosci.* 1981;4:297–300.

Young A, ed. *Functions of the Right Cerebral Hemisphere.* New York, NY: Academic Press; 1983.

Zeki S. *A Vision of the Brain.* London: Blackwell; 1993.

Zola-Morgan S, Squire L, Amaral D. Human amnesia and the medial temporal region: enduring memory impairment following a bilateral lesion limited to field CA1 of the hippocampus. *J Neurosci.* 1986;6:2950–2967.

Index

Note: Page numbers in *italics* indicate figures; page numbers followed by t indicate tables.